The Springer Series on Human Exceptionality

Series Editors

Donald H. Saklofske
University of Calgary, Alberta, Canada

Moshe Zeidner
University of Haifa, Mount Carmel, Israel

For further volumes:
http://www.springer.com/series/6450

Rachel Seginer

Future Orientation

Developmental and Ecological Perspectives

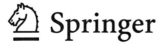 Springer

Prof. Rachel Seginer
University of Haifa
Faculty of Education
31905 Haifa
Israel
rseginer@construct.haifa.ac.il

ISSN 1572-5642
ISBN 978-0-387-88640-4   e-ISBN 978-0-387-88641-1
DOI 10.1007/978-0-387-88641-1

Library of Congress Control Number: 2008939946

Printed on acid-free paper

springer.com

Strong in will to strive, to seek, to find, and not to yield.
(A. Tennyson, 1861, *Ulysses*)

Preface

*By contemporary I mean a present with an anticipated future,
for we must do our best to overcome clinical habits which
make us assume that we have done our part if we have
clarified the past.*

(Erikson, 1968, pp. 30–31).

*The scope of time ahead which influences present behavior,
and is therefore to be regarded as part of the present
life-space, increases during development. This change in time
perspective is one of the most fundamental facts of
development. Adolescence seems to be a period of particularly
deep change in respect to time perspective.*

(Lewin, 1939, p. 879).

I chose to open this book with two excerpts from Erikson's and Lewin's writings because they indicate that future orientation has had its deep roots in psychological thinking, and call readers' attention to the long standing interest in two fundamental issues: the motivational power of constructed future images and their development across age. More specifically, Erikson and Lewin's writings underscore the importance of future thinking for influencing present behavior tendencies, and point out that the ability to think about the future and realize the "scope of time ahead" increase with age, and reach a special developmental significance in adolescence.

Accordingly, this book is on how individuals across the life span construct the subjective images of their future and how researchers drawing on different approaches define, conceptualize and examine the formation of these images, their inter- and intrapersonal antecedents, personality correlates, and effects on behavioral and developmental outcomes. However, while multiple approaches enrich the conceptual foundation and empirical research of any area, inadvertently they also lead to the use of diversified terminology. An incomplete list of terms indexing the construction of future images in current use includes *future orientation, future thinking, future time perspective, episodic future thinking, future self, personal strivings, personal projects, life tasks, considering future consequences, prospective memory, time perspective, possible selves,* and *mental time travel.* Two historical terms have been *futurism* (Israeli, 1930) and *psychological future* (Lewin, 1942/1948).

As biblical wisdom – here illustrated by the story of the tower of Babel – has instructed us, the strength a community draws from the use of one common language is considerably curtailed when its members each uses a different language:

> And the Lord said, Behold, the people is one, and they have all one language;... and now nothing will be restrained from them, which they have imagined to do...let us go down, and there confound their language, that they may not understand one another's speech. (Genesis, Chap. 11, 6–7).

Applied to the scientific scene, diversified terminology emanates from the use of different theoretical approaches that their interface augments shared knowledge and creates new research options. Their cost, however, is limited access to relevant information packaged in different language. Therefore, one aim of this volume has been to give voice to the different approaches, conceptualizations, and ensuing terminologies. Nonetheless, it is plausible that not all approaches – and certainly not all studies – have been registered and included.

As is clear from the title of the book, the work we have been carrying out at the University of Haifa describes the subjective images individuals construct about the future as *future orientation*. By using this term, those of us who do so emphasize the quality of future orientation as an active engagement in future thinking and future-related behavior that facilitates acquaintance with prospective events, experiences, and options and makes the future psychologically closer, more real, and amenable for planning.

The capacity for orienting to the future is innate and its early expressions are noted in infancy. However, its form, content and function change with age and as first suggested by Lewin, its capacity for self-direction becomes more pronounced in adolescence, as transition-to-adulthood and adult roles become more tangible and getting ready for them a normative expectation. This is probably why for psychologists, writers, educators and parents future orientation is related to adolescence more than to any other developmental period and why in addition to Erikson and Lewin, as early as the 1960s several other developmental psychologists (e.g., Douvan & Adelson, 1966; Mönks, 1968) considered future orientation an essential adolescent developmental mechanism. For the same reason interest in adults' future orientation is relatively scant and recent (e.g., Salmela-Aro, Nurmi, Saisto, & Halmesmäki, 2001; Salmela-Aro & Suikkari, 2008; Wilf, 2008). Until recently it was right to say that even fewer researchers have been studying the future orientation of old-age individuals (Cottle & Klineberg, 1974; Lang & Carstensen, 2002; Nurmi, 1992). However, interest in the neuropsychology of memory and questions about similarities and differences between the neuropsychology of remembering and expecting ("prospective memory") has added several studies (e.g., Addis, Wong, & Schacter, 2008; Spreng & Levine, 2006).

Main Issues

These emphases have led to several questions about the development of future orientation, its antecedents and outcomes. Although the book addresses future orientation across the life span, its main focus is on adolescence and emerging adulthood. Thus, following review of the developmental origins of future orientation (How and when does future oriented thinking emerge?), the book examines the intrapersonal underpinnings of future orientation (Do adolescents varying in self-evaluation, control beliefs, or defensive pessimism differ in their construction of future orientation?), its gender specificity (Can we identify feminine and masculine future orientation?), and the extent to which interpersonal relationships with parents, siblings and peers shape it (Do adolescents experiencing high positive parenting, close sibling relationships and peer acceptance construct their future orientation differently than do adolescents experiencing less positive parenting, close sibling relationships and peer acceptance?). Finally, the effect of future orientation on developmental outcomes is examined, asking: Do adolescents with high future orientation scores do better at school? Do adolescents and emerging adults adjust better to new situations and experience a higher sense of identity and intimacy?

Related to each of these questions is the issue of culture. While initially the question has been how cultural settings affect the construction of future orientation, as future orientation models have become more elaborate and findings accumulated, the question guiding our research has been rephrased and we now ask what aspects of future orientation are more or less susceptible to cultural influences, and whether the effect of future orientation on developmental outcomes is culture specific?

Plan of the Book

The main issues of future orientation delineated above are discussed in detail in the following eight chapters. Although each chapter is devoted to one specific issue, the five chapters (3–7) focusing on factors affecting the development of adolescents and emerging adults' future orientation and its outcomes keep a similar structure. Each of these chapters (or their main sections) consists of three parts: conceptualization of the construct under consideration, propositions about the relations between that construct and future orientation, and its empirical examination.

Chapter 1 presents the conceptual framework of future orientation. Its first part delineates the evolvement of the future orientation construct. This part discusses three topics that differ both conceptually and chronologically: early conceptual analyses, the athematic and thematic approaches, and finally multivariate approaches whose development has built on knowledge accumulated from earlier research. The second part presents four interfacing approaches that like the future orientation construct examine the effect of future thinking on behavior and pertain to the motivational, goal, personal dispositions and possible selves approaches.

Chapter 2 describes future orientation in the first three developmental periods: infancy, early, and middle childhood. Its first part reviews research on the evolvement of future orientation in infancy, experimentally assessed by several indicators of visual anticipatory behavior; its second part addresses the development of young children's sense of the future as manifested in controlled experiments and naturalistic interaction with adults (particularly mothers). The third part relates to the development of future orientation during the elementary school years by examining children's hopes and fears narratives and their changing character from fantasy to reality-based themes.

The aim of Chapter 3 is to examine how self and personality characteristics affect the construction of future orientation. Drawings on their pertinence to future orientation three self dimensions and three personality characteristics are included. The self dimensions pertain to self esteem and self agency as two aspects of individuals' generalized sense of self-worth, and the self schema of loneliness, and personality characteristics relate to primary and secondary control, defensive pessimism and strategic optimism. The effect of each on future orientation is examined in the context of culture and gender.

Chapter 4 focuses on sex differences. It opens with review of the three main approaches to gender differences – evolutionary psychology, social role theory and socialization of gender roles – and their explanations of the extent, origins and underlying processes, reviews psychological literature on gender effects on future orientation and presents recent analyses of the effect of social and cultural context on future orientation gender differences and similarities. These analyses draw on data collected from Israeli-Arab adolescents as an instance of a society in transition from traditionalism to modernity and particularly on the future orientation of Israeli-Arab girls describing how they construct a future that intertwines the traditional (i.e., being a devoted wife and mother) and the modern (i.e., pursuing higher education and career).

Chapter 5 is the first of two chapters focusing on the construction of future orientation in the context of interpersonal relationships. Specifically it examines how parenting affects future orientation by relating to three issues. The first two pertain to parent-adolescent relationships and parental beliefs about adult roles as experienced by adolescents. The third issue concerns similarity and association between adolescents' and parents' future orientation. Each of these issues is addressed in terms of multiple cultural settings indicating cross cultural commonalities and differences. In particular, the chapter shows that across different cultural settings the link between parenting and future orientation is mediated by global self evaluation and indicates the validity of the parenting-future orientation mediating model for both industrial and transition to modernity youths.

Chapter 6 describes the effect on the construction of future orientation of two adolescent contemporaries: siblings and peers. The effect of these interpersonal relationships and the confluence of parents, siblings and peers on future orientation is examined within modern and transition to modernity cultural contexts showing particularly three important findings. That the effect of relationships with siblings and peers like the effect of parenting on future orientation is not a direct one but rather mediated by the self; that parenting, relationships with siblings, and relationships with peers each has a net effect on future orientation, and that the mediating function of the self and the net effect of all three interpersonal relationships apply to different cultural settings.

Chapter 7 examines the effect of future orientation on five developmental outcomes relevant to adolescents, emerging adults, and midlife adults: academic achievement for adolescents, identity and intimacy for emerging adults, and adjustment to transition (military service) for emerging adults, and midlife men (early retirement). Finally, the Summary and Conclusions chapter (Chap. 8) consists of three parts. The first summarizes the book by relating to five issues pertaining to the conceptualization of future orientation, and developmental, personality antecedents, interpersonal antecedents, and cultural factors affecting it. The second part indicates directions for future research, and the third part discusses the path from theory to action, particularly addressing the use of accumulated knowledge on the antecedents and outcomes of future orientation for promoting educational outcomes and helping adolescents and emerging adults to secure a better future.

Altogether, the aim of this book has been to present an integrated description of future orientation research across the life span, particularly addressing the expression and developmental outcomes of future orientation and four factors underlying its construction: personality, gender, close interpersonal relations, and culture. Hopefully, this volume is not a summary but rather an overture, out of which additional new research directions will emerge.

Haifa, Israel   R. Seginer

Acknowledgements

Even when it bears the name of a single author, a book is seldom the project of one person. Research reported in this volume was carried out over a period of 15 years with my students whose theses, dissertations, and co-authored papers are cited in its various chapters. Sami Mahajna, Inas Margieh, Maha Suleiman, and Hiam Tannous helped me understand the meaning of being adolescent in the Israeli Palestinian-Arab community, Hoda Halabi-Kheir and Rabiaa Hssessi in the Israeli Druze community, and Shlomit Dekel in the chabad ultra-orthodox Jewish community. Ruhama Nakash and Nurit Toren-Kaplan contributed to our knowledge by studying the future orientation of adolescents who immigrated from former Soviet Russia.

Eti Ablin, Sarit Berkman, Sigal Guter, Efrat Lilach, Michal Noyman, Simona Sharoni, Ronit Schlesinger, and Shirli Shoyer studied the future orientation of adolescents and emerging adults, focusing on interpersonal and personality antecedents and developmental outcomes. While much of our work focused on adolescents and emerging adults, the work of Yehuda Gelberg reached out to the future orientation of children as young as 2nd, 4th and 6th graders, and Ronit Shalev and Michal Wilf each opened a door to the future orientation of adults undergoing meaningful – though different – personal experiences: the loss of a child killed in action (Shalev) and adjustment to civilian life after 25 years of professional military service (Wilf).

The borderless world of academic pursuit introduced me to four colleagues whose valuable help and true friendship is here gratefully acknowledged. Catherine Cooper with whom I have had many face-to-face, transatlantic telephone conversations, and electronic dialogues about future orientation, identity, and cultural diversity, Jari Nurmi with whom the early version of the three component future orientation model has been developed, Gisela Trommsdorff who hosted me at her University of Konstanz lab, and since our first meeting over 20 years ago has shared her vast knowledge and provided constructive comments in our numerous get-togethers, telephone conversations, and e-mail encounters that have always been instructive, warm, and supportive. My friend Ad Vermulst of the University of Nijmegen introduced me to the unwritten secrets of successfully running Structural Equation Modeling and has extended his knowledge and support since.

Ruth Linn and Moshe Zeidner my colleagues and friends from the University of Haifa, both gave their help and support. Moshe's help at the initial stages of the writing project and his good and friendly advice along the entire process have been invaluable. Work on this book has been interrupted twice by events beyond my control. I am grateful to Judy Jones of Springer and to Don Saklofske and Moshe Zeidner, co-chairpersons of the editorial board, for their patience, support, and encouragement.

Sami Mahajna, Shirli Shoyer, and Sandra Zukerman – three former students who became dear friends and appreciated colleagues – have been particularly helpful. Sami has been a liaison with the local Arab-Palestinian community and a perceptive interpreter of cultural changes and developmental processes among adolescents and their families. Shirli has helped me in all phases of this project, did excellent work, gave good advice, and nothing has ever been difficult for her to carry out. Sandra did the statistical analyses with deep understanding and keen ability to overcome obstacles, and like Shirli, and together with her has always been there when the need aroused. Finally, most warmly and lovingly, I thank my family, and particularly Ido, for their patience and support.

Contents

Chapter 1
Future Orientation: A Conceptual Framework

"Would you tell me, please, which way I ought to go from here?"
"That depends a good deal on where you want to Get to" said
the Cat
"I don't much care where-" Said Alice.
Then it doesn't matter which way you go" said the Cat.
"-so long as I get somewhere" Alice added as an explanation
"Oh, you're sure to do that" said the Cat, "if you only
Walk long enough." Lewis Carroll, Alice in Wonderland

To paraphrase the dialogue between Alice and the Cat, it is their constructed image of the future that directs individuals when each of them – like Alice – ponders "which way I ought to go from here?" And it is the "where you want to get to" that guides their behavior, but not all of it. Because, just as future orientation is about where one wants to get and the ways she or he ought to go, it is also about destinations one fears to reach and routes she or he should avoid. Moreover, as research reported in this and subsequent chapters shows not all future thinking is goal directing; some of it – like Alice's "-so long as I get somewhere" – consists of future images that do not aim at or lead to specific plans, goals, or hopes.

Thus, a basic assumption underlying future orientation research has been that the 'where' and 'where not' as well as the 'ought' and 'ought not' are subjective. Their construction results from the interplay between individuals' needs and their interpretation of the values, socio-economic reality and developmental opportunities afforded by their socio-cultural setting (Seginer, 2008).

The importance of future orientation. The relevance of future orientation for individuals' behavior and development has been postulated by psychologists and intuitively understood by lay persons. Lewin (1942/1948) who used the term "psychological future" was among the first psychologists to recognize that:

The picture presented by this "psychological future" seldom corresponds to what actually happens later...But, regardless of whether the individual's picture of the future is correct or incorrect at a given time, this picture deeply affects the mood and the action of the individual at that time. (Lewin, 1942/1948, pp. 103–104)

As attested by the frequent use of future metaphors in promoting both commercial and public interests, the power of the future has been particularly

R. Seginer, *Future Orientation*, The Springer Series on Human Exceptionality,
DOI 10.1007/978-0-387-88641-1_1, © Springer Science+Business Media, LLC 2009

recognized by the advertising business community. "Don't wait for the future go find it", "Where there is care there is future", "You never actually own a Pateck Phillipe [a Swiss made watch], you merely look after it for the next generation", and "The future isn't something you travel to, it's something you build up" are just several examples of the use of future metaphors in advertisement.

Not unlike other areas of scientific inquiry, researchers have used different terms to describe the images individuals develop about the future: future time orientation, future time perspective, possible selves. Conversely, "future orientation" has been used to describe such aspects of future-related issues as temporal extension (i.e., how far into the future individuals think) (Teahan, 1958), a sense of continuity between the past, present and future (Marko & Savickas, 1998), and attitudes toward the future (Nuttin & Lens, 1985).

Six approaches to future orientation. Future orientation has been addressed by different approaches, whose emphases complement each other and jointly contribute to our understanding of the How Why and What of people's prospective thinking.

In particular, at present six psychological fields share interest in future orientation: human motivation, self theories, personality, cognitive processes, neuropsychology, and human development. Human motivation researchers view the future as the time zone in which goals, plans, and hopes are located and hence consider the subjective construction of future orientation an important aspect of behavior (Nuttin & Lens, 1985), particularly relevant to academic achievement (Raynor & Entin, 1982). Self theorists draw on James's (1890/1950) *possible selves* to describe the projection of the self into the future and its motivating power (Markus & Nurius, 1986; Oyserman & Markus, 1990). For personality researchers, considering the future is a stable personality characteristic that facilitates planning, encourages academic achievement, protects against risk taking behaviors (Zimbardo & Boyd, 1999), and prompts resilience (*morale*) in times of threat and strife (Lewin, 1942/1948).

Cognitive psychologists (Tulving, 1985, 2005) focus on the parallel nature of memory and future thinking as processes involving reliving the past and pre-living the future (Suddendorf & Corballis, 1997), and neuropsychologists study the commonalities and differences of the neurological processes underlying them. Finally, developmental research has shown that future orientation is relevant to each period from infancy to adulthood and old age. However, developmental tasks taking place in adolescence such as identity formation (Erikson, 1968) and bridging childhood and adulthood (Douvan & Adelson, 1966; Lewin, 1939) have made future orientation especially pertinent to this period (Nurmi, 1993, in press). In fact, the work and ideas of Douvan and Adelson, Erikson, and Lewin prompted the future orientation research carried out since, although with greater attention to contextuality.

Thus, a considerable part of the research reviewed in the various chapters of this volume examines individual differences emanating from age, gender, personality characteristics, and relationships with parents, siblings, and peers in the context of socio-cultural diversity. Emphasis on the effect of cultural factors on adolescents' future orientation leads to another contextual factor pertaining to a rising number of adolescents the world over who experience *double transition* created by a reality in which personal and social changes co-occur.

The multiple definitions of future orientation. Although it can most generally be described as individuals' tendency to engage in future thinking, the various approaches to future orientation led to multiple conceptualizations ranging from *extension* to *personality* characteristics, from *athematic* to *thematic* models, and from *uni-* to *multidimensional* constructs. This volume considers all approaches; however, the one viewing future orientation as *the images humans develop regarding the future, as consciously represented and self-reported* prevails and directs much of the discussion. Initially, this approach drew on the understanding that, as important as athematic qualities like extension into the future and personality inclination for future thinking are, the themes or content of future thinking and the affective tone underlying it are essential aspects of future orientation.

Future orientation and autobiography: equivalence and dependence. The thematic approach prompted an awareness of the similarity between future orientation and autobiography (Seginer, 2005). Like autobiography, future orientation takes place in the present, and like it consists of 'traveling in time' (Suddendorf & Corballis, 1997) to tell a personal dynamic life story comprising those experiences, events and interpersonal relationships individuals deem important. Most important of all, like autobiography, future orientation is subjectively constructed and thus gives meaning to one's life. A recent psychological study shows that across time autobiographical memory and future thinking reciprocally affect each other (Sutin & Robins, 2008) and neuroscience research (Dudai & Carruthers, 2005) points out the dependence of future thinking on autobiographical (episodic) memory (Tulving, 2002). Specifically, it shows similarity between brain networks activated remembering the past and imagining the future (Schacter & Addis, 2007).

Given the multiple approaches to future orientation and related constructs, this chapter consists of two main sections. The first reviews the evolvement of future orientation research from its early beginnings in the 1930s to the present. The second part addresses four interfacing approaches that examine similar issues but draw on different conceptual frameworks and use different terminology. The four approaches address future orientation by emphasizing its motivational, self, goal, or personality perspectives.

The Evolvement of Future Orientation Conceptualization

Early Psychological Analyses

Contemporary conceptualizations of future orientation can be traced back to the early work of three behavioral scientists: Frank (1939), Israeli (1930, 1936a) and Lewin (1939, 1942/1948). Each brought to the study of future orientation a different approach. Israeli – the first among them to publish his work on future orientation – was an experimental psychologist whose work was driven by his belief in the importance of "harnessing the future to present goals" (Israeli, 1930, p. 121) and his disappointment of its neglect in psychological inquiry. Frank was a social philosopher mainly concerned with the development and meaning of future thinking, and Lewin regarded the "psychological future" as part of the life space.

Nevertheless, their analyses commonly address three issues related to the conceptualization of future orientation and its motivational and developmental functions. One pertains to the simple basic observation that both its construction and its behavior regulation function take place in the present. The second relates to future orientation as domain specific so that individuals construct their image of the future by relating to different domains, and the third concerns the content, or themes, of these domains which may be personal or social, realistic or ideal, and reality-based or fantastic.

Israeli's pioneering work. Israeli's interest in the study of the subjective meaning of the future led him to experiment with different methods ranging from estimates of future events (e.g., divorce rate) to hypnotic imagination of the future and its description by individuals from different social groups. Consequently, his studies addressed the subjective importance of the future relative to the past and present (Israeli, 1933a), judgment of future criticism of the past (Israeli, 1933b), and the construction of future autobiographies (Israeli, 1936b).

His assessment of future autobiography involved an elaborate procedure in which participants from different social groups were instructed to write their autobiographies by looking back from 1935 to 1932 through 1975 to 1970. Although he should be credited with developing the future autobiographical concept and underscoring the importance of context, his elaborate methods were deemed impractical and replaced by other simpler methods (reviewed in a subsequent section on thematic approaches).

Frank's contributions. Although seldom acknowledged, Frank (1939) should be remembered for introducing to future orientation research two novel ideas. The first pertains to the concept of *extension* which describes how far into the future individuals project their thinking. As discussed in greater detail in a subsequent section of this chapter, Frank provided extension with its theoretical underpinnings and has been the first to consider the importance of *optimal* distance to the future (not too close, not too distant) for goal directed behavior.

His second contribution relates to early human development. Like contemporary researchers (see Chap. 2) Frank believed that some form of future orientation can be identified in infancy. Moreover, underlying his analysis have been two assumptions: that as early as infancy, future thinking indicates cognitive ability, and that the onset of "human career" is marked by the regulation of physiological functions whose two essential characteristics are acceptance of values and consideration of future consequences. Thus,

> The transformation of naïve behavior into conduct involves the acceptance of values, or, more specifically, necessitates value behavior and time perspective wherein we see the individual responding to present, immediate situation-events (intra-organic or environmental) as point-events in a sequence *the later or more remote components of which are the focus of that conduct* [*italics added*]. (Frank, 1939, p. 295).

Lewin's contributions. Lewin's influence on future orientation research is no doubt the greatest. Like Frank and Israeli, he was concerned with the motivational power of future orientation as directing present behavior. However, while their analyses of this function of future orientation were theoretical, Lewin tested his propositions in experiments linking level of aspiration to performance and in qualitative analysis linking future orientation to morale (Lewin, 1942/1948).

No less important is his introduction of future orientation to developmental thinking. Although known for his influence on social psychological and personality thinking, Lewin started his career working with Stern (Kreppner, 1994). Assuming development is marked by the individual's ability to extend further into the future and increase "...the scope of time ahead" (Lewin, 1939, p. 879), he used his interest in adolescent development to illustrate his field theory and its applications to social psychological issues (Lewin, 1939). Of special interest to him had been adolescent transition as an opportunity for widening the life-space, and particularly its geographical, social, and temporal dimensions. In Lewin's words:

> Adolescence seems to be a period of particularly deep change in respect to time perspective...Within those parts of the life-space which represent the future, levels of reality and irreality are gradually being differentiated...In other words, [in adolescence] one has to "plan": to structure the time perspective in a way which is in line both with one's ideal goals or values and with those realities which must be taken into account for a realistic structuring of the plane of expectations. (Lewin, 1939, p. 879).

Thus, Lewin's foremost contribution has been the conceptualization of future orientation as the joint product of person (*ideal goals or values*) and environmental (*those realities which must be taken into account*) factors and its inclusion in life space. Given the developmental emphasis of this book, it is also worth mentioning that Frank and Lewin have each applied his interest in future orientation to developmental periods that continue to attract future orientation researchers to date: early development and adolescence.

Athematic Approaches to Future Orientation

Several researchers approached research on future orientation assuming that underlying its construction is a generalized aptitude to think about the future. Because it considers only the structural dimensions of future thinking and not the events, experiences, and other objects of which future thinking consists, this research is best described as athematic. In fact, it subsumes several approaches that focus on either structural characteristics of the constructed future life space or on personal dispositions to consider the future and orient behavior toward it regardless of situations, settings, or life domains.

Although the two foci differ in several respects, they commonly reflect a stable circumstance-free tendency toward the future. The structural characteristics of the future life space pertain to two qualities: *extension* into the future and *representation* of the future relative to the representation of the present and the past in one's narratives. The dispositional approaches relate to individuals' inclination to think about the future (or avoid it) as a global *personality* characteristic. However, as discussed below, for some and particularly for Frank, extension to the future and personality inclination to think about the future are interdependent.

Future time extension. A basic premise of the extension approaches has been that regardless of the themes, events, or objects that occupy the *future life space*, how far into the future individuals extend their thinking is a significant psychological issue. The rationale for examining it has drawn on the work of Frank on optimal future orientation as a necessary condition for instrumental behavior. Frank contended that:

> The more remote the focus of his time perspectives, the more he will exhibit preparatory or instrumental behavior that uses the present only as a means to the future; the more immediate the focus the more he will exhibit consummatory behavior and react naïvely and ignore consequences. This he may also do if the future focus is so remote that it loses all potency over the present. (Frank, 1939, p. 298).

In all, extension research has been concerned with three issues: the psychological processes underlying extension to the future, its developmental underpinnings, and its demographic and psychological correlates.

The *psychological processes* underlying extension to the future are cognitive and motivational. For some, like Frank (1939), extension to the future reflects individuals' generalized aptitude to think about the future and thus serves as an indicator of *cognitive abilities*. For others, led by Nuttin (Nuttin, 1984; Nuttin & Lens, 1985), future oriented thinking is prompted by *motivational* forces. An extended future time perspective, Nuttin and Lens contended, allows for a larger number of future objects to be represented and for long-term goals to be set. However, to maintain the reality anchor of such long-term goals individuals initiate a chain of sub-goals which act as end-means sequences linking the present to the distant goal object.

For *developmental* psychologists the ability for prospective thinking develops in infancy in response to the delay of satisfaction of basic needs. Using different explanations, both the psychoanalytic and the Piaget cognitive development approaches assume that the development of the notion of time in general and of future orientation in particular have been related to feeding experiences.

According to psychoanalysis, the notion of time emanates from the infant's *frustrations* due to postponement of gratification. Thus, anticipation for later gratification results in the conscious development of expectancy, time sense and vocabulary consisting of words like "now", "today", "tomorrow", and "in a few days" that finally develop into an abstract notion of time expanding from the past into the future (Wallace & Rabin, 1960). In a similar though more positive vein, Piaget (1955) described the development of future expectancies as part of the process of *adaptation* to the need-satisfaction delay which results in the accommodation of a time schema.

The *demographic and psychological correlates* of extension into the future have been examined by several researchers. While agreeing on its conceptualization as "...the forward expanse of time over which future images of the self are projected..." (Lessing, 1972, p. 464) and its assessment as the distance between the present and the future (the time – or age – assigned to the future event), their terminology and to some extent measurements differed. Thus, extension has been described as *prospective time span* (Epley & Ricks, 1963), *temporal distance* (Ekman & Lundberg, 1971), *time-span of stories* (Kendall & Sibley, 1970), *length of future time perspective* (Lessing, 1968), *extension of future time perspective* (Lessing, 1972) or *protension* (Wohlford, 1968).

Their findings, mostly due to diverse operational definitions and dissimilar respondents, are in low agreement. Nevertheless, some trends are visible indicating that extension is negatively related to age (9–15 years of age) (Klineberg, 1967; Lessing, 1972), modernity (vs transition to modernity) (Poole & Cooney, 1987), delinquency (Barndt & Johnson, 1955; Stein, Sarbin, & Kulik, 1968), stealing (Brock & Giudice, 1963) and anxiety (Epley & Ricks, 1963), and positively related to life satisfaction (Lessing, 1972), mental health (Lessing, 1968), optimism (Teahan, 1958), empathy and interpersonal involvement and academic achievement (Epley & Ricks, 1963; Teahan, 1958).

Nonetheless, Frank's (1939) contention about optimal extension has been reiterated by more contemporary researchers (Mischel, Grusec, & Masters, 1969), indicating that, regardless of its valence (positive or negative), as extension increases and reaches the distant future, its effect decreases.

Orientation to the future, present and past. Given that time is continuous and today is the past of tomorrow and the future of yesterday, the question about the interrelatedness of the past, present, and future orientations in fact drew only little attention from researchers. The first to examine it had been Israeli. Interested in the relative importance of the future relative to the past and the present Israeli (1933a) assessed the value of the three time divisions (past, present, and future) among college students majoring in different subjects and found that the majority of students (94%) considered the future more important than the past, but only a minority (30%) considered the future more important than the present.

However, comparison of the three time divisions can take different approaches. Assuming that the temporal space is a closed system, Rokeach and Bonier (1960) examined future orientation by assessing the proportion of representation of future themes relative to past and present themes in response to TAT cards. Their findings show that both closed and open mind individuals include more present than past and future responses, but closed mind include more future responses than do open mind individuals. Their explanation that closed mind individuals experience higher anxiety level and ". . . feel more compelled to project into the future the outcomes of events taking place in the present." (p. 373) conflicts with theoretical implications of the effect of anxiety, particularly anxiety about the future (Zaleski, 2005) and may nevertheless be explained by their use of the TAT methodology.

When interest in the relations between time divisions has been rekindled (Zimbardo & Boyd, 1999), conceptualization and assessment have become more elaborate and past and present orientations treated as representing each two perspectives. The past relates to its positive and negative aspects and the present to hedonistic and fatalistic expressions. The future scale emphasizes goal setting ("when I want to achieve something, I set goals and consider specific means for reaching these goals"), planning ("I believe a person's day should be planned ahead each day"), and being punctual ("I meet my obligations to friends and authorities on time").

However, the association between the future time perspective and each of the present and past scales is relatively low (ranging from $r = .12$ to $-.29$) and with the exception of past-positive are negatively associated. Is the negative relation between present and future inevitable? Not according to Sheldon and Vansteenkiste (2005) who base their analysis on how the present is conceptualized.

Specifically, they contend that, while hedonism is antithetical to future orientation by emphasizing immediate pleasure at the expense of future benefits, and fatalistic present is antithetical to future orientation by holding a pessimistic viewpoint that extends to the future, other aspects of the present may be positively related to the future. One such conceptualization of the present according to Sheldon and Vansteenkiste pertains to individuals' conscious awareness of their true self that researchers describe as *mindfulness* (Brown & Ryan, 2003). However, to date the relation between the mindful-present and future orientation has not yet been published.

Yet another approach to the relation between time zones has been developed by Shirai (Shirai 2002; Shirai & Beresneviciene, 2005). Taking as his point of departure the subjectively preferred time zone, Shirai has been asking his respondents their reasons for preferring one over the two others. These data allow him to distinguish between two types of future and present orientations: negative and positive. Positive present and future are each related to the other time zone indicating the instrumentality of the present for achieving future goals and hopes while negative present and future are not subjectively connected to the other time zone. Moreover, Shirai's findings show the cultural meaning of preferred time zone. Thus, the prevalence of present orientation in the Japanese culture is reflected in the higher preference for the present by Japanese college students than by Belgian and Lithuanian students.

Future orientation as a personality characteristic. The contention that future orientation develops into a stable personality characteristic drew on two grounds. The first is *motivational*, maintaining that inherent in future orientation is a mechanism of self-reinforcement that leads to the gradual development of a personality characteristic. Gjesme described it as:

> *a general capacity to anticipate, shed light on and structure the future*, including a cognitive elaboration of plans and projects and reflecting the degree of concern, involvement and engagement in the future. This capacity is assumed to manifest itself whenever there is a certain value and/or valence associated with the potential future plan or event, i.e., an individual's future time orientation is *aroused* and manifests itself as a function of the *anticipated* valence or importance of the future tasks, events, or activities. (Gjesme, 1983, p. 452).

This approach in fact represents a personality by situation approach (Mischel, 1968) by which a personality attribute is manifested only under certain conditions that might be intra-personal, interpersonal, or sociocultural.

Using this approach, researchers working in the Research Center for Motivation and Time Perspective in Leuven, Belgium conceptualized the future time perspective (FTP) as consisting of two aspects: the *dynamic* and the *cognitive* (De Volder & Lens, 1982; Husman & Shell, 2008; Nuttin and Lens, 1985). While, according to their conceptualization, the cognitive aspect pertains to the instrumental value attributed to each future object, and hence is domain specific, the dynamic aspect of future time perspective pertains to the person's *disposition* to attribute high valence or value to more distant future objects, regardless of their thematic nature. Thus, individuals with long future time perspective experience a future object such as hope, plan or goal in the distant future as psychologically closer than do individuals with short future time perspective and maintain the value of distant reward or goals more than do individuals with short future time perspective.

Three other dispositional approaches that pertain to consideration of future consequences (Joireman, Anderson, & Strathman, 2003; Strathman, Gleicher, Boninger, & Edwards, 1994), self appraisal of one's capability to reach future goals (Snyder et al., 1991), and the future dimension of time perspective (Goossens, Luyckx, Lens, & Smits, 2008; Sircova et al., 2008; Worrell & Mello, 2007; Zimbardo & Boyd, 1999) are described in a subsequent section about interfacing approaches.

The Thematic Approach

Underlying the thematic approach has been a basic premise that the future – much like the present and the past – is not an empty temporal space (Nuttin & Lens, 1985). Whereas time itself can be grasped as an abstract notion, time zones (or time divisions as they are alternatively referred too) – past, present, and future – are imagery-based and defined by their content. The richness of human experience and diversity of viewpoints are also manifested in the multiple domains subsuming this content. Thus, whereas the categories used by different approaches may vary, they all consist of multiple thematic domains.

Initial research. The thematic approach draws on three early analyses. Israeli's (1936b) and Gillespie and Allport's (1955) future autobiography, and Cantril's (1965) analysis of human concerns. Although all shared an interest in the themes included in the constructed future of various social and cultural groups, their work emanated from different approaches and its objectives influenced by the historical period in which it had been carried out.

As noted earlier, Israeli's research was prompted by his interest in the social psychology of time and particularly in the motivational underpinnings of future thinking and realization. His publication of *some aspects of the social psychology of futurism* (Israeli, 1930) was the first to report future orientation research. The work of Cantril and of Gillespie and Allport took place in the post World War II era. Guided by their concern about international understanding and commitment to world peace, both research projects consisted of multinational comparisons. For Gillespie and Allport (1955) the question was not embedded in theoretical considerations but rather in the scientists' social responsibilities to world community. Thus, they asked:

Do young people in *different countries* view their futures in essentially the same way? If we find a uniformity of peaceful ideals and intentions we may have reason to hope for a better world. If however, we find little uniformity, we must try to delineate the chief national differences. They may be so striking that we shall be forced to affirm the existence of diverse national characters and perhaps abandon the hope that advances in communication and growing similarity in educational practices are creating a single world community. (Gillespie and Allport, 1955, p. 3).

In the spirit of the early 1960s in the United States, Cantril (1965) was responding to a situation in which "responsible government officials are today turning more frequently to the social scientist for insights into the nature and solution of the problems with which they are confronted." (Cantril 1965, p. 3). His judgment was that what social scientists could provide the political system with was information about "what people want", which he described as "concerns".

As a sociologist he thought that a full range of human concerns should include hopes and fears in both the personal and the national levels. While the distinction between the personal and the national (or collective) has been followed only seldom, the work reviewed in subsequent chapters indicates that the conceptualization of future orientation in terms of hopes and fears has become the standard. From a psychological point of view, underlying it has been the theoretical advantage of viewing future orientation as having both *approach* (i.e., hopes) and *avoidance* (i.e., fears) motivational qualities (e.g., Mönks, 1968).

For reasons which have to do with the sociology of scientific research more than with explicit scientific considerations, the use of athematic and thematic approaches followed a chronological path. Thus, the 1950s and 1960s future orientation studies applied mainly the athematic approaches (with the exception of Mönks' thematic analysis) and among them particularly the extension methods, and research from the 1980s on (Greene, 1986; Nurmi, 1987, 1989; Poole & Cooney, 1987; Pulkkinen & Rönkä, 1994; Seginer, 1986a; Trommsdorff & Lamm, 1980) employed the thematic approach.

Data collection and data analysis. In research using this approach data are collected by open-ended means consisting of essays in which respondents describe their life in the future (Gillespie & Allport, 1955; Mönks, 1968) or questionnaires (see Appendix) in which respondents list their hopes and fears (Nurmi, 1987; Seginer, 1986a; Trommsdorff & Lamm, 1980) and analysis is carried out in two steps. In the first each narrative unit (the smallest meaningful phrase) is coded into its compatible prospective life domain (e.g., education, work and career); in the second, the *density* score of each respondent's prospective life domain is calculated as the ratio of the number of domain specific narrative units/total number of narrative units. The analysis is carried out separately for hopes and for fears. To illustrate, if a child lists 10 hopes narratives, three of which were coded as pertaining to education and schooling, her hopes education and schooling density score is 3/10 = 0.30; if the total number of her prospective life course categories (summing up the schooling and education, military service, work and career, and marriage and family domains) is 6, the density score of this overarching category is 0.60.

Analysis of data collected in Israel from different groups such as Arab, Druze, Jewish ultra-orthodox girls, and Jewish urban and kibbutz girls and boys yielded eight prospective life domain categories that have maintained their consistency across the years (Seginer, 1986a, 2005). These domain categories, their description and sample narratives are presented in Table 1.1. Subsequent analyses showed they can be grouped into two sets of overarching categories: prospective life course vs existential categories, and core vs culture specific categories.

The prospective life course and existential categories. Because respondents are encouraged to write everything that comes to their mind, they include in their protocols both prospective and atemporal events and experiences. The first pertains to events related only to their subjective future and described as the *prospective life course*. For adolescents this overarching category consists of three core domains: higher education, work and career, and marriage and family. The second relates to events that apply as well to their past and present and described as the *existential* category. It draws its name from the meaning of existence as *continuance in being* and consists of domains pertaining to self concerns, leisure, significant others, and collective issues (i.e., society and state).

The validity of this a priori grouping has been substantiated by data collected in Israel that show they differ across three dimensions. One, the *future life space* (i.e., all future related narratives) of children is characterized by a larger share of existential narratives than those of adolescents (Gelberg, 1996). Second, the tendency to list prospective life course narratives is positively associated with several indicators of psychological well-being such as self esteem, optimism, and intimacy (Seginer, 2005).

Finally, underlying the two empirical differences listed above is the nature of the two categories. Content analysis shows that the prospective life course narratives are task-oriented and self-guiding, whereas the existential narratives, and especially those related to self concerns, address non-specific experiences, mood and emotions (e.g., "that I will have good/prosperous life") and lack self-guiding. Bandura's comment regarding goals is applicable here too: "Goals do not automatically activate the self-influences that govern motivation and action. . .General goals are *too indefinite and noncommitting* [*italics added*] to serve as guides and incentives" (2001, p. 8). Such "abstract desires and wishes" will, however, gain influence on behavior when ". . .translated into goals that can be achieved by behaving in particular ways" (Lawrence & Dodds, 2003, p. 520). Thus, it is not just any form of thinking about the future that is facilitating development, but one of specific instrumental nature.

Altogether, research employing the thematic approach has been descriptive. Consequently, it has been mainly concerned with group differences between girls and boys (Seginer, 1988b), lower and middle class (Trommsdorff & Lamm, 1980; Lamm, Schmidt, & Trommsdorff, 1976), younger and older adolescents (Nurmi, 1987), and different ethnic and national groups (Poole & Cooney, 1987; Nurmi, Poole, & Seginer, 1995; Seginer, 1986a). These comparisons led to the distinction between the common core and culture-specific domains.

Core and culture-specific domains. Despite different physical conditions, cultural orientations and beliefs about adult roles, adolescents growing up in different

Table 1.1 Future orientation domains

Domain	Themes	Sample narratives	
		Hopes	Fears
School and graduation	Examinations, grades, academic track and majors, graduation certificate, school atmosphere	Complete my high school requirements; move to a better school; A in Physics	That I flunk final exams; I will not be admitted to the science program
Military service	Motivation, quality and duration of military service; specific unit and type of service preferences	Be admitted to an elite unit; be exempted from military service; to have a meaningful military service; that I won't waste my time	That I will waste my time in military service; serve far away from home; not be admitted to preferred unit; I'll be harmed while in military service
Higher education	Admission to college or university; preferred major; academic achievement and graduate degrees	To get a high grade in the psychometric exam [equivalent to ACT]; to study chemistry at Tel Aviv University; be accepted to the psychology program and obtain graduate degrees in psychology	I will not have enough money to continue my education; that I will not be accepted to the program I always wanted to attend; that my parents will not allow me to study at a university away from home
Work and career	Statements regarding job, occupation, and profession	Become an architect; I would like to be a lawyer; a job that will earn me money and high social position; find a job	That I will not become a lawyer (because I am not a good student); be unemployed; my family will not allow me to get a job
Marriage and family	Future spouse (romantic partner is included here for transition-to-adulthood and adults) and children	To marry my boyfriend Danny; get married; have an understanding husband and wonderful children; have a big family	That I will be childless; that I will not marry the right person; after I get married my husband will treat me harshly; something bad will happen to my children
Self concerns	General statements about self; statements about mood and personality characteristics	To be happy; that people will love me; to be a respectable person; that all my hopes be fulfilled; to be honest; to be courageous; to be a good girl	That I will have an unhappy life; that I will not be the happy and respectable woman I wish to become; many disappointments

Table 1.1 (continued)

Domain	Themes	Sample narratives	
		Hopes	Fears
Others	Parents and other family members peers, friends, romantic partner (if not included in Marriage and family)	That my mother will get her college degree; that my parents will be proud of me; that my father will not die (my mother died of cancer); that my sister will recover from her illness	Terrible things will happen to my mother and father and other family members; that my sister's engagement will be annulled; that my parents will not have enough money to send my brother to college
Collective issues	Statements pertaining to one's community, country, nation, and world affairs	World peace; that we will not have nuclear war; my village will get a new road; my favorite football team will win the cup; that Jews will stop discriminating against Arabs	Nuclear war; the Palestinians will not get their rights; the world will be a bad place for people to live in

socio-cultural settings relate to a common core of four prospective life domains: education, work and career, marriage and family, and self concerns. Beyond these, however, adolescents construct their future according to the norms, values and life conditions prevailing in their social settings.

Thus the individualistic orientations and economic comfort of western societies is reflected in the tendency of Australian adolescents to list leisure narratives (Poole & Cooney, 1987), of Finnish adolescents to list property and leisure activities narratives (Nurmi & Pulliainen, 1991), and of German adolescents to include material comfort narratives (Trommsdorff, 1982). Mandatory military service is reflected in the tendency of Israeli Jewish girls and boys and Druze boys to list military service (Seginer, 2001a) but, hesitant about their Israeli identity, new immigrants from former Soviet Russia and particularly those defining themselves as cosmopolitan Jews list fewer military service hopes and fears (Toren-Kaplan, 1995). Israeli Arab and Druze adolescents, growing up in societies that endorse familistic and collectivist values, also list others (i.e., family members) and the collective (i.e., my village, country, nation) (Seginer & Halabi-Kheir, 1998).

The Three Component Model of Future Orientation

Aware of the narrowness of an approach consisting only of the cognitive representation of the future, two multi-dimensional multiple-step future orientation models have been constructed. The first has been developed by Nurmi (1989, 1991) and consists of three components: motivation, planning, and evaluation. Motivation pertains to interests expressed by the *goals* individuals set for themselves, planning relates to the *plans* and activities individuals intend to employ to attain their goals, and evaluation to the *anticipated success* of materialization of goals as reflected in causal attributions and affect. In their turn, causal attributions are related to individuals' subjective appraisal of their "opportunities of controlling their future" (Nurmi, 1991, p. 6); affect pertains to the "...immediate and also unconscious types of evaluation" (Nurmi, 1991, p. 6) and its valence depends on materialization expectations; success expectations invoke positive emotions such as optimism, and failure expectations arouse pessimism.

The second model has been constructed by Seginer, Nurmi, and Poole (Seginer, Nurmi, & Poole, 1991; Seginer, 1995, 2000, 2005). Like Nurmi's model, it is *generic* (i.e., applies to different life domains) and consists of three components whose links form *multiple steps*. Drawing on earlier theoretical analyses (Nurmi, 1991; Nuttin & Lens, 1985; Trommsdorff, 1983), the three components describe the motivational, cognitive, and behavioral aspects of future orientation and the relations among them. Each component subsumes two or three variables.

As noted above, the model grew out of an earlier conceptualization of future orientation that focused only on the cognitive representation of anticipated events and experiences and rests on the pivotal function of motivational forces for the cognitive representation and behavioral engagement aspects of future orientation. Accordingly, the motivational component affects directly the two other components; it also

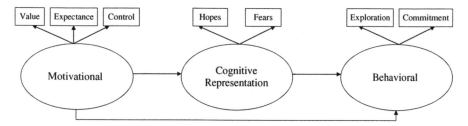

Fig. 1.1 The future orientation three-component model

affects the behavioral component indirectly, via its effect on the cognitive component (Fig. 1.1). It is important to note that the empirical estimate of the future orientation model became possible only as structural equation modeling (SEM) techniques became more accessible to behavioral scientists. The nature of each of the components and the variables subsumed under it are described below.

The motivational component. This component relates to the question of what prompts individuals to think about the future? Or rather, what prompts them to invest in thinking extended into the future? The affinity between future orientation and achievement motivation (Raynor & Entin, 1982) has led several researchers to describe the motivational aspects of future orientation in terms of two concepts initially used for the analysis of achievement motivation: the *value* one sees in future domains, and the *expectancy* of successful domain-relevant outcomes.

Irrespective of achievement motivation, for other researchers the motivational properties of future orientation emanate from the interests (Nurmi, 1991) and needs of the individual (Nuttin & Lens, 1985; Trommsdorff, 1986), value of expected behavior outcomes and the subjective appraisal of their attainability (Atkinson, 1964; Atkinson & Feather, 1966; Austin & Vancouver, 1996; Eccles & Wigfield, 1995; Miller & Brickman, 2004; Raynor & Entin, 1982), and from attributing the fulfillment of personal hopes, plans and goals to *internal control* (i.e., ability and effort) factors (Rotter, 1966; Weiner, 1974, 1985).

Consequently, three motivational variables have been delineated: the *value* of a prospective life domain; *expectance* (i.e., subjective confidence) of materialization of hopes and plans and its affective outcomes (Carver & Scheier, 2001, 2002), and a sense of *internal control* over the materialization of prospective hopes and plans reflected in the person's subjective belief that such materialization depends on her or his skills and efforts. *Value* pertains to the importance and relevance individuals attribute to a prospective domain. Is higher education important for my future life? Is it worth my effort? Will career be beneficial (useful) for my future life? Will family life be central or marginal to my future life?

Expectancy relates to individuals' confidence about the materialization of their domain-specific hopes, goals and plans. As such it also includes the emotional tone and particularly optimism about the materialization of hopes, goals and plans. Thus, expectance is expressed in a sense of being determined to fulfill one's plans about higher education or future career, and be confident about the materialization of hopes, goals and plans, or optimistic about marriage plans.

The inclusion of the *internal control* variable emanated from the social learning theory (e.g., Rotter, 1954, 1966; Weiner, 1972, 1996) contention that expectance consists of both situation-specific and a "generalization of expectancies (GE) from other related behavior-reinforcement sequences" (Rotter, 1954, p. 166) that crystallize into beliefs about the nature of reinforcement as dependent on one's own behavior and characteristics (internal control) or on uncontrollable external factors (external control) (Rotter, 1966). In other words, the internal-external control construct describes the extent to which individuals believe she or he ". . .posses power or lacks power over what happens to him" (Lefcourt, 1966, p. 207) or her in general and regarding goal attainment in particular (Weiner, 1996).

Given that the future is an occurrence not yet experienced, *generalized* expectancies such as the internal and external control beliefs are of special relevance to the study of future orientation. In light of earlier multivariate analyses (Seginer, 2001b) that showed external control did not contribute to the explained variance, this variable has been excluded from the motivational variables. Several recent analyses (Dekel, 2009; Mahajna, 2007; Seginer, Shoyer, & Mahajna, 2008; Seginer, Vermulst, & Shoyer, 2004; Shoyer, 2006) employing structural equation modeling (SEM) linked the value, expectance and internal control variables to a future orientation motivational latent (theoretical) variable.

The cognitive representation component. As long as researchers had been interested only in the thematic aspect of future orientation, the cognitive representation of the future was described in terms of two dimensions: content and valence. Content pertains to the various life domains by which individuals construct the future and valence is based on the assumption that individuals relate to the future in terms of *approach* and *avoidance* as expressed by *hopes* and *fears*. Thus, research focused on domain representations in the hopes and fears prospective life *space*s of different groups. Underlying it has been the assumption that high frequency indicates the salience of a domain.

These issues can be assessed either by open-ended questionnaires and essays or by scalable items in which respondents mark how often they think about higher education, work and career, or marriage and family. Each method has its advantages and drawbacks. On the advantages side, the open-ended method offers respondents' spontaneous representation of the future and informs researchers of the rich expressions by which individuals from different socio-cultural groups represent their future life space. However, its spontaneity is also its disadvantage. Because respondents are free to list what comes into their minds, they may not relate to all prospective domains; the result is a skewed distribution and a great deal of missing data. Conversely, by using Likert scales researchers lose the spontaneity and richness of expression but gain in having their data amenable to testing hypotheses about the intrapersonal antecedents and outcomes of future orientation.

The behavioral component. The *behavioral* component consists of two variables: *exploration* of future options by seeking advice, gathering information, and probing their suitability vis-à-vis the individual's personal characteristics and life circumstances, and *commitment* to one specific option, and can be applied to different prospective domains. Exploration consists of behaviors directed to the outside world and inward to the person her- or himself. Collecting information about higher education or career options, talking to other people and consulting them regarding higher education or career option are examples of outward directed behaviors. Checking whether a certain career fits the person, or how interested one really is in psychology as a major, and imagining oneself living the rest of ones life with ones partner are inwardly directed explorations.

Commitment relates to decision making. Individuals indicating that they have made up their mind about their career, academic major, or getting married, or making serious preparation to enter a career or go to college have made a commitment regarding that life domain. Although common sense, Frost's (1960) *The road not taken* (. . .And be one traveler, long I stood/And looked down one as far as I could/To where it bent in the undergrowth;/ then took the other, as just as fair. . .), and ego identity conceptualization assert that decision follows exploration, in this model the two processes are conceptually and psychologically concurrent and subsumed under the behavioral component.

It is important to note that, although in describing the behavioral component the 'building blocks' of the identity formation conceptualization are being used, the meaning of exploration and commitment in the future orientation and identity formation conceptualizations is different. The difference relates to two issues. First, in the theoretical framework of ego identity, exploration and commitment are the *observable indicators of intrapsychic processes* of identity formation (Marcia, 1993) while in the future orientation conceptualization active engagement in exploration and commitment is assumed to lead toward the materialization of prospective hopes, wishes, and plans. Second, according to ego identity conceptualization, identity statuses are defined by the *combined* presence or absence of explorations and commitment (Cote & Levine, 2002; Marcia, 1993) whereas in the future orientation conceptualization they are treated separately.

Summary. Aware of the richness of the future orientation construct, both Nurmi and Seginer et al. developed multi-dimensional multi-step models. Both models are generic (i.e., may apply to various future life domains), and consist of three components, each indicated by several empirical variables. The components included in Nurmi's model are motivation, planning, and evaluation and those included in Seginer et al.'s are motivational, cognitive, and behavioral. Although drawing on different theoretical underpinnings, they share several common empirical indicators pertaining to success expectations, sense of internal control, and exploration of future hopes and goals. The empirical estimates of the Seginer model and its outcomes are reported in the various chapters of this volume (particularly in Chaps. 3, 5, 6, and 7).

Four Interfacing Approaches

Just as future orientation has lent itself to several conceptualizations resulting in different assessments and research questions, issues related to future thinking have evolved from different theoretical frameworks. Underlying these approaches are two questions related to the effect of future thinking on development, particularly during adolescence, and on behavior. The first question is developmental in nature and concerns the relation between future orientation and identity. It has been initially studied by Erikson (1968) and Marcia and colleagues' (Marcia, Waterman, Matteson, Archer, & Orlofsky, 1993) analyses of *ego identity*, and addressed in a subsequent chapter (Chap. 7) where the relations between future orientation and identity are examined. The second question on the effect of future orientation on various behavioral indicators is addressed by *motivational* (Nuttin & Lens, 1985), *self* (Markus & Nurius, 1986), *goal*, and *personality* approaches. Their conceptualizations, the terms each uses to describe future thinking, and their main findings on the effect of future thinking on behavior are reviewed here.

The Motivational Approach: Future Time Perspective

The motivational underpinnings of future thinking have been discussed in the work initiated by Nuttin (Nuttin, 1984; Nuttin & Lens, 1985) and further developed in the work of Lens and his students and colleagues (the Leuven group) and other researchers (Miller & Brickman, 2004). For these researchers future thinking involves "…human needs that are cognitively processed into goal objects and behavioral projects" (Nuttin & Lens, 1985, p. 18). Underlying this approach has been the consideration of two basic facts: that since early age humans are able to engage in outlining hopes, goals and plans, and that the future is the time where these hopes and fears, goals and plans are located. Consequently, *future time perspective* pertains to orientation "…toward motivational goals in the immediate, the more distant or far distant future" (Lens, 1986, p. 179).

Active/motivational and cognitive/imaginational time perspectives. Their emphasis on the motivational nature of future time perspective led Nuttin and Lens (1985) to draw attention to two different time perspectives: active/motivational and cognitive/imaginational. Two conditions facilitate the development of active realistic future time perspective. Underlying both are mechanisms for maintaining the present-future link. The first is *perceived instrumentality* pertaining to individuals' tendency to perceive behavior carried out in the present as instrumental or leading to the pursuit of a future goal. To illustrate, high school students who work hard at school and obtain high grades in order to be admitted to a high standing college program which will in turn facilitate admission to graduate program in psychology or medical school perceive high school academic achievement as instrumental for career in each of those areas.

The second condition for the development of active motivational future time perspective consists of establishing a *chain of means-end* structure that bridges the time distance between present activity and the motivational object. Thus, the student who perceives the instrumentality of her high school academic achievement for the pursuit of higher education and professional career must initiate a chain of means-ends activities that will maintain the reality value of the distant goal and facilitate its achievement by activities relevant to the attainment of the distant goal. In the case of future orientation related to higher education and career such means-end chains consist of being admitted to a college-bound high school program, working hard and doing well on the academic subjects related to one's aspired college major, and in certain cultural groups also convincing parents of the value of higher education.

The difference between Nuttin and Lens's approach and other related approaches concerns behavior regulation. Specifically, while in their *motivational induction method* only dreams, fantasies and "castles in Spain" represent cognitive or imaginational time perspective which obviously lacks a motivational effect, in analyses carried out in the frameworks of self agency (Bandura, 2001), in possible selves and future orientation the distinction is between specific, concrete, and goal-oriented narratives and those that are not. To illustrate, items like "to be myself", "to succeed in life" (Nuttin & Lens, 1985, p. 194) – coded as positive motivational objects by the motivational induction method – are considered as *self-enhancing* rather than self-regulating by the possible selves approach (Oyserman, Gant, & Ager, 1995), as *abstract desires and wishes* by Lawrence and Dodds (2003), and as representing *existential* rather than prospective life course domains by the future orientation approach (Seginer, 2005).

Perceived instrumentality. Research ensuing from the early work of Nuttin and Lens focused on two questions: the relation between perceived instrumentality and achievement motivation, and the nature of the conditions that facilitate or hinder perceived instrumentality. Underlying the first question has been the assumption that future time perspective is indicated by perceiving the instrumentality of present behavior for reaching a future goal (Simons, Vansteenkiste, Lens, & Lacante, 2004). Its examination shows that perceived instrumentality *is* linked to academic achievement even among low achieving students placed in vocational schools (Creten, Lens, & Simons, 2001).

The question about facilitating (or hindering) conditions focused on two issues. The first pertains to individuals' *attitudes* toward the future (positive vs negative) and the second to the nature of the perceived instrumentality process as *extrinsic or intrinsic*. Examination of the first issue led to the conclusion that although perceived instrumentality has a positive effect on several behavioral indicators, this effect is moderated by attitudes toward the future and the nature of the present task. According to one early study (Van Calster, Lens, & Nuttin, 1987) perceived instrumentality has a positive effect on academic motivation and achievement only for individuals holding positive hopeful attitudes toward the future.

Extrinsic and intrinsic perceived instrumentality. The seemingly extrinsic nature of perceived instrumentality as a process by which present activities are motivated by their association with future valuable goals raised questions about its consequences for task vs performance orientation (Lens, Simons, & Dewitte, 2002). Demonstrating that perceived instrumentality also has intrinsic characteristics, researchers (Simons, Dewitte, & Lens, 2000) asked whether the effect of extrinsic and intrinsic perceived instrumentality is enhanced or hindered by intrinsic or extrinsic regulation conditions? To study it, the authors developed three experimental situations in which perceived instrumentality is operationalized in terms of the utility value of present behavior for future goals and regulation as emanating from extrinsic or intrinsic motives.

The three experimental conditions were: extrinsic perceived instrumentality–extrinsic behavior regulation (studying hard to become an engineer to avoid living in a poor neighborhood), intrinsic perceived instrumentality–intrinsic behavior regulation (studying hard psychology to become a good psychologist), and extrinsic perceived instrumentality–intrinsic behavior regulation (to develop oneself by reading about computers for no obvious future goal but rather for developing one's general knowledge).

When respondents were asked to think about themselves in each of the situations and evaluate the extent to which these situations would arouse task and performance goals, the findings showed that the extrinsic perceived instrumentality (motivation)–extrinsic regulation condition aroused more performance orientation than the two other conditions. Even more instructive, however, has been the finding that under conditions of intrinsic behavior regulation, the goal orientation prompted by extrinsic perceived instrumentality is very similar to the goal orientation relevant to intrinsic perceived instrumentality.

Thus, the authors conclude, "extrinsic motivation may lead to an adaptive goal orientation if the extrinsic motive is personally meaningful" (Simons et al., 2000, p. 349). A subsequent study (Simons et al., 2004) highlights the relevance of intrinsic behavior regulation: when activity is framed in terms of future extrinsic goal, its effect on performance is weaker than that of having no future goal at all.

Summary. The motivational approach – in which future thinking is described as *future time perspective* – draws on the assumption that, to satisfy their needs, humans must form goals and develop goal-achieving behaviors. Given that goals are placed in the future and behavior used as *means* for achieving a specific goal occurs in the present, behavior must be *perceived as instrumental* to the achievement of the goal and the association between goals – particularly those placed in the distant future – and behavior serving as means for achieving it must be maintained by a *chain of means–goals*. Moreover, although instrumentality is often interpreted as indicating extrinsic motivation, future time perspective research has shown that perceived instrumentality has also intrinsic characteristics and that such instrumentality reaches more adaptive goal orientation when intrinsically regulated.

The Self Approach: Possible Selves

The possible selves construct draws on the self theory and particularly on work of several of the founding fathers of psychology. James (1910) distinguished between the "immediate present me" and the "potential social me" and Mead (1934) posited that individuals generate potential selves by a process that starts with considering several courses of action, judging them against the responses of others, and drawing on these reactions as they design future actions.

The possible selves construct. Underlying the possible selves construct are three basic assumptions on the nature of the self: the self is a *multifaceted* phenomenon

(Markus, Cross, & Wurf, 1990; Markus & Wurf, 1987), self representations pertain to *all time divisions* (past, present, and future), and the self has *motivational* capacities that instigate goal directed behavior (Markus & Ruvolo, 1989). Drawing on James's idea of "potential selves" as reflecting the person's potential, possible selves ". . .pertains to how individuals think about their potential and about their future." (Markus & Nurius, 1986, p. 954). Such thinking applies to three aspects of the self: the ideal self (what a person would like to become), the real self (what she or he could become) and the feared self (what one is afraid of becoming), as each is expressed by the person's aspirations, hopes, goals, and fears.

Possible selves are generated in the context of individuals' socio-cultural settings and historical periods. Once formed, they have three main functions: motivational, evaluative, and simulation. Specifically, possible selves act as incentives for future behavior, provide individuals with an opportunity to evaluate the now selves in terms of their future aspirations, hopes and fears, and facilitate the materialization of future hopes and plans by allowing the person to imagine the action and resources needed to accomplish the task (Cross & Markus, 1990). By imagining different scenarios, individuals may also evaluate the likelihood of materializing their plans, hopes, or goals (Markus, Cross, & Wurf, 1990).

Initially, this theoretical framework generated two lines of research: the validity of the possible selves construct and the embeddedness of possible selves in personal and social context. Each is described below.

Examining the validity of the possible selves construct. To test the validity of the possible selves construct (Markus & Nurius, 1986), respondents were presented with a list of positive, negative and neutral attributes pertaining to five categories: general qualities, life style possibilities, general abilities, occupational possibilities, and the opinion of others on the person. Next, they were requested to respond to those items by considering whether the item described them now, in the past, could ever be considered as a possible self, and how probable and desirable that possible self had been for them.

Analysis of their responses showed that individuals use more of these items to describe their possible selves than their past selves, to think about themselves in the future more often than in the past, and tend to endorse positive more than negative descriptors ("positive bias"). The effect of possible selves on affective-motivational states beyond the effect of the now self is demonstrated for three dependent variables: self esteem, negative affect, and hopelessness.

Assessing possible selves' embeddedness. A second question posited by early possible selves research has been the extent to which the cognitive representation of goals, hopes, fears, and plans that bridges the present and the future *is embedded* in social and personal conditions. To examine this question, respondents were requested to write down three expected selves and three feared selves. These data allowed Oyserman and Markus (1986, as cited in Markus & Nurius, 1986) to posit two hypotheses about possible selves of delinquent and non-delinquent adolescents.

The first hypothesis addresses the themes by which youths from the two groups describe their possible selves. Underlying it is the assumption that possible selves reflect adolescents' reality so that the nature of the delinquents' possible selves is more negative than that of the non-delinquents. Their findings confirm the hypothesis for the feared but not for the expected possible selves: the feared possible selves of the delinquent youths relate to criminality themes whereas the possible selves of the non-delinquents are more diverse and less negative.

The second hypothesis concerns the role of balanced possible selves in predicting delinquency. Underlying it is the assumption that balanced possible selves augment motivation to achieve a desired end state by (1) alerting the person who developed a hoped for possible self (e.g., getting a job) to the ill effects of a feared possible self (e.g., stay out of job) and (2) by providing the person imagining a feared possible self with a hoped for possible self that indicates a "way out" of the feared self. Together, or separately, the two processes energize and direct behavior toward achieving the desired self (Oyserman & Markus, 1990).

Applied to delinquent and non-delinquent adolescents, Oyserman and Markus predicted that non-delinquents will list more balanced possible selves than will delinquents. Their findings show that 81% of the non-delinquents but only 38% of the delinquents had at least one balanced possible self (Oyserman & Markus, 1990); nonetheless, balanced possible selves do not predict delinquent behaviors, such as self reported theft, aggression, vandalism, and truancy (Oyserman & Saltz, 1993).

An extended possible selves model. Prompted by findings showing that balanced achievement-related possible selves and academic achievement are positively related, and informed by Cantor's (Cantor & Kihlstrom, 1987) social intelligence conceptualization and its emphasis on strategies, Oyserman and her associates (Oyserman, Bybee, Terry, & Hart-Johnson, 2004; Oyserman, Bybee, & Terry, 2006; Oyserman et al., 1995) extended the possible selves model by including in it *strategies* that mediate the hoped for possible self and its desired outcome. However, like researchers studying other similar constructs, possible selves' researchers posited that not all possible selves are equipped or accompanied with strategies for obtaining hoped for possible selves and avoiding feared possible selves. When they are, they *self regulate* behavior; however, when they are not their function merely serves *self-enhancement.*

Thus, future orientation research reviewed earlier that led us to distinguish between the prospective life course and existential domains and suggest the former are behavior instigating and directing and the latter – by being general – lack these qualities, points to a similar distinction. Oyserman et al.'s studies indeed demonstrate the effect of the self regulatory academic possible selves, but not of the self enhancing possible selves, on improved academic achievement and other related educational outcomes such as preparing homework, classroom participation, and summer school referral (negative effect).

Summary. The possible selves construct anchors the discussion on future oriented thinking in self theory, contending that the selves individuals wish for themselves, consider possible and desire *not* to have are part of the self system and are activated within the working self. Their main function is to bridge the present and the future and their main advantage is that they are relatively free of reality and hence may prompt coping with stresses and challenges whose success seem improbable to the outside observer. Like the future orientation construct, the possible selves conceptualization is domain specific, relates to both desired (ideal) and feared future, distinguishes between goal-directed and non-goal directed future, and, like the future time prospective approach, emphasizes the importance of understanding the importance of the instrumentality of present domain-specific behavior for attaining future goals.

Personality Goal Approaches

The goal approach to personality grew out of criticism voiced by several researchers (Cantor, 1990; McAdams, 1996) about the limited usefulness of traits for understanding human behavior, and the ensuing relevance of goals that unlike traits, are contextualized, provisional, and relate directly to human experiences of success and failure (Karoly, 1993). By emphasizing intentionality, goal approaches in fact address the future oriented aspects of personality. Nonetheless, although for a time goals were considered as new units of analysis in personality psychology which serve as an alternative to the trait approach (Little, 1989), presently traits and goals are two distinct levels of personality (Cantor, 1990; Little, 2006; McAdams, 1996). Cantor (1990) described the two levels as the "is" and the "does" of personality, and Little (2006) describes the second level – or tier – as personal action constructs (PAC).

The three approaches presented here study personality by using cognitive units of analysis that focus on the examination of everyday phenomena as hierarchically structured, intentional and hence future oriented, and embedded in social-cultural and historical contexts (Little, 1989; Pervin, 1989; Zirkel & Cantor, 1990). However, drawing on different theoretical frameworks, they ask how individuals organize their everyday activities in the present and the future (*personal projects*), define their goals across different life settings and developmental periods (*personal strivings*), and develop suitable strategies for pursuing age and culture appropriate life tasks (*life tasks*).

Personal Projects. The conceptualization of personal projects drew on the importance Murray (1959) attributed to the study of *serials*– that is, to the temporal aspects of human behavior – rather than to momentary decontextualized activities which have been the focus of much psychological research. In translating Murray's serials into a researchable construct, Little (1987, 2007) focused on the intentional, ecological and systemic contexts of action and coined the term personal projects, described as ". . . self-generated accounts of what a person is doing or is planning to do" (McGregor & Little, 1998, p. 494). Extended into the future, personal projects are inter-related so that each serves as part of a system of commitments and concerns (Little, 1987) generated in response to the person's social and historical circumstances, and their cognitive, motivational-affective, and behavioral aspects are intended to direct the person into obtaining future goals.

Like other goal approaches, personal projects are idiosyncratic, generated by each individual for her- or himself and may range from very specific such as "doing macramé plant hangers" to noble projects like "coming to terms with my faith" (Little, 1983, p. 293). However, its assessment is not merely idiographic; it also involves nomothetic methods pertaining to the coding of the personal projects in terms of 12 content categories, and the appraisal of each personal project by respondents in terms of relevant dimensions pertaining to self benefit, fun, efficacy, integrity, support (McGregor & Little, 1998), stress, and progress (Salmela-Aro, Vuori, & Koivisto, 2007).

Using this methodology, personal projects data can answer both theoretical and practical questions. In one study (McGregor & Little, 1998) happiness and meaning were assessed by respondents' self ratings of their personal projects showing they serve both symbolic and instrumental functions and consequently can promote both meaning (via the integrity aspect of personal projects) and happiness (via the efficacy aspect of personal projects). Overall, empirical findings indicate that engagement in meaningful, well-structured, efficacious, other-supported, and not too stressful personal projects have a positive effect on psychological well being (Little, 2000). Personal projects methods can also be used to describe the needs of individuals and target groups (e.g., new immigrant adolescents, depressed students) and hence serve as a basis for providing individual psychological help and planning intervention programs.

Personal strivings. As Little's personal projects conceptualization draws on Murray's concept of serial program, Emmons' (1989, 1996) personal strivings conceptualization draws on Floyd Allport's (1937) "teleonomic trend". Allport used this term to describe behavioral tendencies that reflect what the person is trying to do, or the purpose she or he is trying to fulfill. For Emmons (1999) the conceptualization of personal strivings as "what a person is trying to do" conveys three important elements: their goal base, action orientation, and meaning giving that personal strivings acquire by reflecting on personal choices. Altogether, personal strivings direct individuals ". . .toward particular outcomes and away from others" (Emmons, 1999, p. 29). While personal strivings are idiographic, they are stable and can be described by a set of categories commonly shared by many individuals.

The empirical study of personal strivings consists of five basic questions. The first pertains to the list of personal strivings that individuals generate in response to the stem sentence "I typically try to_____ ", and the second to ways for materializing each of 15 personal strivings respondents outline. The third issue concerns the evaluation of each striving in terms of dimensions like valence, commitment, probability of success, effort, and difficulty. The fourth issue concerns strivings interdependence, i.e., the extent to which success on each striving facilitates or hinders the achievement of each of the other strivings, and results in average instrumentality or conflict (1/instrumentality) scores (Emmons, 1989). Finally, the fifth question concerns the emotional cost of each striving, measured by reporting how *unhappy* individuals are after materializing each striving (ambivalence). Empirical findings show that conflict and ambivalence are associated with poor psychological and physical well-being (Emmons & King, 1988), and abstract strivings are associated with depression and considered harder to achieve than concrete strivings (Emmons, 1992).

Life tasks. Like personal projects and personal strivings, life tasks (Cantor & Langston, 1989; Cantor, Kemmelmeier, Basten, & Prentice, 2002; Cantor, Norem, Langston, Zirkel, Fleeson, & Cook-Flannagan, 1991) are self-generated, intentional, and hence behavior guiding, and pertain to everyday experiences. Their particular contribution to the understanding of human behavior stems from two of their characteristics: they represent interplay between the culturally common and the personally unique, and have developmental relevance.

On the collective side, life tasks are shaped by cultural demands, particularly those applying to age and gender. Thus, individuals are commonly driven by pursuit of universal life tasks like identity, intimacy, control, and power, and students, particularly as they leave home and start college, are engaged in tasks like "being on my own", "getting good grades", and "establishing a future direction" (Cantor & Kihlstrom, 1987). On the personal side, however, individuals differ in how they interpret each life task and hence in their strategies for solving problems or challenges each task presents.

Thus, life tasks are contextualized in the socio-cultural setting and age-graded expectations. The developmental relevance of life tasks has another aspect: during transition periods "...the demands and constraints are often made (painfully) clear... [and] the individual becomes especially aware of his or her role in shaping personal life tasks" (Cantor & Kihlstrom, p. 170). Consequently, Cantor and her associates chose the undergraduate years as the period in which they conducted much of their research and focused on such life tasks as intimacy pursuit (Cantor, Acker, & Cook-Flannagan, 1992), independence (Zirkel & Cantor, 1990), achievement and interpersonal relationships (Cantor, Norem, Niedenthal, Langston, & Brower, 1987), and the balance between personal identity and group participation (Cantor et al., 2002).

As applies to the other goal constructs, assessment begins with listing of life tasks which respondents rank in order according to importance and code into at least one of six consensual college life-task categories (e.g., getting good grades, making friends) and specify plans for dealing with these tasks. Finally, respondents are asked to rate each consensual dimension on 11 meaning dimensions such as importance, enjoyment, challenge, and absorption.

By employing these as well as other measures, Cantor and her colleagues demonstrated how adolescents and emerging adults develop personal strategies for solving the problems posed by age graded and culturally defined life tasks such as dating relationships (Cantor & Sanderson, 1998), making friends (Cantor & Harlow, 1994) and forging personal identity (Cantor et al., 2002), and how these strategies direct everyday behavior undertaken toward goal pursuit in situations conducive to that pursuit.

Summary. Given that goals are located in the future, all goal approaches address action guiding future orientated thinking. The life task approach differs from the others by emphasizing context and multidimensional nesting. Three aspects of the context are particularly emphasized in the work of Cantor and her colleagues: the sociocultural setting, the developmental period and age graded expectations, and the situations suitable for goal pursuit. Obviously, the three dimensions are not independent of each other. Instead, cultural orientations define age graded expectations and the appropriateness of situations for goal pursuit by individuals according to their age, gender, and social role.

Personal Dispositions Approaches

As evident from the literature reviewed thus far, future-related constructs are multidimensional and vary in their conceptual foci. Applied to the dispositional approaches, at least three emphases can be identified: future-related thinking, self appraisal, and behavioral manifestations. The *thinking* aspect specifically concerns weighing the future against the present by considering the distant outcomes of current behavior (Anderson & Wood, 2005; Strathman et al.,1994).

The *appraisal* aspect relates to evaluating one's goal-related capabilities (Snyder et al., 1991), specifically pertaining to two expectancies: outcome and efficacy. Both expectancies refer to individuals' beliefs about behavior-outcome contingency. However, outcome efficacy relates to the belief that a performed behavior will result in a *particular* outcome, described as the *pathway* component of the hope model while efficacy expectancy pertains to individuals' confidence in their ability to perform behaviors that will lead to *desired* outcomes, described as the *agency* component of the hope model.

The *action* aspect studied by Zimbardo and Boyd (Zimbardo and Boyd, 1999; Boyd & Zimbardo, 2005) pertains to goal setting, planning ahead, and meeting deadlines as well as to their dispositional correlates reflected in behaviors like weighing costs and benefits, resisting temptations, and being punctual. Underlying these approaches are two assumptions: (1) that each describes a relatively stable personal disposition that influences and predicts how individuals will act across a range of daily activities, and (2) that these dispositions are measurable. As pointed out by Zimbardo and Boyd regarding past, present, and future time perspectives, dispositions develop gradually:

> When a tendency develops to habitually overemphasize one of these three temporal frames when making decisions, it serves as a temporal cognitive "bias" toward being past, future, or present oriented. When chronically elicited, this bias becomes a dispositional style or an individual-differences variable, that is characteristic and predictive of how individuals will respond across a host of daily choices (Zimbardo and Boyd, 1999, p. 1272).

Consequently, each conceptualization has been translated into a research tool whose reliability, discriminant and construct validity, and effect on everyday behaviors above and beyond other related psychological constructs have been demonstrated. These behaviors apply particularly to risk taking, health related behaviors, and academic achievement. Thus, research on the effect of *consideration of future consequences* shows its negative effect on aggression (Joireman et al., 2003) and its positive effect on environmental and health related behaviors above and beyond the effect of individual differences measures such as conscientiousness, hope and optimism (Strathman et al., 1994).

In a similar vein, Zimbardo and Boyd's (1999) *future time orientation* measure is related to students' sexual behavior so that those scoring higher on future orientation are less involved in sexual relationships, and among those having had sexual intercourse, future orientation is related to behaviors indicating preventive exposure to HIV (Rothspan & Read, 1996). Finally, hope (Snyder et al., 1991) is positively related to students' selection of more difficult goals above and beyond the effect of optimism and high school GPA, and to students' university GPA above and beyond high school GPA.

Summary

The four interfacing approaches presented in this chapter share with the future orientation research an interest in the effect of future thinking on behavior. The motivational approach pursued by the Leuven group brings to the fore the effect of future goals on present behavior which is perceived instrumental for the pursuit of these goals, particularly emphasizing the differential effect of intrinsic and extrinsic goals on achievement motivation. The goal approaches are concerned with mapping out individuals' goals and characterizing their attributes and behavior prompting qualities, and the personal dispositions approaches address issues related to future-related thinking, self appraisal, and behavioral manifestations of being concerned with the future.

Finally, the possible selves approach is anchored in self theory positing that the selves individuals wish for themselves, consider possible, and desire *not* to have are part of the self system and their main function is motivational: to bridge the present and the future. While earlier researchers were concerned by the irreality of future orientation, the possible selves approach contends that, by being relatively free of reality, possible selves may prompt coping with stresses and challenges.

In all, review of the four interfacing approaches brought to the fore similarities among them as well as their unique contribution to the understanding of future thinking. All approaches have an idiographic component supplemented by nomothetic approaches pertaining to the characterization of each future-related unit (be it task, personal project, personal striving, or possible self). However, while all approaches assess subjective value and expectancy, some also assess accessibility, costs, and attainment strategies.

Chapter 2
The Evolvement of Future Orientation: Infancy Through Middle Childhood

Although especially relevant to the adolescent period, the capacity for orienting to the future is innate, identified in early infancy, and – as already noted in Chap. 1 – underlying it are neurophysiological processes generated in the cerebral cortex (Brunia & Boxtel, 2001; Wentworth, Haith, & Karrer, 2001). However, interacting with other innate abilities (such as memory and language), interpersonal experiences, and cultural values its expressions vary with age. Given that much of this book applies to adolescence and emerging adulthood, the key questions addressed in this chapter pertain to the developmental periods from infancy to middle childhood. Specifically they ask what are the early indications of future orientation in infancy, how do language, memory, and interpersonal factors in early childhood affect the notion of future and future thinking, how do various aspects of future orientation develop in middle childhood, and how do they change their expression, scope, and instrumentality?

Future Orientation in Infancy

For Haith and his colleagues, the early precursors of future orientation can be identified as early as at the age of 2 months in the form of anticipation of events indicated by *eye movements* and assessed in laboratory experiments (Adler & Haith, 2003; Haith, 1994; Haith, Benson, Roberts, & Pennington, 1994; Haith, Wentworth, & Canfield, 1993). Three main considerations led to the selection of the eye movement rather than of other non-verbal indicators present at birth, or shortly afterwards (Haith, 1994; Reznick, 1994): that the indicator is closely related to the relevant perceptual systems, controllable from birth, and fast. Eye movements also have the advantage of being responsive to auditory stimuli, stable over the life span, and easily recorded.

The assessment of infants' future orientation. The prototypical experiment examines infants' visual anticipation by performing the following procedure. Babies are presented with pictures, using one of two sequences: *regular alternating* and *irregular sequence*. The regular alternating sequence consists of repetitious picture presentations in which an image appears at one location, disappears, and reappears in another location.

R. Seginer, *Future Orientation*, The Springer Series on Human Exceptionality, DOI 10.1007/978-0-387-88641-1_2, © Springer Science+Business Media, LLC 2009

In the standard visual expectation paradigm (VExP) experiment (Haith, 1994) pictures are shown repeatedly one to the right and one to the left of a visual center, separated by the same duration of interstimulus interval (ISI), and infants' future orientation is defined in terms of two behavioral criteria: anticipatory fixation (prior to appearance) to the side on which the picture is expected to appear, and reaction time (RT). The control condition consists of the same paradigm and stimuli but the duration of the ISI and the location of the pictures are random and hence unpredictable. Running this experiment, Haith, Hazan and Goodman (1988) demonstrated that, when provided with regular left-right presentation sequence, 3.5 months old babies anticipate the visual image more accurately (assessed by percentage of anticipations) and faster (assessed by reaction time) than do babies in the control condition.

Infants' anticipatory behavior: How early? How generalizable? To show that these findings indicate infants' capability for anticipatory behavior, Haith and his colleagues had to answer three additional questions. How *early* can anticipatory behavior be identified? What conditions *facilitate* (or hinder) infants' anticipatory behavior? Can anticipatory behavior formed at one time and task be *generalized* to another time and a related task?

In a series of carefully designed experiments, Haith (1994, 1997) showed that, when presented with the basic L-R design, 2-month old babies are able to anticipate spatial location. Nonetheless, visual anticipatory behavior is moderated by task demandingness. Thus, whereas by 2 months babies can anticipate only the basic design, by 3 months of age their capability improves so that they can anticipate series of up to two events (L-L-R-R design) occurring in the same location. Similarly, designed experiments demonstrate that as early as 2 month of age, stable picture content facilitates higher anticipation rate, and for the 2- but not 3-month old babies, also faster reaction time (Wentworth & Haith, 1992).

In more recent studies Haith and his colleagues demonstrated that 3-month-old infants' anticipatory behavior is facilitated by regularity of content and location of picture. Thus, regularity of content across a class of related but distinct events (i.e., stimuli of the same color but different shape and pattern) (Adler & Haith, 2003) and spatiotemporal regularity by which pictures are presented, as well as inter-event contingency (created by contingency between central picture and peripheral pictures to the left or to the right of the central picture) (Wentworth, Haith, & Hood, 2002) all facilitate infants' anticipatory behavior.

Finally, a crucial question about the anticipatory behavior of infants has been how generalizable is accumulated knowledge to other times and other tasks? Experiments run by Haith and his colleagues (Haith, 1997) showed that, by 3 months of age, infants extended their expectations for several days, and improved anticipation and reaction time of a related task of vertical (rather than the original horizontal) eye movement.

The developmental trajectory of anticipatory behavior. A particularly relevant question for this discussion is the developmental trajectory of anticipatory behavior during the pre-verbal period: does anticipatory behavior grow easier (i.e., higher anticipatory behavior rates) and faster? Can it be manifested under conditions that require overcoming obstacles? Experiments that used the VExP with older babies showed inconsistent trends: RTs went down with age both for 6-month- (Jacobson et al., 1992) and for 8-month-olds (DiLalla et al., 1990). However, percentage of anticipation was higher for the 6- than for the 2- and 3-month-olds, albeit also for the 8-month-old babies. Thus, as babies grow up their anticipatory RT goes down, but toward the last third of the first year, fewer (19.3% and 17% according to Benson et al. and DiLilla et al., respectively, compared to 28.1% of the 6-month-olds) exhibit this behavior.

Contending that these experiments created for the babies an unrealistic environment devoid of competing ongoing stimuli, Reznick (1994) designed an encumbered anticipation experiment in which, during their first year of life, infants anticipated an event that was "potent enough to disrupt attention to an ongoing event" (Reznick, 1994, p. 45). His participants were 4-, 8-, and 12-month-old babies, and the stimulus materials used were two successive panels of red, green and yellow lights and two boxes each housing a mechanically operated cheerleader bear. These materials were obviously considerably different from those used in the standard procedure and its modifications, and their use showed that 4-month-olds were unable to engage in encumbered anticipatory behavior, and 8- and 12-month-olds only rarely. However, for the 12-month-olds, encumbered anticipation occurs more often when the stimulus event is the panels, obviously less interesting than the "cheerleading" bears.

Finally, the question raised by findings on infants' visual anticipatory behavior is what are the adaptive and developmental functions of anticipatory behavior? Why should babies engage in it? On the face of it, such behavior is gratuitous and for the 2- or 3-month-old baby serves no purpose; it does not bring mother any closer or make any of her services – such as food or clean diapers– more available. In light of this, Haith (1994) posited three ways in which infant anticipatory behavior serves adaptation and development: it speeds up information processing (see also Adler & Haith, 2003 on infants' visual anticipation in the service of efficient processing of event information), it may provide the infant with a sense of control, and finally, it serves as the early manifestation of and foundation for future orientation. For future orientation researchers, particularly relevant is the third conjecture positing that by engaging in visual anticipatory behavior infants introduce themselves to the notion and meaning of "future" long before they can verbally demonstrate it.

Future Orientation in Early Childhood

As appealing as Haith's conjecture is the relevance of infants' visual anticipatory capabilities to the future thinking and behavior of older children is at present not known. Moreover, as children acquire language, the theoretical approaches on which future orientation research draws, the research questions investigated, and the indicators used by researchers change. Consequently, the definitions of future orientation and its indicators abound.

Despite diversity of conceptualization and assessment methods, underlying the various approaches is a common understanding that future orientation is about the projection or extension of the self into the future (Moore & Lemmon, 2001) and that beyond infancy its expression and assessment are mainly (though not solely) verbal. Moreover, it cannot be developed without the child's grasp of the concept of time as it applies to order codes and locations in represented time patterns (Friedman, 2005), ability for verbal representation, and discourse socialization (Hudson, 2001, 2006; Nelson & Fivush, 2004).

Given that the development of future orientation in early childhood is contingent on knowledge of time (Suddendorf & Corballis, 2007) through social discourse embedded in cultural context, this section is devoted to three main issues: children's sense of the future, planning behavior, and the socialization of future thinking in mother-child interaction and children's literature.

Children's Sense of the Future

Children's knowledge of the future emerges from their sense of time. Given time continuity, one of their first challenges is to differentiate between already occurred and anticipated events and experiences. This task is challenging not only because tomorrow is the yesterday of the day after tomorrow but also because reconstructing the past and anticipating the future both involve *mental time travel* (Busby & Suddendorf, 2005; Suddendorf & Busby, 2005; Suddendorf & Corballis, 1997, 2007). Hence, this section opens with research on the differentiation between past and future, continues with children's knowledge of future events, and concludes with the evolvement of children's episodic future thinking.

Differentiating between past and future. Although at this age children can use correctly temporal terms associated with the past (*yesterday*) and the future (*tomorrow*) (Nelson, 1996), they still encounter difficulties in differentiating between the two time periods. This tendency has also been noted by Friedman and Kemp (1998) who observed 3- to 6-year-old children attribute their semantic knowledge of "coming soon" to "short time ago". Three reasons may account for this difficulty: the future consists of events that have not yet taken place (Hudson, 2001), children use temporal language before they fully grasp the meaning of temporal terms (Nelson, 1996), and children are distracted by adults' discourse that often changes the location of events from the future to the past (and vice versa). To illustrate, until the event (e.g., Valentine Day, the child's birthday), parents and teachers repeatedly refer to it as occurring in the future ("coming soon") and thus create interference of memory processes that cause children to confuse the recent past with the near future (Friedman, 2000).

Children's knowledge of future events. Children's ability to handle future events develops gradually. This has been demonstrated in a series of experiments by Friedman and his colleagues in which children's knowledge of the future is tested vis-à-vis three tasks: their ability to arrange the temporal order of daily activities, to understand duration (duration knowledge), and estimate future time distances.

Children's ability to arrange the *temporal order* of daily activities (Friedman, 1990) is studied by presenting the children with four cards that depict four daily activities: waking, lunch, dinner, and going to bed. In the first experiment, 3- to

9-year-old children are instructed to order the events within the day forward and backward (reverse order). Findings show that children 4 years or older are able to construct a forward order, and children 5 years or older are also able to construct the reverse order at above chance levels.

While the main purpose of this experiment has been to examine children's ability to arrange activities they practice daily according to their temporal order, the experiment can also examine the extent to which present orientation affects children's temporal ordering of daily activities. Its findings show that only a few children start the sequence of the daily activities from the time of the day in which the experiment take place, but the majority of those who do so are from the 4-year-old age group. Six of the 10 4-year-old participants tested during the morning hours start the *forward* ordering of daily activities with lunch. Thus, not all young children are able to perform the temporal ordering of the daily activities independently of the time of the day in which the task is performed.

In a second experiment, nursery school to third grade children (4–9 years old) are presented with different reference points (e.g., waking in the morning, eating lunch) and asked to judge which of two daily activities comes next going forward and which comes next going backwards in time. Results show that all children are able to judge forward relative order at above chance levels; by first grade they are also able to perform the backward ordering at above chance level.

The third experiment was designed to examine another aspect of children's sense of the future: *duration knowledge*. The task is to judge the length of intervals separating six daily activities: waking in the morning, breakfast, lunch, dinner, bath, and going to bed. The effect of age is observed in the results of this experiment as well. As children (3–9 years old) grow older, their ability to judge the interval between different daily activities becomes more differentiated, more accurate and less varied (as indicated by standard deviations) within each age group. Correlation coefficients between children's judgment and an estimate of the true length of intervals between each two activities go up gradually from 0.21 for the 3- and 4-year-olds to 0.76 and 0.71 for the 8- and 9-year-olds.

To examine children's *estimates of time distance*, Friedman and his colleagues developed a set of experiments in which children's ability to locate correctly *anticipated events* along a future time axis is tested. These experiments show that children are capable of distinguishing between near and distant future events only when they reach the age of 5. By age 7 many children can tell correctly the number of days until the weekend, but not the number of months to a distant holiday. Like the 5-year-olds, they can make only global distinctions regarding the location of future time: events are classified by them either as expected to occur in the near (short time) or in the distant (long time) future (Friedman, 2005).

An instructive exception is their birthday which they can locate much more accurately, *if* it is coming within the next 2 months (Friedman, 2005). By age 10, however, children are able to order events such as holidays or seasons quite accurately, do it not only from a reference point of the present but also from other reference points, and describe distance into the future in conventional units such as months (Friedman, 2000).

Children's episodic future thinking. Just as episodic memory (Tulving, 1972, 1985) pertains to individuals' knowledge of their past experiences, episodic future thinking (Atance & O'Neill, 2001) concerns their ability to *project themselves into the future* and experience personal events before they have happened. To study it among young children, Atance and O'Neill (2005a,b; Atance & Melzoff, 2005) developed an experimental trip task in which children are asked to pretend they are getting ready for a trip and help their parents packing by choosing three of eight items displayed to them. The eight items (such as juice, Band-Aid, and telephone) were selected by the researchers because they satisfy four types of needs: physiological (e.g., hunger), physical (e.g., being injured), emotional (e.g., being bored), and emergency (e.g., needing communication).

The task was designed to satisfy the following criteria: (1) it incorporates the notions of self and future, (2) it involves a novel future event for which children are not expected to hold a script (as is the case in "bedtime" or "getting ready for school"), (3) it may be responded to with uncertainty terms, and (4) it does not require inhibitory control skills. Their findings (Atance & O'Neill, 2005a) show that at age 3, slightly over one third of the children are able to explain their choice of item by referring to a future need and/or its probable occurrence (using "if" or "maybe").

Two findings suggest that these children's ability to project themselves into the future is not related to linguistic ability but rather to non-verbal ability: association with a behavioral indicator (being able to draw a picture children stated they intended to) but not with general language ability (Atance & O'Neill, 2005b). Like other indicators of future knowledge, episodic future thinking improves with age: 4- and 5-year-olds do better on the trip task than 3-year-olds, and 5-year-old are less distracted by semantic associates than are 3- and 4-year-olds (Atance & Meltzoff, 2005). However, while children's episodic future thinking is affected by their ability to anticipate a future need, like in the case of adults, it may also be affected by conflicting current needs (Atance & Melzoff, 2006).

Summary. Although underlying future orientation are motivational, social-cultural, and cognitive processes, research on children's knowledge of the future focuses mainly (if not exclusively) on its cognitive aspects. Within this framework, researchers focus on such apersonal (semantic) aspects of the future like the ability to distinguish between past and future events, to arrange the temporal order of daily activities, understand duration (duration knowledge), and estimate future time distances, as well as their episodic future knowledge describing children's ability to think about personal events they have not yet experienced.

Much of this work agrees that future knowledge does not emerge before children reach the age of 3; some aspects of it – as expressed in their language and behavior – are obtained by age 5 but other aspects (such as order of the months of the year) only at a later age. Overall, children master different future timescales at different ages (Friedman, 2005). However, still missing is an integrated picture that shows how the apersonal and the episodic aspects of future knowledge are related and the extent to which they are affected by motivational and socio-cultural factors.

Two Approaches to Processes Underlying the Development of Future Knowledge

Common to the two approaches discussed here are questions about the early evolvement of future orientation thinking, the age at which children first demonstrate future thinking, and the psychological processes underlying children's expression of future knowledge. While both approaches focus on cognitive processes, Friedman's model assumes knowledge of the future is based on representation of time patterns (Friedman, 2005) while Weist (1989) emphasizes how future knowledge is represented in children's language.

Friedman's model of spatial-like images. The purpose of Friedman's (1990) experiments has been to test three competing explanations. The first is that knowledge of the future can be explained by the *"temporal string"* model (Anderson, 1983) according to which order consists of unidirectional pointers between elements and their successors. The second explanation (Seymour, 1980) posits the possession of what Friedman described as semantic *"locative codes"* that facilitate adults' knowledge of the order of elements (e.g., months) in temporal patterns. The third model, suggested by Friedman, assumes that "the elements of a temporal pattern are represented in the form of *spatial-like images*" (Friedman, 1990, p. 1400) that individuals retrieve whenever engaged in activities requiring knowledge of the future.

Two considerations indicate the advantage of the image model over the other two. One is that all three experiments performed by Friedman can be explained in terms of the spatial-like images model but not in terms of the other two models. The second pertains to results of an introspective study (Schroeder, 1980) in which college students reported they possessed images of the times in a day. These temporal images allow adults and older children to perform "mental time travel" (Suddendorf & Corballis, 1997) which in turn explains how older children and adults can perform backward ordering of future events (Friedman, 2005).

The imagery model can also explain why young children confuse past and future (as demonstrated by their tendency to relate to certain events that already occurred as belonging to the future). If, according to Friedman (2000), 1 week after Valentine day 4- and 5-year-old children tend to locate it in the future rather than in the past, they have *not yet constructed a temporal imagery model.* In its absence, they rely on their memory from the days before Valentine day when adults referred to it as an anticipated future event. However, as children reach age 6 the distinction between past and future becomes clear and both are gradually internalized as parts of the temporal framework (Friedman, 2005).

Weist's theory of temporal systems in child language. Weist's theory (Weist, 1989) describes language acquisition as consisting of a sequence of four temporal systems each characterized by a network of three time concepts: event time, speech time, and reference time. *Event time* pertains to the event described by the speaker, *speech time* refers to the time in which the speaker is producing the sentence, and *reference time* specifies the time of the event ("today", "the day after tomorrow", "when I grow up").

The first temporal system, characteristic of children younger than 1;6 (one-and-a-half years old) is the *speech time system*. At this developmental period language is mainly restricted to the child's immediate perceptual environment and hence children do not differentiate between event time, speech time, and reference time. Instead, both the event time and reference time are bound to speech time. The second period (1;6 to 2;6) is characterized by the *event time system* in which children are able to use two time concepts: speech time and event time. By using both time concepts they are able to relate to past and ongoing events. However, to use Weist's illustration, when at this developmental period children say "Ernie fell off" or "Mummy painted the wall" they use both speech and event times but not reference time (when exactly did mummy paint the wall?). They can also, according to Weist, express desires and intentions and thus orient themselves toward the future, as is illustrated by a 1;10 girl's utterance (translated from the Polish): "Mommy will take it out".

The third period (2;6 to 3;0) is characterized by the *restricted reference time system*. The activation of this system facilitates the use of temporal adverbs ("yesterday", "tomorrow") and temporal adverbial clauses ("when you get back home") that signify the ability to use *reference time*. The fourth period (3;0 to 4;6) is characterized by the *free reference time system*; this system signifies children's ability to manipulate the speech time, event time, and reference time independently.

As the use of reference time becomes more flexible, children are able to use words like "before" and "after" and refer to events located at different points in time. To use Weist's example: "When asked what she had done earlier in the day, Monica (4;5) said: *I just played with something and after that I just walked around a little*" (Weist, 1989, p. 68). Although Weist described the free reference time system as characterizing children as young as 3;0, most research findings suggest that the ability to use three temporal locations, necessary for using freely speech time, event time, and reference time appears only around age 4;0 (Benson, 1994).

If the use of time talk is indicative of cognitive development, then, according to Weist, children's orientation to the future may be expressed earlier than usually considered by researchers. Drawing on observations indicating that Polish children as young as 1;8 can produce sentences like "(I) will bring (something)" indicates, according to Weist, early expression of having a sense of the future. Moreover, "When children express a desire, obligation, or command, they have an expectation which concerns a state of affairs subsequent to speech time" (Weist, 1989, p. 91).

An empirical assessment of Weist's *four temporal systems of child language* adapted his systems to the study of children's (12–42 months of age) future time language (Benson, 1997). Diverting from the convention of experimental or observational procedures, Benson interviewed parents about their child's future language use and encouraged them to supplement their response with examples from the child's talk. Analyses indicated that parents' reports support Weist's developmental systems.

To illustrate, parents of 12-month-old infants said it was "sometimes true" that their child could perform future oriented behavior that corresponds to Weist's first system (e.g., "my child knows how to indicate that she or he wants desired things"). Parents of 42-month-old children said it was "always true" that their child could perform behaviors that correspond to the first stage, and "sometimes true" they could perform behaviors corresponding to Weist's fourth stage ("my child says that some things follow other things").

Altogether, with increased age, children's scores on each temporal system as well as their total scores went up. Thus, although she relied on parents' information rather than on directly observing children, Benson's method captured the developmental sequence of future talk in early childhood and gave additional support to Weist's theory.

Planning Behavior in Early Childhood

As children acquire knowledge of the future and its verbal expression they can engage in more elaborate future oriented behavior such as planning. Its description as consisting of hierarchically ordered behaviors of goal setting and the organization of a sequence of actions intended to achieve the goal (Gauvain, 1999) as well as the execution of these actions indicates that not all aspects of planning are equally future oriented. While planning depends on its development (Benson, 1997), once a goal has been formed and the sequence of necessary actions for achieving it constructed, the execution of plans depends on memory and the development of monitoring skills (Hudson & Fivush, 1991) rather than merely on future orientation processes.

Levels of planning. Research on the planning abilities of young children describes a five level process (Hudson & Fivush, 1991) that builds on children's event knowledge (Nelson, 1986) and proceeds from young children use of their knowledge about events (*generalized event representation*, GER) to creating a sequence of activities related to subgoals in familiar and novel situations. In its earliest stage (Level 0), children make use of their ability for GER in a manner that might be mistaken for early articulation of planning. What distinguishes this from subsequent levels is that, although children have acquired GERs of simple sequences such as daily routines and they use them to anticipate the sequence of familiar routines, they are still unable to meet the event-based planning criterion, namely, to fill in global event slots with goal-appropriate specific instances.

When they reach Level 1 (at about 3 years of age) that consists of a *single goal event planning*, children are able to use their GERs more flexibly and translate a general event into a specific instance of this event. To use Hudson and Fivush's example, when describing their morning routine children are able to fill in the clothing slot with different items, depending on such external circumstances as whether it is a warm or cold day, a school or weekend day.

Level 2 pertains to *multiple event goal planning* indicated by children's ability to attend to two simultaneous event goals and coordinate their planning. Thus, planning a shopping trip, children may plan buying food for breakfast and dinner. At level 3, described as *coordinated event planning*, children form subgoals – each of which has its own spatial-temporal sequence – and arrange them into hierarchical order, and at level 4, pertaining to *novel event planning*, children break down different events and use them to construct new action sequences.

Scripts and plans. While planning is based on general event knowledge, its distinctive feature is its future oriented aspect. Thus, from the point of view of this analysis, the relevant aspects of planning are the ability for goal setting, for relating goals to actions and activities that serve as means for the attainment of these goals, and engaging in preparatory activities. Therefore, studies that compare between scripts – that indicate event knowledge – and plans (Hudson, Shapiro, & Sosa, 1995; Hudson, Sosa, & Shapiro, 1997) and investigate children's advanced preparations and the conditions that facilitate engagement in them (Shapiro & Hudson, 2004) are of particular interest here.

Do children behave differently when asked to tell about a task (*script knowledge*) and when requested to *plan* the performance of such a task? To assess it, Hudson et al. (1995) interviewed 3- to 5-year-old children about going to the beach and grocery shopping by reading to the children examples of either a script or a plan, followed by a request to tell the experimenter what happens when s/he goes to the beach or grocery shopping (script condition), or describe a plan for going to the beach or grocery shopping (planning condition). On a second trial, the experimenter asked each child on the script condition to tell her the first thing s/he *does* as she goes to the beach or grocery shopping, followed by questions on "what do you do next" until the child signaled s/he was done. Children assigned to the planning condition were asked what is the first thing they will *have to do*, followed by questions on "what do you have to do next", until the child signaled s/he is done.

Results of this experiment show that the difference between the production of script and plan is age dependent. Employing the number of actions in a narrative as an indicator of reported information, 3-year-olds are better (i.e., their narratives consist of more action units) at producing scripts than plans whereas 5-year-olds do better on producing plans. Moreover, at this age range, production of plans, but not of scripts, is influenced by age so that 5-year-olds do better than 4-year-olds, and 4-year-olds do better than 3-year-olds.

Assuming that onset actions (e.g., go/drive there) indicate planfulness, their proportion (out of the total number of action units) indicates age differences as well as condition (script vs planning) and event (grocery shopping vs going to the beach) effects. Thus, older children who participate in planning (rather than script) going to the beach (rather than grocery shopping) use more onset actions. Moreover, for children of this age, then, the probability of thinking about future oriented actions depends not only on child characteristics and the nature of the task but also on the nature of the *event*, and particularly on its excitement or familiarity.

Planning novel tasks. Demonstrating the dependence of planning on the generalized event knowledge of children as young as 3 years, research carried out by Hudson and her colleagues made an important contribution. However, since planning more often than not applies to novel tasks, the next issue focuses on how children plan novel events to which generalized event knowledge (based on familiarity with events) cannot be applied. Putting it differently, the question is which factors compensate for the absence of event knowledge? Three factors are particularly relevant here: the first pertains to the *structure* of the event to be planned and the two others to the *what* and *how* of provided information. In other words, the second factor pertains to the content of the information provided by the environment, and the third to *how* such information is being provided.

Event structure. The effect of the event structure was examined in a study (Shapiro & Hudson, 2004) of 3- to 5-year-olds whose task was defined as representing an enabling or a conventional event. Using Abelson's classification of events according to activities leading to the achievement of a superordinate event goal, Shapiro and Hudson defined the *enabling event* as consisting of a task with a sequence of actions and activities which are *logically* temporally invariant (e.g., waking up must be preceded by falling asleep), and the *conventional event* as consisting of a sequence of actions and activities which could in principle be varied, but are *conventionally* performed in an invariant temporal order (e.g., washing hands and eating).

Working with these two kinds of events, Shapiro and Hudson examined whether it is the logical links between activities or their convention that facilitates planning. Their findings show that, although the enabling event task consists of logically invariant temporal order which presumably enables planning, children who participate in this experimental condition make more errors than children who participate in the conventional event task. Shapiro and Hudson's explanation drew on the consequences of making a mistake on each of the two tasks: in the enabling task, one mistake inevitably led to subsequent ones and made the entire planning process more demanding, whereas in the conventional event task, one mistake did not necessarily disrupt the entire planning process and goal achievement.

Information content. To examine how information provided to young children facilitates their planning ability, researchers supplied children with three kinds of information: the end-state (Bauer, Schwade, Wewerka, & Delaney, 1999) or completed example of the project (Shapiro & Hudson, 2004), the initial step, and a sub-set consisting of two of the three-step sequence (Bauer et al., 1999). Findings of this research show that, for preschoolers, not all information has the same facilitating value. At 21 months of age, information about the *end-state* (Bauer et al., 1999) improves planning behavior, is more helpful than the same amount of information pertaining to the *initial step* in the sequence of activities, and does not become more helpful by an additional step (either the initial or the middle step). Thus, in the absence of generalized event knowledge, information about the end-state provided by an outside source is necessary and sufficient to facilitate planning.

Information channels. Transmission of planning-pertinent information is also multi-channeled. It may involve *observation* of another person – usually an adult – preparing the necessary items for executing the plan, *listening* to adults' explanations about necessary preparations (Hudson et al., 1997), or *sharing responsibility* with another individual – a peer or an adult – while working on a planning task.

Experiments testing the effect of these various channels show that for 3-year-olds, but not for others, the listening plus observing has an advantage over the observing-only channel. Work by Rogoff and her colleagues (Gauvain & Rogoff, 1989; Gardner & Rogoff, 1990) show the contribution of shared responsibility – be it with a peer or an adult – to effective planning behavior and particularly to the use of preparatory activities such as advance scanning and to planning behavior effectiveness during a posttest (Gauvain & Rogoff, 1989).

In sum, future orientation is essential for planning for two reasons: goals are located in the future, and acts to be performed are hierarchically ordered. However, planning *behavior* depends on cognitive and interpersonal abilities that develop during early childhood.

Socialization of Future Knowledge

Obviously, underlying the construction of future orientation is a grasp of time concepts that, because of their abstract nature, are socially constructed and can be learned only in the context of social interaction. Specifically, children learn time concepts by listening and actively engaging in conversation about the future.

Mothers' time talk. For most children in the early childhood period, social interaction takes place in the home and particularly with mothers. Nonetheless, research about mothers' time talk is scant and descriptive. The few studies that have been carried out offer a consistent picture about the nature of time talk in general and about the future in particular (Hudson, 2001, 2002, 2006) and in fact explain why interest in these issues is so limited: mothers of 3-year-olds devote only 2% of their total talk to time talk (Norton, 1993). Nonetheless, analysis of their use of future talk has identified three distinct strategies.

First, unlike talk about the past, future talk is *age* dependent. To illustrate, as children grow from 14 to 36 months, mothers' talk about the future increases from 36% to 58% of time talk (Benson, Talmi, & Haith, 1999). Second, mothers' future talk is more *complex* than their talk about the past (which explains age differences in mothers' talk about the future but not about the past). It relates to generalized event knowledge rather than to specific events (that occurred in the past), consists of higher frequency of hypothetical language ("Maybe we will. . .", "Do you think. . ." "Would you like to have. . ."), and refers more often to conventional time markers ("tomorrow", "next week"). Third, mothers' future talk *actively engages children* in thinking about the future and planning and thus provides children with opportunities to learn time concepts and develop knowledge about the future (Hudson, 2002) as well as non-temporal tasks such as shared responsibility (Gauvain, 1999).

Given that as mothers engage their children in future talk they use different conversation styles, the next question is how these styles affect children's contribution to conversation about future events? Examining this issue, Hudson (2006) coded mothers' conversations with their 2.5- or 4-year-old children into categories that described type of utterance (e.g., question, evaluation), temporal frame of reference (e.g., past, future), and temporal reference (e.g., sequence) that were subsumed under three factors: elaborative and advanced language, general and past reference, and repetitive prompts and preferences.

Her findings reiterate earlier findings that future talk develops between 3 and 4 years and is differentially related to mothers' conversation style. While all three affect the contribution of older children to conversation about the future, the contribution of young children is *not* related to repetitive prompts and preferences, and the contribution of older children is more strongly related to the elaborative style than to the other two. However, these findings should be understood in their developmental context. Applying Vigotsky's (1978) *zone of proximal development*, Hudson (2006) suggests that children who have only partial understanding of temporal language benefit from temporal conversation because listening to temporal language in the context of everyday events facilitates their conceptual development.

Guided participation. Are the processes involved in mothers' future talk unique to this specific situation? According to Rogoff's (1990) analysis of cognitive socialization in early childhood, the answer is no. Essentially, mothers' future talk is an instance of guided participation in which mothers involve their child in a process "...in which caregivers and children's roles are intertwined, with tacit as well as explicit learning opportunities in the routine arrangements and interactions between caregivers and children." (Rogoff, 1990, p. 65).

However, for guided participation to be an effective learning opportunity, the interaction between children and caregivers (e.g., parents, siblings, peers, and teachers) must satisfy the condition of *intersubjectivity* (Rogoff, 1990). Underlying it are joint assumptions and shared understandings (Newson & Newson, 1975) that, regardless of their age (Rogoff identified intersubjectivity in a 12-month old baby-mother interaction), make it possible for communication partners to accommodate each other by attending to an aspect brought into focus by the other (Rommetveit, 1985) and take the other person's perspective. However, despite its importance for communication in general and child-caregiver interaction in particular (Newson & Newson, 1975; Riegel, 1977; Rogoff, 1990), to date this aspect of future time socialization has not been studied.

Closest to it have been studies of children's planning effectiveness when the task is carried out alone, with a partner, or when child and partner share decision making (Gauvain & Rogoff, 1989). For 5-year-olds, the greater advantage of shared decision making is explained by its intersubjective nature: as adults guide planning while being tuned and responsive to children's limited ability, they offset the difficulty of planning inherently abstract future events (Rogoff, 1990). However, a recent study (Gauvain & Perez, 2008) shows that compliant children (4–5 years old) gain more from a mother-child joint planning task than do noncompliant children. Their mothers are less directive, share more task responsibility with their children, and adjust more often to the child's learning needs than do mothers of noncompliant children.

Motivational-emotional aspects. Research on socialization of future knowledge in early childhood (like research on adults' guiding behavior in planning situations) has focused mainly on cognitive facilitation, leaving the role of the motivational-emotional aspects of parent-child relationships unexplored. In its absence and in light of future extension of the self on episodic memory, a study of the relation between mother-child relationship and children's autobiographical memory (Cleveland & Reese, 2005) is relevant.

The importance of this study is in partitioning parental behavior into its motivational (autonomy granting) and cognitive (task structuring) aspects and examining their interaction with children's age. Its findings show that maternal structuring is important for the autobiographical memory of all children; maternal support, however, is relevant only for the autobiographical memory of younger children

(40 month old). Given that autobiographical memory serves as the cognitive-experiential basis of episodic future thinking and that the future is inherently abstract, autonomy granting as an index of motivational-emotional support indirectly facilitates the development of future thinking in early childhood and might continue to affect its development at an age that autobiographical memory is affected mostly by cognitive task structuring.

Future Themes in Children's Literature

Although children's literature has treated a variety of themes related to time in general and the future in particular, it has remained an unresearched area. Some of these themes – particularly those related to future thinking – are illustrated here by drawing on Hebrew, German, English, and Russian nursery rhymes, lullabies, and folk stories informally collected to demonstrate their representation in children's literature.

Nursery Rhymes and kindergarten stories. Hello, Hello Daddy (Hello, Hello Aba, in Hebrew, Horen, 1985) is one of first nursery rhyme books read to children as young as 2 years of age. It opens with

Hello, hello
Is this daddy [I am talking to]?
Hello, hello
Is this my lovely boy?
Where are you Daddy?
I am at work
Daddy
What *will* you bring me? (*Italics added*) A present?

From there on the dialog between father and child continues discussing the presents daddy will bring his child, playing with such fantasy-objects as a boat with wheels, a car with wings, or a goat wearing eyeglasses and ending with

No, daddy
A man is wearing glasses
OK my child,
I will bring you a man,
I will bring you. . .Daddy

Other instances of introducing children to future thinking can be demonstrated in nursery rhymes and children's stories about daily routines, bedtime, visiting the family, and the amazing process of growing up.

One story illustrating how slow the process of growing up seems to young children is the Journey to Age Four (Orlev, 1985/2005):

Maya was everyday three years old, three and a little, three and a little more, three and a quarter, three and a half, but wanted very much to be four. So...Maya asked her father when she is going be four.

Dad laughed and said: "in half a year's time"

"Is this a long time?"

"Very long" said dad, "a full half year"

"Tomorrow?" asked Maya

"No", said dad, "many tomorrows"

Lullabies. The wish to grow up (which at the end of a day or in the middle of a sleepless night may be shared by parent and child) is often emphasized in lullabies.

Hush, L'il Baby

Hush, l'il baby, don't say a word

Mama's gonna buy you a mockin'bird.

If that mockin'bird don't sing

Mama's gonna buy you a diamond ring

If that diamond ring turns brass,

Mama's gonna buy you a looking glass

.... gets broke

.... billygoat.

.... don't pull,

.... cart and bull

.... turn over

.... dog named Rover

.... won't bark

.... horse and cart.

.... fall down,

Then you'll be the sweetest li'l baby in town.

While the American lullaby addresses universal experiences set in the future, a Hebrew lullaby from the pre-State of Israel pioneering era interweaves the spirit of its time (the value of working the land) with traditional lullaby themes.

Sleep well my child sleep well

...Tomorrow we start anew

Tomorrow daddy will go out to plow...

When you grow up

The two of you together will go out to the fields.

Middle childhood stories and literature. The movement of the moon around earth and its cyclical nature was introduced to me by my Russian born and raised grandmother who told me a folk story from her childhood about why the moon does not wear trousers.

One day, many, many years ago the moon wanted to get himself trousers. So he
   went to the tailor and said
"Mr. Tailor could you please make me a pair of trousers?"
"Of course" said the tailor "let me take your measurements and come back next
   week to try it on."
The next week when the moon came to try them on his trousers they were much
   too small.
"Never mind" said the tailor, "I will fix it for you. Come back next week to try it
   on"
The next week, however, the trousers were again too small, and the tailor said
"Don't worry Mr. Moon I will fix it for you. Come back next week"
The next week the trousers were too big. This time, the tailor lost his patience. He
   said
"Mr. Moon, stop changing your figure. I can't make you trousers if you keep
   growing bigger and smaller all the time"
"I can't" said the moon. "This is my nature"
"If so" said the tailor "you can't wear trousers. They will never fit you."[1]

Finally, in the nineteenth century, German school age children were introduced
to the horrible future consequences of bad behavior by the *Struwwelpeter* collection
of stories by Heinrich Hoffman (a German pediatrician who wrote these stories as a
Christmas gift for his son), translated into English by Mark Twain (1845/1935). Of
particular interest to us is the story about Augustus who would not have his soup.
As shown below, this story outlines the progressive course – day by day – of the
future consequences of not eating soup:

The Story of Augustus who not have any Soup

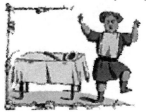

Augustus was a chubby lad;
Fat ruddy cheeks Augustus had;
And everybody saw with joy
The plump and hearty healthy boy.
He ate and drank as he was told,
And never let his soup get cold.
But one day, one cold winter's day,
He threw away the spoon and screamed:

---

[1] Just as this volume was ready to be sent out to the publisher, a new children's book in which
the moon is described in the feminine (Hebrew has one masculine and one feminine name for the
moon) had been published, acknowledging its folk story basis: Naor, L. (2008). *Simla hadasha
lalevana [the moon has a new dress]*. Tel Aviv: Modan

"O take the nasty soup away!
I won't have any soup to-day:
I will not, will not eat my soup!
I will not eat it, no!"

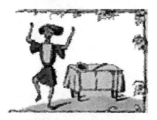

Next day! now look, the picture shows
How lank and lean Augustus grows!
Yet, though he feels so weak and ill,
The naughty fellow cries out still
"Not any soup for me, I say!
O take the nasty soup away!
I will not, will not eat my soup!
I will not eat it, no!"

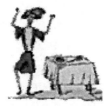

The third day comes. O what a sin!
To make himself so pale and thin.
Yet, when the soup is put on table,
He screams, as loud as he is able
"Not any soup for me, I say!
O take the nasty soup away!
I won't have any soup to-day!"

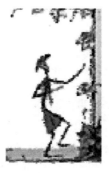

Look at him, now the fourth day's come!
He scarce outweighs a sugar-plum;

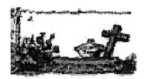

He's like a little bit of thread;
And on the fifth day he was-dead.

Summary. Given that time concepts are socially constructed, socialization of future knowledge needs to be examined at both the individual and the cultural levels, asking how the mother-child dyad and culture facilitate the development of future concepts. Review of the *mother-child setting* studies suggest that, possibly because in early childhood mothers devote only a small part of their total talk to time talk, research on future orientation socialization is scant and focuses on the cognitive aspects of mother-child communication. Extant research shows that mothers' talk about the future differs from their talk about the past. Specifically, their future time talk is more complex, age dependent, and engages the child in guided participation. At present, research has been focusing mostly on the cognitive aspects of knowledge of the future while its motivational-emotional and social underpinnings await further research.

Its relevance notwithstanding, representation of future themes in *children's literature* has not been investigated by developmentalists. In its absence, in this chapter excerpts from lullabies, nursery rhymes and kindergarten and school age stories illustrate the age-gradedness and pertinence of children's literature to the acquisition of future knowledge. Probably due to the inherently abstract nature of the future, its meaning and related time concepts are introduced by different genres in early childhood. Conversely, literature for school age children emphasizes the value of future thinking and the importance of considering future consequences. In light of the relevance of guided participation and adult-child intersubjectivity, one question for future research is the effectiveness of adult-mediated electronic literature, as may be the case in TV or DVD watching.

Future Orientation in Middle Childhood

Narrating the future is founded on the integration of cognitive abilities underlying time knowledge (i.e., order codes, location in represented time patterns and duration), verbal fluency, and the ability to produce a coherent story. This section addresses the development of this ability in middle childhood; however, to trace its early beginnings the discussion draws on some informal observations and interviews of *kindergarten* children that in the absence of systematic research may serve as basis for future research.

Early Expressions of Hopes and Fears

At age 3, Anat was discussing with her mother what she will need to do when she grows up so she could buy herself all those fancy shoes she saw displayed at the shoe store window as the two made their daily walk to Anat's daycare center. Telling her mother she will earn money by working, she reflected on the cognitive process, explaining to her mother: "You have to imagine how it's gonna be".

At age 5;10 in the summer before he entered 1st grade, Yuval understood the *future* as "something that will happen when I grow up" and when asked for an example added "when I will be 1st grader". However, his narrative of the future oscillated between the near future (1st grade) and adulthood and demonstrated that although he was familiar with adult roles he was still unable to apply order and duration concepts to his narrative of the future. Thus, he hadn't made up his mind whether he wanted to be a swimming or Karate coach, wanted to have an apartment for himself, his wife and children but thought this would happen when he is in military service (that for Israelis takes place between the age of 18 and 21). Although he could express it only in concrete terms, Yuval did understand the meaning of gradual advancement. When asked what one had to do to become a Karate coach he said "to be in Karate, the most important thing is your outfit. I have a yellow belt; Eiran (his older brother) has a purple belt. But to be a coach you must have a black belt."

In a similar manner, Yoav (5;9) understood what future meant and he too spoke about it by oscillating between school and adult career as an astronaut who would fly a spaceship to outer space. He also knew what one should do in order to become an astronaut: "[you have to make sure] that our spaceship won't blow up on us on the way to Earth. . .that it won't go down because that's where gravity is". For him – as for his age mate Yuval – what one needed to become an astronaut was "to buy a suit, to buy shoes, to buy a suit, to buy shoes, to buy everything".

Obviously, while able to use terms like gravity and spaceship return to Earth, like Yuval, Yoav did not fully distinguish between the party costume and the adult career role. As the interview continued it was clear that Yoav's notions of past and future, hopes and fears were still being developed. Thus, when asked what else he would like to be (when he grows up) he answered: "to be [working] in the electricity company, to be a TV actor, to work in the zoo, to be. . .a photographer, to be a policeman, to take care of foxes, and that's it".

Interviewer: And when will you do it?
Yoav: Now
Interviewer: Now? Can you do all these things now?
Yoav: No, not exactly. When I grow up. When I am a daddy. When I will be working.
Interviewer: Is there anything you fear about in the future? Something you don't want to happen?
Yoav: Oh, yes. That Earth will not be turning too fast.
Interviewer: What will happen then?

Yoav: We will all be dead.
Interviewer: What else?
Yoav: That my family and everyone I know will disappear from this world.
Interviewer: Do you know what is Hope, Yoav?
Yoav: Oh, yes. Hope is something else.
Interviewer: Right. What is your hope for the future?
Yoav: To be that one with the dolphins.
Interviewer: What, the trainer?
Yoav: Yes. The one who gives them food and all that.
Interviewer: And when will you be a dolphin trainer – before or after you go to
   school?
Yoav: You must go to school first.

At age 5, careers are gendered and Noa (5;0) wants to be an actress because
she will be seen on television, and because "...it is more interesting than being
just a model or a dancer". While interviews with kindergarten age children show
that future talk is laden with fantasy, and depends on their gender, experiences, and
whether or not they had older siblings – who like Yoav's siblings talk about school
and help him form the impression that school is "studying and boring classes and
200 intermissions which are great fun..." – they fit Friedman's (2000) findings that
at this age children still confuse past and future.

However, it is very clear that they have grasped the notion that the self is continuous over time and extends into noncurrent events (Moore & Lemmon, 2001;
Nelson, 2001). Thus, although children may be acquainted with the concepts of
fears and hopes, and with "fears" more than with "hopes", their expressions arise
from fantasizing on persons and events that come to their mind, like the explosion
of the Columbia space shuttle that took place more than 2 years before the interview
with Yoav but was inscribed in his memory.

The Construction of Future Hopes and Fears in Middle Childhood

Observations like those described above prompted the question of how early children construct a realistic prospective life image that underlies their charted future
trajectory, and how extensive is it? Although only sparsely investigated, the studies
that did take place show several meaningful findings.

Age differences in hopes and fears for the future. In one study (McCallion &
Trew, 2000) 5- to 9-year-old Northern Ireland children were interviewed about
their hopes and fears regarding school and job. Responding to the Possible Me
Tree interview schedule (Day, Borkowski, Punzo, & Howespian, 1994), children
listed their hopes and fears for the future. Analysis showed that the number of
responses about school and job grow larger with age both cross-sectionally and
longitudinally (T2 assessment took place 1 year after T1). Regarding school,
these children's hopes and fears narratives refer mainly to school achievement

and reflect their understanding of the future value of school learning. In a similar vein, the mean number of career responses is age-related both cross-sectionally and longitudinally, even though younger respondents are able to express a future career aspiration, and career preferences remain stable over a 1-year period.

A cross sectional study of hopes and fears. In another study carried out in Israel, Gelberg (1996) asked 2nd, 4th, and 6th grade girls and boys to list their hopes and fears for the future in an open-ended questionnaire. This questionnaire (described in detail in Chap. 1) instructs respondents to list their hopes and fears for the future in two separate sections and write down how old they expect to be when each hope or fear becomes relevant (see Appendix).

To make sure respondents were familiar with the normative order of social roles such as being high school students, serving in the military, getting a job, and starting a family, after completing their hopes and fears questionnaire the children were requested to answer a questionnaire in which they had to write down what individuals usually do at age 15, 18, 22, 25, 30, 50, and 70. Gelberg found that, even among 2nd graders, children were familiar with the normative sequence of social roles. This allowed him to continue with his analysis of all three age groups using the procedure and thematic categories initially developed for the analysis of hopes and fears narratives expressed by adolescents ranging in age from 9th grade to high school graduation (Seginer, 1992a).

Following the procedure detailed in Chap. 1, Gelberg's analysis consisted of two steps: (1) coding the children's responses into one of seven categories: schooling and higher education, military service, work and career, marriage and family, self concerns, significant others, the collective (inter-judge reliability = 92%), and (2) computing *density* and *specificity* scores. As noted in Chap. 1, *density* scores pertain to the number of domain specific narratives/the total number of narratives ratio for hopes and fears, respectively, for each domain and overarching category. *Specificity* scores pertain to the mean of the specificity ratings for each domain. They are produced by assigning each narrative a score ranging from 1 (low specificity) to 3 (high specificity). To illustrate, "to get married" is scored 1, "to have a big wedding party" or "to get married and live happily" is scored 2, and "to get married and have three beautiful children" is scored 3.

The hopes and fears of 2nd graders. For 2nd graders, much like for the 5-year-olds described earlier, the future is understood as the time yet to come and events yet to be experienced, but the content of these yet unlived events is drawn from both reality and the world of fantasy. Thus, their hopes include reality-based narratives like "To own a car", "To be rich", "To have a big house", "I hope my friend and I will continue to be friends", "I want to be a dancer", and a mature view like "When I complete my military service I will study to become a medical doctor because in my opinion this is a good job" (listed by the son of a medical doctor), as well as fantasy narratives like "I will fly to the moon", "I will want to stop growing up", "I will have lots of rings", "I will be a princess". These narratives are also illustrated in the children's drawings (Figs. 2.1 and 2.2) that represent both concrete though stereotypic images (a girl draws herself as a beauty queen and a boy as a jungle

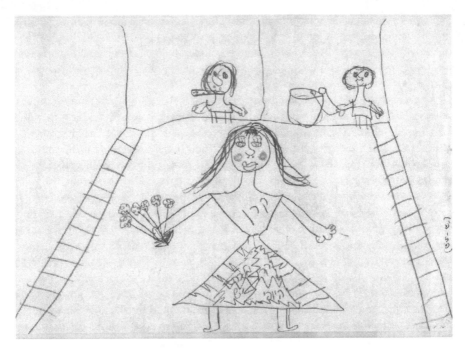

Fig. 2.1 My future by a 2nd grade girl: beauty queen

ranger) and the uncertainty of the future (a girl who wrote next to her drawing of black and pink hearts "I see hearts of light and darkness").

Their fears too are split between reality and fantasy, illustrated by reality-based fears like "my house will be broken into and my money and car stolen", "dogs will chase me", "I don't want to work in the garbage", "I will be hurt", and "shortly after the army [i.e., completing military service] I will not be accepted to be a doctor because maybe I am not suitable for the job". Their fantasy fears include "I will be afraid of crocodiles", "I will be eaten by a bear", "A monster at night", "I will become a Ninja turtle".

Age differences. Overall, age differences are reflected in the density scores of the prospective life course and existential domains and in the content of narratives, and only to a lesser extent in their specificity scores, mainly because the specificity measure turned out to be inappropriate for the analysis of the fantasy narratives. Thus "to be superman and fly high above the city" is a high specificity but obviously low reality narrative. This is also illustrated in the children's drawings (Figs. 2.3 and 2.4). Fourth graders imagine themselves as professionals: a girl draws herself with a lawyer's cap and a boy adds a balloon in which he says over the phone: "Yes; and please bring the insurance files. Tomorrow I am going to Haifa." He also adds that he sees himself as a quite successful lawyer or insurance agent. As they get to 6th grade, girls draw themselves as university students, and kindergarten and school teachers. One girl (Fig. 2.5) sees herself in the theater (left side of the drawing) but

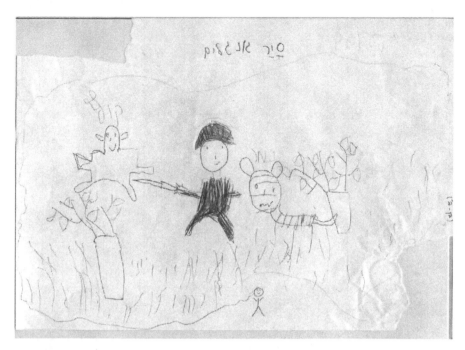

Fig. 2.2 My future by a 2nd grade boy: jungle ranger with a monkey to his left and a tiger to his right

also as having a family (right side of the drawing). Boys draw themselves at home, having the good life (a swimming pool next to the house), in romantic relationship, but as 2nd and 4th grade boys in soccer (Fig. 2.6).

As Figs. 2.7 and 2.8 illustrate, the prospective life course domains are age-related; the exception is work and career. This domain, more than that of education, military service, and marriage and family, is as represented in the prospective life space of 2nd as in that of 4th and 6th graders. Considering the high salience of military service in the life of Israelis and the fact that over 90% of the children have been growing up with their biological parents, these findings suggest, nevertheless, that the world of adults is more easily accessed via the domain of work and career than via military service, higher education, or marriage and family.

Analysis of the density scores of the fears domains show no age differences. This conclusion changes when the unit of analysis is the prospective life course overarching category and density scores are calculated for both hopes and fears. Then, significant age differences are found showing that, with age, the density scores of the prospective life course domains grows higher and of those of the existential domains grow smaller. However, the structure of these differences for the hopes and the fears aspects differs. The hopes score of 4th graders is significantly different from that of 2nd graders whereas their fears score is significantly different from that of 6th graders. In other words, for hopes the divide is between the 2nd and 4th grades and for fears between the 4th and 6th grades.

Fig. 2.3 My future by a 4th
grade girl: lawyer

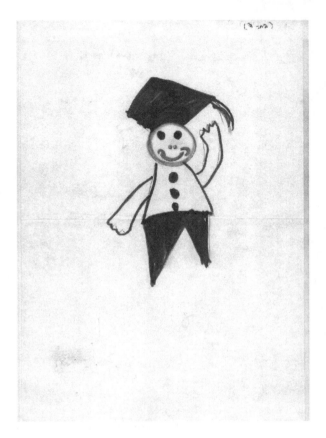

The explanation of the differential age differences for *hopes* and *fears* draws
on two considerations. The first pertains to the *developmental* tendencies and the
second to specific *cohort* effects.

Developmental tendencies. Although studies carried out with different socio-
cultural groups (e.g., Mönks, 1968; Nurmi, 1987; Seginer, 1988a,b,c) and with girls
(Seginer, 1992a) and boys (Berkman, 1993) indicate that adolescents and adults
produce more hopes than fears narratives, young children understand the meaning
of fear better than the meaning of hope; however, by 4th grade they have a good
grasp of what is meant by hopes. Thus, the greater difficulty individuals encounter
in processing negative information as well as across age avoidance of fear-arousing
events, especially those not yet experienced, are not strong enough to counteract the
primordial sense of fear with which young children are familiar.

Cohort differences: the effect of unique events. The analysis of the three age
groups revealed an interesting finding: of the three groups, the *collective issues* score
of 4th graders was considerably higher than that of both 2nd and 6th graders. In
fact, they scored higher than any other Israeli Jewish group assessed in recent years
and also differed in their content: many of them related to Saddam Hussein and

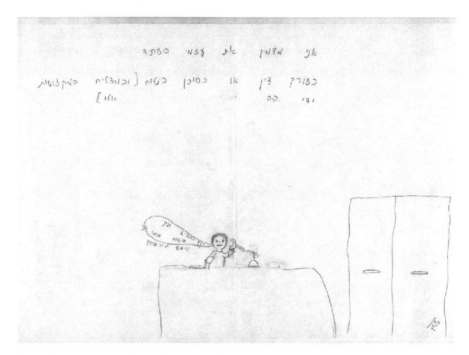

Fig. 2.4 My future by a 4th grade boy: "a quite successful lawyer or insurance agent"

the 1991 Gulf war when Israel was under the attack of Iraqi Scud missiles, schools were closed and uncertainty prevailed. Although the war took place 3 years earlier, its effect on the 4th graders who were then in 1st grade had been lasting and expressed in fears like "we will have a war", "Saddam Hussein will start a war on Israel", "a war in which the Iraqis and the Moslems will throw Katyusha rockets on us", but also others like "Planet Earth will explode", "we will have an earthquake".

Given that all respondents experienced the war – the 2nd graders as 4-year-olds and the 6th graders as 3rd graders – the question has been why the Gulf war left a stronger impression on the 4th graders than on the two other age groups? The answer draws on the work of Elder (Elder, 1974, 1986; Elder, Caspi, & Burton, 1988; Elder, Modell, & Parke, 1993) and Stewart (Stewart & Healy, 1989) showing that age moderates the effect of historical events on children, adolescents, and adult development so that the same social event – be it war, economic crisis, or the rise of women's movements – has different effects on individuals' development.

Applied to the present findings, 2nd graders were too young at the time of the Gulf war, and the 6th graders had some understanding of the war situation. However, the 4th graders were in 1st grade and experiencing both a personal change and the stress shared by all Israelis resulting from where and when the next Scud would hit and whether the threat of chemical and biological weapons would come true. Three years later, for some children the memory of war – which was threatening all, but for them also disrupted entrance to 1st grade – was reflected in how they constructed

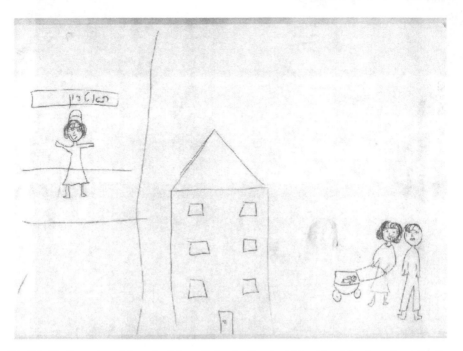

Fig. 2.5 My future by a 6th grade girl: multiple roles/family (*right side of the picture*) and theater career (*left*)

the future. Though the numbers are small and hence only indicative, this tendency suggests that memory affects not only the cognitive aspect of future orientation but also its emotional tone.

Gender differences. Although gender differences are traced in the narratives of 5-year-olds, they continue to develop with age (Fig. 2.9a–d): by 4th grade, girls are more oriented to education and boys to work and career. However, the greater interest of girls than of boys in marriage and family is indicated only by 6th graders. The tendency identified for age differences whereby fears are less differentiated by age than hopes is also true for gender differences. Nevertheless, 6th grade girls are more concerned with education and with marriage and family than are 6th grade boys.

Consequently, when the domains subsumed under the prospective life course and existential categories, respectively, are summed up, gender differences reach statistical significance for fears but not for hopes, with F $(1,270) = 4.60$ p < 0.05 and 5.84, p < 0.05 for the prospective life course and existential categories, respectively.

By focusing on age and gender differences we may be overlooking *similarities* between younger and older children, girls and boys. One such similarity is found for the *self concerns* category of all three age groups and two genders. Although its density score goes down from 47% of the hopes' prospective life space for 2nd grade boys to 21% for 6th grade girls and from 70% of the fears' prospective life

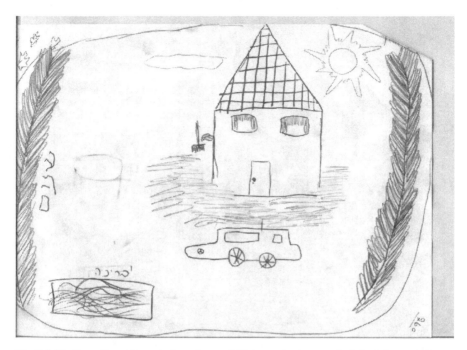

Fig. 2.6 My future by a 6th grade boy: the good life/peace (*written on the left of the page*), home, car and swimming pool

space for 2nd grade boys to 35% for 6th grades girls, overall this domain is more intensely represented in the children's prospective life space (indicated by the total number of hopes or fears) than any of the other future domains (31% of the hopes' and 51% of the fears' prospective life space pertain to self concerns).

In a similar vein, the work and career domain is more intensely represented in the boys' prospective life space than any of the other prospective life course domains (i.e., schooling and education, military service, marriage and family). Girls, however, change preferences as they reach 4th grade and the primacy of work and career in 2nd grade is replaced by marriage and family also maintained by 6th grade girls.

Future orientation and academic achievement. The age-related shift from existential to prospective life course narratives raises a question regarding the processes which facilitate this tendency as children move from 2nd to 4th and 6th grade. Specifically the question is whether the evolvement of a reality based prospective life course dominated future orientation is related to children's *cognitive-intellectual* abilities? Drawing on Greene's (1986) findings that future orientation is not related to cognitive development as defined by formal operations, and the non-availability of standardized achievement tests in Israel, Gelberg estimated intellectual ability in terms of academic achievement, positing that prospective life course density scores are positively associated and existential domains density are negatively associated with academic ability.

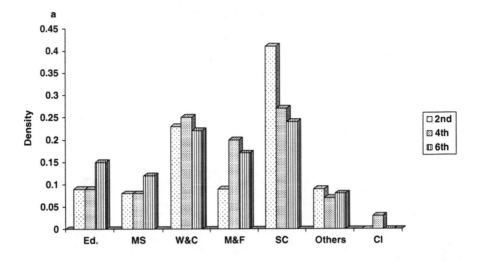

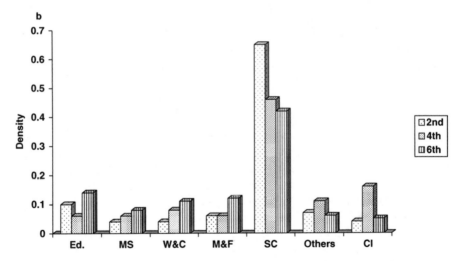

Fig. 2.7 Hopes and fears age differences: 2nd, 4th and 6 grades. **a** Hopes. **b** Fears. Ed = Education, MS = Military Service, W&C = Work and career, M&F = Marriage and family, SC = Self concerns, CI = Collective issues, density scores pertain to the domain specific/total number of narratives

His findings show that Grand Point Average (GPA) is more strongly and consistently related to the future orientation of 6th than of 2nd and 4th graders. Thus, analysis of the hopes density scores showed that for 6th graders the representation (i.e., the density score) of the education domain is positively related to GPA ($r = 0.24$, $p < 0.05$) while the representation of collective issues and the overall existential domains representations are negatively related to GPA ($r = -0.23$, $p < 0.05$ and -0.36, $p < 0.01$, respectively).

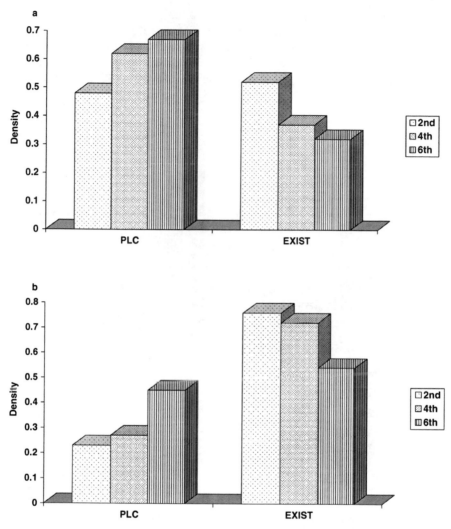

Fig. 2.8 Hopes and fears age differences: 2nd, 4th, and 6th grades. **a** Hopes. **b** Fears. PLC = Prospective life course, EXIST = Existential domains

The validity of these findings is supported by three other findings showing (1) that for 6th graders the *specificity* score of the education domain is positively related to GPA ($r = 0.45$, $p < 0.01$), (2) that the total number of hopes narratives is positively related to GPA ($r = 0.20$, $p < 0.05$), and that (3) nevertheless none of the other prospective life course domains (i.e., military service, work and career, marriage and family) nor the total density of prospective life course domains are related to GPA. Thus, the consistent effect of higher education future orientation on academic achievement found for culturally diverse adolescents (Chap. 7) can already be traced among 6th graders.

Future orientation and self esteem. Based on the basic premise that a sense of continuity is inherent to the meaning of self (Erikson, 1968; James, 1890; Markus & Nurius, 1986) and that as children grow up self-evaluation becomes the standard that directs behavior (Harter, 1999; Higgins, 1991), Gelberg examined the relation between a short version of the self-esteem scale (Coopersmith, 1967) and the density

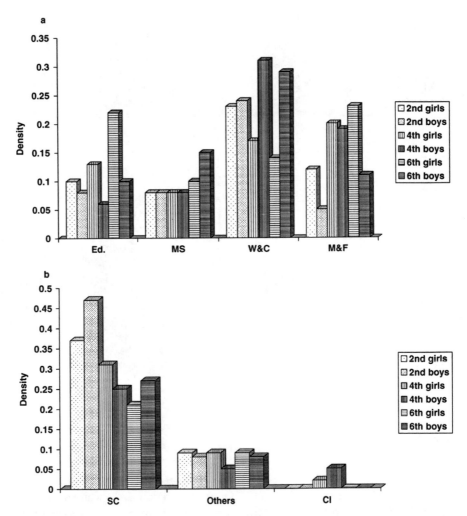

Fig. 2.9 Hopes and Fears Gender Differences: 2nd, 4th and 6th grades. **a** Hopes/prospective life course domains. Ed = Education, MS = Military service, W&C = Work and career, M&F = Marriage and family, SC = Self Concerns, CI = Collective Issues, density scores pertain to the domain specific/total number of narratives. **b** Hopes/existential domains. SC = Self concerns, CI = Collective issues. **c** Fears/prospective life course domains. **d** Fears/existential domains. SC = Self concerns, CI = Collective issues. Density scores pertain to the domain specific/total number of narratives

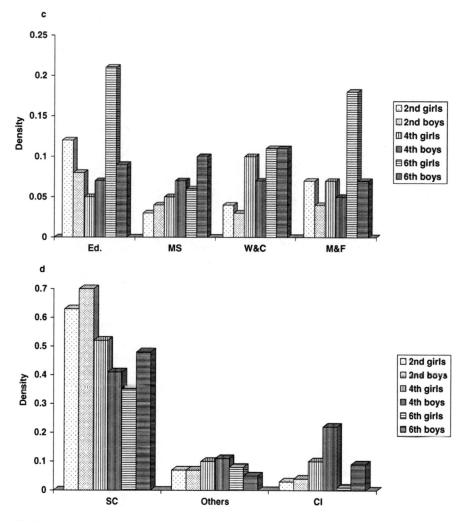

Fig. 2.9 (continued)

of each domain as well as the density of the two overarching categories: the prospective life course and the existential domains.

His hypothesis that the relation between self-esteem and future orientation will gradually build up is confirmed. While for 2nd graders self esteem and future orientation are not related, self-esteem is positively related to the density of the prospective life course overarching category for the 4th ($r = 0.24$, $p < 0.05$) and 6th graders ($r = 0.33$, $p < 0.01$) and negatively related to the existential category of both age groups ($r = -0.21$ and -0.22, $p < 0.05$ for 4th and 6th graders, respectively). For 6th graders, but not for the younger age groups, self-esteem is related also to the education ($r = 0.28$, $p < 0.05$) and self concerns ($r = -0.30$, $p < 0.01$) domains.

Summary: future orientation in middle childhood. Although 2nd graders are acquainted with the notion of the future and with the sequence of age-graded social roles, their narratives about the future differ from those constructed by 4th and 6th graders in being less realistic and hence less goal-oriented, behavior guiding and unrelated to academic ability (GPA) and self-esteem. This budding ability develops between 4th and 6th grades, so that when children reach 6th grade, investment in prospective life course is positively related to self esteem, and the school and education hopes – but not those pertaining to other domains – are positively related to academic achievement.

Summary: Future Orientation from Infancy to Middle Childhood

The accelerated cognitive and social-emotional development characterizing the period between infancy and middle childhood leads to different research questions and future orientation indicators suitable for each age group. Thus, infancy researchers focus on visual anticipatory behaviors and show that the first evidence of anticipatory behavior is identified as early as 3 months of age. Although its relevance to children's and adolescents' future orientation has not been empirically established, these researchers conjecture that, by engaging in visual anticipatory behavior, infants introduce themselves to the notion and meaning of "future" long before they can verbally demonstrate it.

Early childhood researchers focus on three future orientation issues: children's notions of time in general and of the future in particular as reflected in controlled experiments and naturalistic conversations, planning behavior, and future orientation socialization. In addition to studies of mothers' socialization strategies, the prevalence of future orientation themes in nursery, kindergarten, and school children's literature has also been demonstrated. In middle childhood, as children enter school the focus has been on their ability to extend the self into the future by generating hopes and fears for the future. This research, though limited in scope, shows that, whereas the hopes and fears of 2nd graders oscillate between fantasy and reality, they already show gender differences, that by 4th grade future orientation is reality based, and by 6th grade larger part of it is devoted to the prospective life course and directly related to self esteem. Moreover, the school and education domain, but not other domains, is associated with academic achievement, thus indicating that as children reach early adolescence they perceive the instrumentality of academic achievement for attaining educational goals.

Chapter 3
Future Orientation in Personality Contexts

Though initially lured to describe personality tersely as "what a man really is", in writing what is considered today as the first exposition on personality, Allport defined personality as "...the dynamic organization within the individual of those psychophysical systems that determine his unique adjustments to his environment" (1937/1949, p. 48).

Thus, as Allport has introduced the concept of trait to personality psychology, his influence on contemporary personality theories has been much broader. He understood personality as multidimensional and emphasized the importance of the relations (organization) among its different dimensions and thus preceded Cervone (2005), viewed these relations as changing and as responding to context (time, place, and other aspects of the environment) and thus preceded Mischel (Mischel, 2004; Mischel & Shoda, 1995), and considered adjustment to the environment as involving both mastery and passive adaptation and thus preceded Bandura (1997, 2001), Mischel (1968) and other social-cognitive personality theorists.

It is his contention that "personality *is* something and *does* something" (p. 48) that inspired Cantor (1990) to describe personality aspects in terms of "having" and "doing", and led Briggs (1989), Cantor (1990), Little (1996, 2006), and McAdams (1996) to distinguish between *levels* of personality so that level I subsumes nonconditional dispositional trait theories like the Big Five and level II pertains to social cognitive aspects of personality. In this chapter the focus is on level II personality constructs. Specifically, it reviews the effect on future orientation of each of the following: self esteem and self-agency, psychological empowerment, primary and secondary control, loneliness, defensive pessimism and strategic optimism. Although psychological convention considers personality and cognition as two separate research domains, this chapter also includes at its end a short section reviewing the scant research on the effect of cognitive abilities on future orientation.

To present the rationale underlying the relation between each of the self and personality constructs and future orientation, the subsequent sections open with a conceptual analysis of the personality construct in question and proceed with examining its relation to future orientation. Also common to all is a contextual approach substantiated by empirical analyses that show how life domain, age, gender, and ethnicity moderate the effect of each personality construct on future orientation.

R. Seginer, *Future Orientation*, The Springer Series on Human Exceptionality,
DOI 10.1007/978-0-387-88641-1_3, © Springer Science+Business Media, LLC 2009

Self Esteem and Self Agency

The Self: A Conceptual Framework

Today, several decades after the cognitive revolution in psychology, the importance of the self in guiding individuals' behavior is widely recognized as is the contribution of the early work of Cooley (1902), James (1890), and Mead (1934) to understanding human functioning attested by the voluminous research on the development of the self and its effect on various aspects of behavior. In this section those self aspects deemed pertinent to future orientation are reviewed.

As the pivotal role of the self in processing incoming information and guiding behavior first introduced by James (1890/1950) has been maintained in contemporary research (e.g., Harter, 1996; Markus, 1977; Marsh & Hattie, 1996; Rosenberg, 1965), in particular three specific issues are deemed relevant: the distinction between the I and the Me as two central aspects of the self, the domain specific and global models of the self, and the evaluative nature of self representation and hence the greater pertinence of self esteem than of self concept to the explanation of behavior and development.

I-self and Me-self. The distinction between the I-self and the Me-self (James, 1890) conveys the multiple functions of the self. As the subjective knower, the I-self's functions are to organize and interpret the person's experiences and consequently to construct the Me-self whose function is to represent the self as known. Each consists of multiple components. The *I-self* consists of self-awareness of one's internal states, one's responsibility for learning about the self, keeping its boundaries and consequently generating the Me-self authorship, self-continuity across time, and self-coherence across conditions and experiences (Harter, 2003). However, despite its important functions and following James, the I-self has been regarded as elusive (Harter, 1999) or rather as a hypothetical construct and not intended for empirical research.

Domain specific and global self. Representing the self as known, the Me-self consists of specific domains by which individuals organize this knowledge, but can also be represented in its totality as *global* self. However, while James (1890) described the Me-self as consisting of the *material, social* and *spiritual* selves, contemporary researchers describe it as more differentiated and related to relevant aspects of current life (e.g., academic, social/interpersonal, physical/body image).

The ability to differentiate between various domains of the self and integrate them into a global self-representation depends on the cognitive development underlying the I-self (Harter, 1999, 2003). By middle childhood – and even more so as they reach adolescence – children develop the ability to evaluate themselves by relating both to specific aspects of their functioning such as their schooling, sports performance, or interpersonal relationships with family and peers (domain-specific self evaluation) and to their overall worth (global self esteem or self worth).

As initially indicated by James, reiterated by contemporary researchers (Harter, 1999; Rosenberg, 1979, 1986) and empirically corroborated in several studies, global self esteem is weighted by the subjective importance of each specific domain.

Thus, across data collected in the United States and other countries (mainly European), the correlation between domains adolescents consider important, such as physical appearance, is high (*rs* range between 0.52 and 0.80) and much higher than the correlation between domains adolescents consider as unimportant, such as athletic competence (*rs* range between 0.23 and 0.42) (Harter, 1999). It is for this reason in particular that the practice of creating a global self esteem measure by summing up domain specific self evaluations has been criticized (Harter, 1999). Obviously, the use by researchers of domain-specific, global or both conceptualizations depends on the objective and theoretical framework of each study.

Self concept and self esteem. The distinction between self concept and self esteem draws on James's observation that, as individuals consider their self, they in fact engage in a two-step process. They *perceive* the self and *evaluate* it, just as they do with respect to other persons and objects. However, the process by which individuals evaluate the self differs from how they evaluate other objects and relates mainly to comparison against standards they establish about those aspects of the self deemed important. Thus,

> Our thought, incessantly deciding, among many things of a kind, which ones for it shall be realities, here chooses one of many possible selves or characters, and forthwith reckons it no shame to fail in any of those not adopted expressly as its own. I, who for the time have staked my all on being a psychologist, am mortified if others know much more psychology than I. But I am contended to wallow in the grossest ignorance of Greek...So our self-feeling in this world depends entirely on what we *back* ourselves to be and do. It is determined by the ratio of our actualities to our supposed potentialities; a fraction of which our pretensions are the denominator and the numerator our success: thus, Self-esteem = Success/Pretensions (James, 1890/1950, vol. 1, p. 310).

The Effect of the Self on Future Orientation

Initially, the relevance of the self to future orientation drew on the temporality of the self and its representation in relation to the past, present, or future (Lens, 2006; Nuttin, 1984; Nuttin & Lens, 1985; Rosenberg, 1979). This premise underlay research on adolescents' identity (Coleman, Herzberg, & Morris, 1977) in which present and future self-evaluation are compared and on possible selves (e.g., Markus & Wurf, 1987) as "representation of the self in the future" (Markus & Nurius, 1986. p. 954).

However, based on the conceptualization of future orientation as domain specific hoped-for and feared-of images of the future and consisting of multiple components, self-evaluation and future orientation are treated as two separate constructs. Research on their relations has been guided by two premises. One pertains to the central role played by the self in organizing incoming information and guiding wide range of behaviors ranging from academic achievement to competitive sports and from social skills to depression (Harter, 1999), and the other to the observation that as children develop into adolescents their behavior is guided by the self rather than directly by parental behavior (Harter, 1999; Higgins, 1991). Hence, research presented here assumes that the self serves as an antecedent and examines its effect on future orientation in both bi- and multi-variate models.

Of the multiple manifestations of the self, this section reviews the effect of those self constructs deemed relevant to adolescents' tendency to orient themselves to the future: self agency, self stability, and global self esteem.

Self-Agency and Future Orientation

Self-agency. The self-agency construct has been developed in the context of infancy development. Stern (1985) identified *self-agency* as one of four self-experiences comprising the infant's core self and described it as consisting of a sense of volition, control, and overall authorship over one's acts, and Harter applied this definition to children and adults and described self-agency as a sense of authorship over one's acts, thoughts and emotions (Harter, 1999). Empirical research has operationalized *self-agency* as the person's sense of self-dependence, control and responsibility over her or his acts. Although much of the research on self-agency has been carried out in clinical settings (e.g., Kim & Cicchetti, 2006; Putnam, 1994; Westen, 1993), this conceptualization is particularly appropriate for describing adolescents' self as reflected in their sense of self-governance and responsibility.

Self-agency and future orientation. The relation between this aspect of the self and future orientation draws directly on the definition of self-agency and the assumption that the sense of self authorship is not limited to one's acts in the present but also extends to acts in the future. Thus, the hypothesis has been that of the three future orientation components; self-agency is more closely associated with the behavioral component of future orientation empirically indexed by *exploration* and *commitment*. Empirical analyses (Chaps. 5, 6, and 7) of data collected from Israeli Jewish 11th graders confirm this hypothesis but indicate its domain specificity. Thus, self-agency is associated with the behavioral variables pertaining to higher education and work and career future orientation domain (rs ranging from 0.25 to 0.31, $p < 0.001$) but not with behavioral variables pertaining to the marriage and family domain. Contrary to prediction, we additionally found that self-agency is also related to the motivational variables pertaining to the work and career and marriage and family domains (rs ranging from 0.22 to 0.39, $p < 0.001$). However, multivariate analysis (Seginer, Vermulst, & Shoyer, 2004) showed that, while the direct relation between self-agency and the motivational variables pertaining to the work and career and marriage and family domains is maintained, the relation between self-agency and the behavioral component of future orientation is only indirect and mediated by the motivational component.

Self-Stability and Future Orientation

Self-stability pertains to the experienced stability of individuals' sense of self competence (Alsaker & Olweus, 1992) and, like in the case of Israeli adolescents' self-agency, shows that for Israeli emerging adults the relations between self-stability and the motivational variables of work and career (rs ranging from 0.37 to 0.39), family and marriage (rs ranging from 0.18 to 0.27), and higher education (rs ranging from 0.24 to 0.30) are higher than between self-stability and the behavioral variables pertaining to these domains (rs ranging from 0.11 to 0.25 for work and career, 0 to 0.16 for marriage and family, and 0.15 to 0.23 for higher education) (Guter, 1995). However, findings of a study of Australian and Finnish adolescents' future orientation (Nurmi, Seginer, & Poole, 1995) that showed positive but lower relations between self-stability and exploration and commitment (behavioral variables) in the higher education and work and career domains (rs = 0.19 to 0.21, p < 0.01) suggest the relations are moderated by contextual factors.

Self-Esteem and Future Orientation

The notion initially developed by James (1890/1950) that self-esteem – as the evaluative aspect of the self – has two functions is still valid. One is to provide a sense of self-satisfaction (Rosenberg, 1979) and the other is to induce various behaviors intended to maintain one's self esteem (Tesser, 1988). The decision to estimate the effect of self evaluation on future orientation by employing a global rather than a domain-specific construct drew on the assumption that, since future orientation pertains to prospective roles *not yet experienced*, a global self esteem is more relevant to it than domain-specific self image (Seginer et al., 2004). Thus, research on the self antecedents of future orientation treats future orientation as domain specific and self esteem as global.

Self-esteem and future orientation components. As future orientation is conceptualized in terms of a multiple-component construct, the effect of self-esteem on each of the three future orientation components is presented below.

The relation between self-esteem and the *motivational component* draws on three considerations. The first relates to the premise that, being an indicator of emotional health (Grotevant, 1998), self-esteem makes it possible for individuals to attend concomitantly to current as well as future oriented tasks (Melges, 1982). The second pertains to the nature of the variables subsumed under the motivational component, i.e., the value, expectance, and internal control as both conceptually and empirically related to self evaluation, and the third draws specifically on the value-expectancy proposition that positive self-evaluation has a direct bearing on the value of the task and the person's task-specific success expectancy (e.g., Eccles, Adler, & Meece, 1984; Wigfield, 1994).

Data collected from Israeli Jewish 11th graders support this proposition when tested on four life domains: higher education (Seginer, 2005), military service (Shoyer, 2001), work and career, and marriage and family (Seginer et al., 2004), all showing moderate associations. Thus, individuals valuing themselves also value the tasks they perform (value), and their sense of self-worth prompts success expectations (expectance) and internal control attributions (Eccles & Wigfield, 2002; Weiner, 1974).

Studies specifically focusing on expectance reiterated the effect of the self on future orientation. One study (Zeira & Dekel, 2005) focused on the relation between three adolescent self image scales (emotional tone, mastery of the external world, and social relationships) (Offer, Ostrov, Howard, & Atkinson, 1988) and the subjective probability of the occurrence of events (expectance) pertaining to normative (education, military service, economic independence, marriage and family) and non-normative (deviant behavior) life events among Israeli adolescents (10th to 12th graders). Its findings show that all three measures are positively related to the two adult roles events (economic independence and marriage and family) and negatively related to deviant behavior. However, only the mastery aspect of self-image is positively related to the education domain.

Another study of American adolescent girls and boys (Knox, Funk, Elliott, & Bush, 1998) indicated that girls' expectance more than boys' expectance is contingent on their self esteem (as assessed by the global self competence scale, Harter, 1982). Specifically, this study reported that whereas for boys self esteem is related only to the materialization of the interpersonal possible self, for girls self esteem is related to the subjective likelihood of the materialization of four possible self domains: education, occupation, material or financial, and interpersonal relationships.

The relation between self-esteem and the *cognitive representation* component of future orientation draws on one specific consideration and one common to all three components. Underlying the specific consideration is the conceptual affinity between self-esteem as the *present* subjective self-representation and the cognitive component as the *prospective* self representation. The consideration common to all three future orientation components and mentioned above relates to self-esteem as one aspect of emotional health (Grotevant, 1998) which thus affords individuals to attend to both present and future issues (Melges, 1982).

As reported in Chap. 2, data on the association between self-esteem and self representation of the future (the cognitive component) show that, as children reach middle childhood and are able to engage in self evaluation, self-esteem is positively associated with future orientation (Gelberg, 1996; Seginer, 2005; Seginer, Dan, & Zeliger, 1998), and the association grows stronger as children enter early adolescence (rs ranging from 0.20 for 4th graders to 0.33 for 6th graders). Thus, as children's self-esteem becomes more integrated, its association with the cognitive core of future orientation becomes stronger. Among adolescents, self esteem has been related to future representation of two domains: education (Malmberg & Trempala, 1997; Nurmi & Pulliainen, 1991), and occupation (Malmberg & Trempala, 1997).

Finally, the relation between self-esteem and the *behavioral component* of future orientation is based only on the consideration, common to all three future orientation components, that self-esteem affords individuals with enough inner strength to deal simultaneously with present and future issues. However, findings show only low positive relations between global self esteem and exploration and commitment to prospective education and occupation (Nurmi et al., 1995; Seginer et al., 2004; Shoyer, 2006).

Self-esteem and the three future orientation components: summary. While research on the relations between self-esteem and the three future orientation components is scarce, extant data show that these relations are moderate to low, but more strongly associated with the motivational variables than with the cognitive and behavioral variables. Nonetheless, when examined in multiple-step models that also include adolescent relationships with parents, siblings and peers (Chaps. 5 and 6), the role of self-esteem as mediating the effect of interpersonal relationships and its direct effect on the motivational component and via it on the cognitive and behavioral components is clearly and consistently shown.

The subjective awareness of the motivating forces of self-worth and its relevance to youth orientation to the future is resonated in Walt Whitman's poem:

Afoot and light-hearted I take to the open road,
Healthy, free, the world before me,
The long brown path before me leading wherever I
   choose.
Henceforth I ask not good-fortune, I myself am good-
   fortune,
Henceforth I whimper no more, postpone no more,
   need nothing,
Done with indoor complaints, libraries, querulous
   criticisms,
Strong and content I travel the open road. (Whitman, 1892/1983, p. 119).

The Self-Schema of Loneliness

Self-Schema

The self-schema (Markus, 1977) is another construct based on James's (1890) conceptualization of the self as the organizer and interpreter of individuals' experiences. Like James and many contemporary researchers of the self, Markus has been interested in self-knowledge. Particularly concerned with its cognitive aspects, she (Markus, 1977, 1983) contended that self knowledge consists of multiple self-schemata and that individuals differ in the extent to which they integrate certain experiences into a distinct self-schema or remain aschematic.

However, unlike James and contemporary researchers like Harter and Rosenberg, Markus does not suggest a global evaluative self schema. Instead, underlying the self-schema construct is the idea that self-schemata organize information concerning *specific* aspects of the self; such as dependence vs independence, sex roles, and creativity. Assuming that loneliness is another self-schema particularly relevant to adolescent development and the construction of their future orientation (Seginer, 2001b; Seginer & Lilach, 2004), this section focuses on the rationale and findings regarding the relations between loneliness and various aspects of future orientation.

Loneliness

Loneliness is a familiar phenomenon described as the negative affective reaction to one's appraisal of social relations as lacking. Conceptually, loneliness consists of two components: *cognitive* representation of the self as experiencing wanting social relations and *emotional* negative reaction to it. Its cognitive representational aspect reflects accumulated experiences consisting of both specific occurrences and generalizations across time and situations that self researchers have identified as responsible for the construction of self knowledge. Underlying individuals' negative emotional reaction to loneliness is a thwarted universal need to belong and to establish stable social bonds with caring others (Rotenberg, 1999). While the need is one, the negative affective reactions to its obstruction are many. Among them are despair, depression, boredom and self-criticism (Rubenstein & Shaver, 1982; Wiseman, 1997).

Adolescent loneliness. The centrality of peer relationships for adolescents and reports regarding the prevalence of loneliness among adolescents (Goossens, 2006; Rubenstein & Shaver, 1982) notwithstanding, adolescent loneliness has not been widely studied. Existing research describes lonely adolescents as passively sad and turned inward (Van Buskirk & Duke, 1991), experiencing greater stress (Cacciopo et al., 2000) and high levels of social anxiety (Goossens & Marcoen, 1999), and suffering from behavioral problems including peer rejection and victimization (Boivin, Hymel, & Bukowski, 1995), shyness and social withdrawal problems (Kupersmidt, Sigda, Sedikides, & Voegler, 1999). While those analyses describe adolescent loneliness as uni-dimensional, Sippola and Bukowski (1999) have suggested a dual model which emphasizes that separation can apply not only to others but also to the self. Thus, lonely adolescents have a sense of being separated from others (parents, peers) and alienated from the self which results in feelings of divided self.

Loneliness and Future Orientation

To examine the effect of loneliness on future orientation, Seginer and Lilach (2004) examined three hypotheses pertaining to the domain specificity of the loneliness-future orientation relations, gender differences, and the confounding effect of depression. Contending that the effect of loneliness on future orientation varies according to the theme and distance of each prospective domain, their analyses focus on four domains defined in terms of *relational* and *instrumental* themes and *near* and *distant* distances: interpersonal relationships (relational/near), marriage and family (relational/distant), higher education (instrumental/near), and work and career (instrumental/distant).

Given that loneliness is a self-schema of interpersonal relationships, that the relational future domains are more pertinent to loneliness, and that nearness increases the *reality value* of the domain (Nuttin & Lens, 1985), Seginer and Lilach's prediction has been that loneliness will have a stronger effect on future orientation variables applying to the *relational* than to the instrumental domains, and to the *near* than to the distant domains. Consequently, the prediction has been that loneliness is more strongly related to social relations than to marriage and family and the two instrumental domains. However, this relation could take one of two directions: guided by their *self-schema of loneliness*, lonely adolescents would score lower on

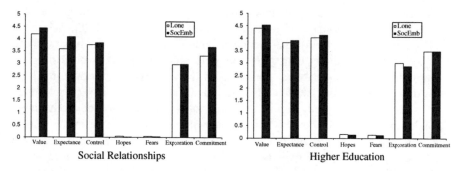

Fig. 3.1 Future orientation variables means scores for social relationships and higher education domains

the relational than on the instrumental domains; motivated by a *need to compensate* their poor present social relationships they would score higher on the relational than on the instrumental domains. Data collected from Israeli Jewish 11th graders show that lonely adolescents score lower than socially embedded adolescents on the social relationships domain, but only on the *motivational* future orientation variables. Figure 3.1 illustrates these findings for social relationships and higher education, indexing the near future instrumental domain. Moreover, their expectance scores are lower than those of the socially embedded adolescents on all four future life domains but particularly (and significantly) on the two relational domains. Thus, lonely adolescents have less confidence in the materialization of hopes, wishes and plans regarding the relational than the instrumental domains. Conversely, the socially embedded adolescents' expectance scores were similar (Fig. 3.2).

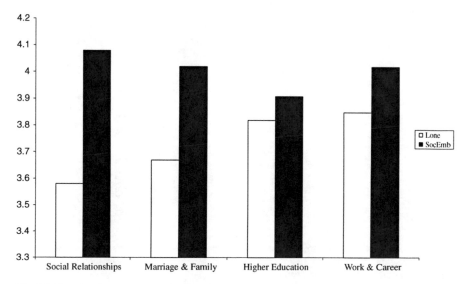

Fig. 3.2 Expectance mean scores for four future orientation domains

Loneliness and future orientation: gender differences. Based on gender differences in the experience of loneliness (Koenig & Abrams, 1999; Wiseman, Guttfreund, & Lurie, 1995), the second hypothesis has been that, because boys express greater loneliness than girls and girls score higher than boys on relational domains, in the relational domains, and particularly in the social relationships domain, lonely boys will score lower on all future orientation variables than will lonely girls. This prediction is borne out but applies only to one motivational variable: expectance. Specifically, lonely boys have *less* confidence in the materialization of hopes, wishes and plans (expectance) regarding the relational than the instrumental domains, and socially embedded boys have *more* confidence in the materialization of hopes, wishes and plans regarding the relational than the instrumental domains. Conversely, all girls (lonely as well as socially embedded) have similar confidence in the materialization of hopes, wishes and plans regarding relational and instrumental domains (Fig. 3.3).

Loneliness, depression, and future orientation. Based on earlier findings on the relations between depression and loneliness (Abramson, Metalsky, & Alloy, 1989; Csikszentmihalyi & Larson, 1984; Koenig, Isaacs, & Schwartz, 1994; Van Buskirk & Duke, 1991; Wiseman, 1997), Seginer and Lilach's third hypothesis has been that the effect of loneliness on future orientation is confounded by depression. However, results show that for this adolescent community sample, the domain specific effect of loneliness on the motivational variables of future orientation stands for itself and is not affected by depressive tendencies.

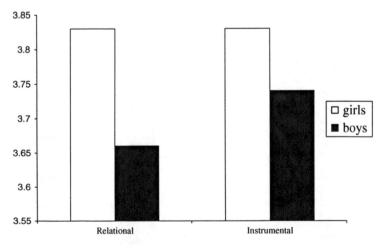

Fig. 3.3 Relational and instrumental expectance mean scores: lonely girls and boys. Relational domains = social relationships (near), marriage and family (distant). Instrumental domains = higher education (near), work and career (distant)

Loneliness and Future Orientation: Summary

This study has taught us three lessons. The first is that the effect of adolescents' loneliness on future orientation is not all-encompassing and that the emotional distress accompanying it does not – as suggested by Melges (1982) – block future oriented thinking as a whole. Instead, it is specific to the *relational* domains and to the *motivational* future orientation variables. The second relates to gender differences. Lonely girls use relational future orientation as compensation for their present condition whereas lonely boys construct a relational future consistent with their present sense of loneliness.

Thus, boys are more vulnerable to loneliness (Koenig & Abrams, 1999; Page, 1990; Russell, 1996; Wiseman et al., 1995) but their greater tendency to spend time alone (Larson & Richards, 1991), lower inclination to form close friendships (Sharabany, 1994; Sharabany, Gershoni, & Hofman, 1981), and reluctance to admit feelings of loneliness all suggest the lower value and lesser probability of materialization of hopes they attribute to prospective social relationships. Girls, on the other hand, who have a greater need for close relationships, protect themselves by granting high probability to improved social relationships in the future.

Our third lesson relates to the distinction between mild and severe loneliness. Although these findings support the social cognitive approach to loneliness that depicts it as a form of self representation or *self schema*, they must be evaluated in light of the relative mild loneliness manifested by community (rather than clinically) lonely adolescents who participated in this study, as well as in other studies (e.g., Russell, Peplau, & Cutrona, 1980; Wiseman, 1997). Thus, while mild loneliness has domain-specific effects as the ones reported in this analysis, a severe form of loneliness may spill over and affect future orientation variables applying to all domains. It also reiterates the relevance of loneliness intensity, whether described as transient vs chronic loneliness (Koenig & Abrams, 1999) or mild vs severe loneliness.

Psychological Empowerment

By its name, empowerment is required by those lacking power. Therefore it is only natural for the notion of empowerment to be developed in the context of community work where the question has been how individuals of low economic, social and educational resources can obtain access to those means necessary for gaining control over their outcomes.

Psychological empowerment. Of the multiple solutions to the question of how the needy gain access to necessary means, psychologists have focused on psychological power, contending that through it individuals may obtain available resources and community services and thus develop a sense of psychological (or self) empowerment. However, what makes up psychological empowerment varies according to the setting and the situation. Indeed, as noted by Zimmerman (1995) and summarized by Perkins and Zimmerman:

> As an open-ended construct, psychological empowerment takes on different forms in different contexts, populations, and developmental stages and so cannot be adequately captured by single operationalization, divorced from other situational condition (Perkins & Zimmerman, 1995, p. 573).

Nonetheless, psychologists now tend to agree that psychological empowerment is multi dimensional, pertaining to issues of *self competence*, knowledge about one's *social setting* and the individuals, institutions, norms and values governing it, and the *action* individuals need to take in order to achieve their goals, labeled as intrapersonal, interactional, and behavioral components of psychological empowerment, respectively. The *intrapersonal* component pertains to beliefs about the person's competence, the *interactional* component relates to individuals' understanding of the socio-political context without which control-directed actions cannot be successfully accomplished, and the *behavioral* component concerns the action individuals use or know they need to use in order to achieve control over their outcomes (Zimmerman, 1995, 2000).

Psychological Empowerment and Future Orientation: The Case of Israeli Arab Girls

The relevance of psychological empowerment to future orientation was first conjectured by Mahajna (2000). His interest in the effect of psychological empowerment on future orientation was prompted by cumulative observations that, in their future orientation hopes and fears narratives, Israeli Arab girls more than Israeli Arab boys and Israeli Jewish girls and boys regard higher education as a means for developing an independent career and thus gaining control over their lives.

This has also been true of girls who grow up in rural areas and attend an all-girl Islamic high school. While their narratives differ from those of Arab boys and Jewish girls and boys both in the number and content of higher education themes, of particular interest is the content of their narratives which shows higher *specificity* of the educational and career options considered, *desire for personal control* over the materialization of hopes and aspirations, and *comprehending the sociopolitical system as means for facilitating or obstructing* the materialization of those hopes and aspirations and knowing how to handle them.

The correspondence between these features and the dimensions defining psychological empowerment led to the conjecture that Israeli Arab girls have been interweaving their educational and career future orientation with themes of psychological empowerment.

Themes of psychological empowerment in future orientation narratives: empirical evidence. To test this conjecture we conducted secondary analysis on the hopes and fears narratives expressed by close to 300 Israeli Arab girls (age 16–18) who attended the same rural all-girl Moslem high school and participated in a study on the family context of adolescent future orientation (Seginer & Mahajna, 2004). This content analysis identified narratives pertaining to all three dimensions of psychological empowerment. Specifically, *intrapersonal* empowerment is expressed by narratives like

I believe no obstacle in the future will prevent me from continuing my education (10th grader, No. 015).

Education is the only weapon I have in this world (10th grader, No. 017).

Every girl in this world sets herself a promising future. I am like that. My first step toward the future is high grades (11th grader, No. 110).

People should plan their future because otherwise they may have to cope with unexpected obstacles that will thwart their plans (11th grader, No. 57).

I am very convinced and determined to continue my education (12th grader, No. 168).

A good student, there is no reason why she won't become a physician or a lawyer (12th grader, No. 188).

Interactional empowerment and concerns about its want are expressed by narratives like

It is plausible that all my dreams will remain stored in the canister of values and norms, because it is not proper for a woman to either study or work. Everything in our society is forbidden on account of religion (10th grader, No. 006).

My plans for the future are not my property because I always have to consult my parents who have a strong influence on me (10th grader, No. 071).

I hope my family will support me both financially and psychologically all the way through [my higher education] (11th grader, No. 121).

I hope my fiancé will help me in all respects so that I will be able to fulfill my dream to study at the university (11th grader, No. 139).

In five months time I am getting married and worry about the obstacles [incurred by it] that will prevent me from continuing my education. I am also worried about becoming a mother at such a young age (12th grader, No.184).

I hope to continue my education by attending a [local] college or university. One cannot break away from getting married. This is a vital issue in our life, but should take place at a specific time: neither earlier nor later (12th grader, No. 231).

Behavioral empowerment is expressed in narratives like

To do well in the matriculation exams and in the psychometric tests [state-wide university entrance examinations]. After that I could continue at the university; therefore it is important to get as many good grades as possible (10th grader, No. 016).

In addition, we identified narratives that *combined* intrapersonal and interactional empowerment. This is illustrated in narratives like

I hope to become a medical doctor. I am very determined to achieve this goal; this is why I invest so much in studying. As to marriage now I am not concerned about it. Its turn will come only after I fulfill my educational objectives (10th grader, No. 56).

I have many hopes but the most important among them is higher education because "education is a weapon in woman's hand". I hope to God to send me a man who encourages women's education. I think I don't have a hope more important than this one (11th grader, No. 117).

I want very much to study chemistry at Tel Aviv University. But tradition won't allow me to do that. Therefore, I am registered at a college [near her home]. But when I grow up and am able to take care of myself, I will take a graduate degree at the university (12th grader, No. 179).

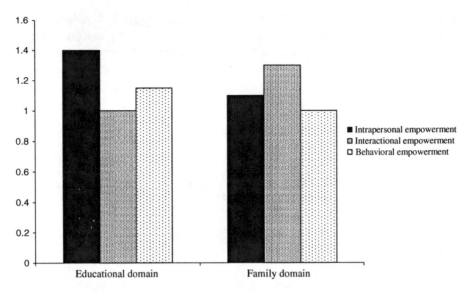

Fig. 3.4 Three aspects of self empowerment: domain mean scores

Overall, the future orientation narratives of these Israeli Arab girls contain more intrapersonal than interactional themes, and behavioral themes are considerably fewer than both. However, when the frequency of the three themes is analyzed separately for the educational and family domains, their domain specificity becomes clear. The educational domain elicits mainly intrapersonal empowerment whereas the family domain mainly interactional empowerment (Fig. 3.4).

Intrapersonal and family antecedents of psychological empowerment. Our analysis also shows that girls who interweave hopes and fears for the future with psychological empowerment themes score higher on both self-esteem and perceived fathers' beliefs about women's roles as traditional (i.e., they perceive father as expecting early marriage and oppose higher education) (Fig. 3.5). Under these

Fig. 3.5 The net effect (β) of self esteem, father's traditionality, and academic achievement on number of psychological empowerment narratives (*r*s in parentheses)

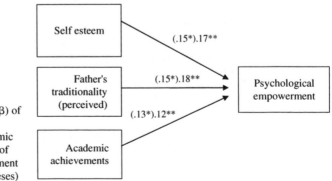

Table 3.1 Correlation coefficients (r) between three psychological empowerment dimensions and two future orientation domains: Arab girls

		Empowerment		
		Intrapersonal	Interactive	Behavioral
Higher education				
Motivational var	Value	0.32***	0.29***	0.14*
	Expectance	0.35***	0.27***	0.10
	Control	0.26***	0.25***	0.08
Cognitive var	Cognitive rep	0.43***	0.41***	0.18**
Behavioral var	Exploration	0.26***	0.32***	0.14*
	Commitment	0.34***	0.32***	0.15*
Marriage and family				
Motivational var	Value	0.04	0.03	0.04
	Expectance	0.06	0	−0.04
	Control	0.12	0.12	0.06
Cognitive var	Cognitive rep	−0.17*	−0.21***	0
Behavioral var	Exploration	0.08	0	0.08
	Commitment	−0.06	−0.06	0.07

*p < 0.05
**p < 0.01
***p < 0.001

conditions, intelligent, self confident girls who hold high educational goals but cannot expect their fathers to support their educational aspirations can rely only on their inner resources.

Psychological empowerment and future orientation. Our next question has been whether in addition to being intertwined with future orientation hopes and fears each of the three dimensions of psychological empowerment is also directly linked to future orientation. We returned to the same school (but not to the same students) and assessed girls' sense of psychological empowerment and future orientation. Our findings (Table 3.1) clearly show that the effect of each of the three dimensions of psychological empowerment on future orientation is domain specific.

In particular, each of the three dimensions has an effect on each of the three components of *educational* future orientation but only on the cognitive representation of *family* future orientation. Moreover, the effect of psychological empowerment on the cognitive representation of the marriage and family domain is *negative*: the lower their sense of psychological empowerment the more often they think about getting married and having a family. Thus, girls' low sense of psychological empowerment drives them to think about their prospective marriage and family life as a domain in which life will be guided by others: their father who will arrange the marriage for them and their husband who will dominate their life from then on. This interpretation is supported by the future orientation *fears* narratives of these girls. Specifically, when listing their fears regarding marriage and family dependency on or control by others is a major theme:

I am concerned about my marriage. I am afraid my marriage will not be successful and I will find out my husband is not the person I thought him to be. I am afraid he will betray his promise about continuing my education (12th grader, No. 169).

I am afraid my future husband will not be responsive to my needs (12th grader, No. 183).

Regarding my marriage, I am afraid my future husband will be a religious person who will abide by the prevailing [religious] values and norms which will guide his conduct, and I will not find out about it before getting married (12th grader, No. 235).

As a counterpoint, one girl expressed a high self empowerment in dealing with her prospective marriage. At age 17 she wrote:

Regarding marriage, I am afraid of marriage problems. Therefore, I keep myself busy with acquiring knowledge about marriage and family life and the secrets of happy marriage (11th grader, No. 113).

The Cultural Context of Psychological Empowerment and Future Orientation

Our next question has been whether psychological empowerment is particularly relevant for Israeli Arab girls growing up in a religious and traditional settings, or is it also associated with the future orientation of Israeli Jewish adolescents growing up in a western setting who at the age of 17 enjoy a fair amount of independence. Our findings show both cultural commonalities and differences. As indicated in Table 3.2, for both cultural groups psychological empowerment is more relevant to instrumental (higher education and work and career) than to relational (marriage and family) domains; however, possibly for different reasons. While Arab girls are aware of and accept their dependence on the power of family men (father, brothers, future husband) over their lives, particularly regarding marriage and family issues, for the Jewish adolescents these issues belong to a more distant future and thus of lesser concern.

Nevertheless, cultural differences are more clearly shown in the relations between psychological empowerment and future orientation regarding the marriage and family domain. Thus, whereas for the Arab girls psychological empowerment is related only to the cognitive representation of marriage and family, and as indicated above this relation is negative, for the Jewish girls psychological empowerment is positively related to the motivational variables. Jewish girls with high sense of psychological empowerment value marriage and family more than the low psychological empowerment girls, expect their hopes, goals and plans will materialize, and believe in their ability to control it. This tendency is also found among Israeli Jewish boys for whom the value and sense of internal control over marriage and family are significantly related to psychological empowerment. Related to some distant point in their future, psychological empowerment makes a difference for the value, expectance and sense of control over marriage and family (motivational component) but not to the more concrete cognitive representation (thinking about) and behavioral domains (taking action toward).

Table 3.2 Correlation coefficients (*r*) between three psychological empowerment dimensions and two future orientation domains, A. Jewish girls, B. Jewish boys

		Empowerment		
		Intrapersonal	Interactive	Behavioral
A				
Higher education				
Motivational var	Value	0.40***	0.36***	0.28**
	Expectance	0.25***	0.24***	0.05
	Control	0.34***	0.43***	0.22**
Cognitive var	Cognitive rep	0.16***	0.23**	0.14
Behavioral var	Exploration	0.21***	0.28***	0.13
	Commitment	0.29***	0.17*	0.08
Marriage and family				
Motivational var	Value	0.18*	0.18*	0.24***
	Expectance	0.29***	0.19**	0.14
	Control	0.17*	0.13	0
Cognitive var	Cognitive rep	0.03	0.04	0.01
Behavioral var	Exploration	0.03	0.01	0.05
	Commitment	0	0.05	0.11
B				
Higher education				
Motivational var	Value	0.62***	0.36***	0.32**
	Expectance	0.34***	0.12	0.20**
	Control	0.56***	0.37***	0.23***
Cognitive var	Cognitive rep	0.16***	0.15*	0.07
Behavioral var	Exploration	0.33***	0.34***	0.11
	Commitment	0.34***	0.20**	0.15*
Marriage and family				
Motivational var	Value	0.32***	0.29***	0.12
	Expectance	0.14	0.14	0.02
	Control	0.34***	0.30***	0.18*
Cognitive var	Cognitive rep	0.02	0.03	0.08
Behavioral var	Exploration	0.03	0.06	0.13
	Commitment	0.12	0.14	0.08

*$p < 0.05$
**$p < 0.01$
***$p < 0.001$

Summary: Psychological Empowerment and Future Orientation

Like self-esteem, psychological empowerment emphasizes individuals' sense of self worth. However, while self-esteem describes global self beliefs, psychological empowerment pertains to individuals' ability to overcome social barriers by enlisting inner resources, be acquainted with the social system, and learn behavioral strategies for overcoming societal hurdles toward goal achievement.

Its relevance to future orientation was first suggested by Mahajna (2000) who conjectured that to maintain high hopes and overcome high fears about higher education Israeli Arab adolescent girls – who grow up in a cultural setting ambivalent about women's education and emancipation – must draw on inner resources that psychologists described as psychological empowerment. Secondary analysis of the hopes and fears narratives expressed by Israeli Arab rural girls identified psychological empowerment themes that corresponded to the three empowerment dimensions: intrapersonal, interactional, and behavioral.

The contextuality of psychological empowerment is reflected in the differential relations between its three dimensions and future orientation variables applied to instrumental (higher education, work and career) and relational (marriage and family) domains. For Arab girls as well as for Jewish girls and boys, empowerment is more strongly related to the instrumental than to the relational domains, and the behavioral dimension least related to future orientation. Thus, it is how adolescents appraise their self competence and what they know about their social environment rather than what needs to be done that prompts the motivational, cognitive, and behavioral components of future orientation. Finally, while first identified in the hopes and fears narratives of Israeli Arab girls, psychological empowerment is as relevant to the future orientation of Israeli Jewish girls and boys as it is to the future orientation of Arab girls.

Defensive Pessimism and Strategic Optimism

Defensive Pessimism

Defensive pessimism (Norem, 2008; Norem & Cantor, 1986a,b; Showers, 1992) is a *cognitive strategy* used in specific achievement-related situations by high achieving individuals whose strong desire for success is combined with high fear of failure (Cantor, Norem, Niedenthal, Langston, & Brower, 1987; Norem & Cantor, 1986a,b; Showers, 1992). To overcome their anxiety (Norem & Chang, 2002) and protect themselves against threats to self-esteem (Norem & Cantor, 1986a) or sense of self worth (Martin, Marsh, & Debus, 2001a,b, 2003) defensive pessimists lower their expectations for upcoming performances, and show rational planning of academic tasks (Eronen, Nurmi, & Salmela-Aro, 1998). Consequently they score as high on academic achievement as do strategic optimists (Eronen et al., 1998; Norem & Cantor, 1986a,b; Sanna, 1996), and over time their school engagement increases and depressive symptoms decrease (Maatta, Nurmi, & Stattin, 2007).

In other words, defensive pessimism serves as an *anticipatory strategy* employed by individuals in situations arousing both desire for success and fear of failure (e.g., final examination). Its activation entails two presumably contradictory processes, aimed at overcoming anxiety and maintaining high performance level: *setting one's expectations* at an unrealistically low level, and *mobilizing* the self by prompting the person "...*to think about and plan for the upcoming event*" (Showers & Ruben, 1990, p. 386, *italics added*).

Defensive pessimism and goal directed behavior. Especially pertinent to the relations between defensive pessimism and future orientation are findings showing that defensive pessimists prepare themselves for an upcoming performance by engaging in anticipatory thoughts about the task (Sanna, 1996) and in 'thinking through' processes which, according to researchers, *motivate* the construction of scenarios containing both positive and negative outcomes and the means for reaching and avoiding them, respectively (Norem & Illingworth, 1993).

Can "expecting the worst" and constructing negative outcome scenarios (or worst case scenarios, Cantor & Norem, 1989; Miceli & Castelfranchi, 2002) lead to positive goal directed behavior? According to Showers (1992), for defensive pessimists who go through the multiple step process described below the answer is *yes*. Guided by their tendency to strive for high achievement and be threatened by possible failure, defensive pessimists engage in a dual process by which they construct negative outcomes scenarios which they counteract by plans intended to thwart those ill effects, and thus curb anxiety, raise their self confidence, and consequently prompt behaviors intended to avoid failure and facilitate goal attainment. Moreover, their high need for success combined with high internal control lead defensive pessimists to "accurate planning and persistent effort" (Miceli & Castelfranchi, 2002, p. 349).

Testing her hypotheses in an experimental setting that emphasized negative possibilities for an upcoming task (negative-focus condition), Showers (1992) found that, without lowering their expectations, under these conditions defensive pessimists perform better than under conditions emphasizing positive possibilities (positive-focus condition), but nonetheless pay an emotional price: their task performance is followed by negative feelings. By carrying her experiment one step further, Showers could show that defensive pessimists participating in the negative-focus condition list more positive thoughts than do defensive pessimists who participate in the positive focus condition. Thus, information about negative consequences prompts positive thoughts that lead to preparation and planning and consequently to higher performance.

Strategic Optimism

As a personality strategy, optimism applies to setting high performance expectations and avoiding scenarios which entail negative outcomes. Whereas defensive pessimism is an *anticipatory* strategy, optimism is a *post-hoc* strategy. Like defensive pessimists, individuals employing optimistic strategies rely on their good past experience, but unlike defensive pessimists they use these positive experiences to set high expectations, and impending events arouse in them positive affect (Eronen et al., 1998) and a sense of being in control (Cantor, Norem, & Brower, 1987).

Relevant to the relation between optimism and future orientation is strategic optimists' tendency to protect their self-esteem retrospectively, after experiencing failure (Norem & Cantor, 1986a; Norem & Illingworth, 1993; Showers, 1992). In other words, while defensive pessimist are *prefactual* and prepare themselves before performing the task, optimists are *counterfactual*, and defend their self-worth by engaging in retrospective downward ("things could be worse") thinking (Sanna, 1996) only if unsuccessful. This may also explain why, when failure is perceived as one-time event, optimists respond with positive affect, but when expecting another similar failure-resulting task in the future, experience reduces positive affect (Sanna, 1996).

Strategies and Dispositions

Defensive pessimism and optimism as personality *strategies* differ from pessimism and optimism as personality *dispositions* in two ways (Norem & Cantor, 1990; Norem & Illingworth, 1993): dispositions – but not strategies – are associated with depressive tendencies, and strategies – but not dispositions – are domain specific, so that defensive pessimism and optimism concerning academic performance and social behavior are relatively independent of each other (Norem & Cantor, 1986a; Showers, 1988). In addition, empirical findings show that defensive pessimists employ more effective coping practices than do dispositional pessimists (Showers & Ruben, 1990) and score lower on anxiety, neuroticism, and fear of negative evaluation (Norem & Illingworth, 1993).

Future Orientation and Defensive Pessimism

Drawing on the conclusion that defensive pessimists and strategic optimists use different temporal patterns (Sanna, 1996) and on the conceptualization of defensive pessimism as an anxiety management strategy employing *prospective thinking*, Seginer (2000) examined the links between defensive pessimism and strategic optimism and future orientation.

Empirical testing of the relations between defensive pessimism, strategic optimism, and future orientation. The main objective of this study has been to investigate the defensive pessimism/optimism-future orientation links, as they apply to the three components of future orientation and two life domains. With this aim, two issues, leading to four predictions, were examined.

First, the *domain specificity* of the links between defensive pessimism and optimism and future orientation. Accordingly, the prediction was that *academic* defensive pessimism and optimism is associated with prospective education (future orientation higher education domain), and *social* defensive pessimism and optimism with prospective military service (future orientation military service domain). Note that military service has both an achievement oriented and social correlates. However, the significance attributed in the military to leadership, camaraderie, unit cohesion and morale (Gal, 1986) led to emphasizing the social functions of military service.

Second, links between defensive pessimism and strategic optimism and *the three components* of future orientation. The prediction that defensive pessimists will score higher on the motivational and the cognitive components drew on the assumption that defensive pessimists are more concerned about the future consequences of their behavior and hence on the nature of the motivational and cognitive components. Specific to the *motivational* component is that defensive pessimists employ this strategy for pursuing *important* (i.e., of high value) goals (Norem & Chang, 2002) and have a high sense of control over the materialization of domain-specific goals (Cantor & Norem, 1989; Norem & Cantor, 1990). However, the complexity of the defensive pessimism construct as combining high drive to success and protection against failure makes it difficult to predict whether or not defensive pessimism is related to expectance.

Findings showing that defensive pessimism is associated with greater production of negative and positive outcomes scenarios (Norem & Cantor, 1986b; Showers & Ruben, 1990) are pertinent to predictions regarding positive links between the *cognitive* component of future orientation and defensive pessimism. Findings showing that individuals who score high on *optimism* focus on the task rather than on its consequences (Cantor & Norem, 1989; Showers & Ruben, 1990) suggest that individuals who score high on strategic optimism will score higher on the *behavioral* component of future orientation, i.e., on exploration and commitment.

These considerations led to three predictions. First, *academic defensive pessimism* will be associated with the *motivational* and *cognitive* components of prospective *education* and *academic optimism* will be related to the *behavioral* variables of prospective *educational* future orientation but not of prospective military service. Second, *social* defensive pessimism will be linked to the *motivational* and *cognitive* variables of prospective *military service* future orientation, and *social optimism* will be linked to the *behavioral* variables of *military service* future orientation but not of prospective education. Third, given that strategic and dispositional pessimism (depression) may be confounded (Cantor & Norem, 1989; Nurmi, Toivonen, Salmela-Aro, & Eronen, 1996; Showers, 1988, 1992; Showers & Ruben, 1990) and that strategic defensive pessimism mobilizes the self to overcome anxiety, by controlling for depressive tendencies (indexed by self criticism) and self efficacy (Blatt, D'Afflitti, & Quinlan, 1976; Blatt, Hart, Quinlan, Leadbeater, & Auerbach, 1993) the effects of both the defensive pessimism and optimism strategies on future orientation will become smaller.

Findings. These hypotheses were tested on data collected from 103 Israeli Jewish students of high academic standing who responded to the future orientation questionnaires battery (see Appendix) and the defensive pessimism questionnaire (DPQ; Norem & Cantor, 1986a) applied to the academic and social situations.

Although the hypotheses were only partly confirmed, findings of this study shed important light on the nature of future orientation and defensive pessimism and on the relations between them.

Specifically, findings show that strategic optimism affects the behavioral variables, but contrary to hypotheses, defensive pessimism does not affect the cognitive component, and strategic optimism – but not defensive pessimism – affects the motivational variables, and particularly the *value* of each domain. Moreover, social optimism affects the behavioral variables pertaining to both higher education and military service, thus refuting the hypothesis that the effect of these personality strategies is domain specific.

The relations between defensive pessimism, strategic optimism, and future orientation: conclusions. Though rejecting two of the three hypotheses derived from the conceptual analysis of the relations between defensive pessimism and strategic optimism (respectively) and future orientation, this study suggests three important conclusions. First, while self esteem, self agency, and loneliness are associated with the *motivational* aspects of future orientation, optimism is associated mainly and consistently with its *behavioral* aspects. Second, although both constructs – i.e., the personality strategies and future orientation – are domain-specific, the relations between them are not. Third, the relation between strategic optimism and future orientation fits with findings pertaining to other self constructs correlates of future orientation and planning orientation research (Eronen et al., 1998). Together, these findings show that future orientation is associated with psychological well being, of which strategic optimism is one indicator.

Overall, this analysis hones the difference between future orientation and defensive pessimism as two modes of future oriented thinking. Defensive pessimism serves mainly as *protection against possible negative outcomes*, and future orientation as a *basis for setting and pursuing prospective goals*. Consequently, future orientation facilitates adolescents' development in general as well as their responses to both social change (Seginer & Halabi-Kheir, 1998) and personal change (Seginer & Schlesinger, 1998). However, given that defensive pessimists are committed to fulfilling their expectations by 'doing what they ought to do' (Miceli & Castelfranchi, 2002), their chances of materializing their hopes, plans and goals are higher but incur emotional costs.

Primary and Secondary Control Orientations

Primary and Secondary Control: Conceptual Framework

Control is a behavior-outcomes contingency construct. When individuals gain desirable outcomes and avoid undesirable outcomes by deliberately altering existing conditions they hold control over the outcomes of their behavior. When they *believe* they have these capabilities, their condition is described as perceived control. Although some research has shown the negative consequences of perceived control, mainly resulting from a mismatch between environmental affordance and individuals' control capabilities (Evans, Shapiro, & Lewis, 1993), much of psychological research has indicated the beneficial effects of control behavior and control beliefs on phenomena ranging from academic achievement to physical health and psychological well-being, across the life-span.

Until the work of Rothbaum and Weisz (Rothbaum, Weisz, & Snyder, 1982; Weisz, Rothbaum, & Blackburn, 1984) the basic premise had been that the person is the *agent* of control and the environment – physical and social – its *target*. Drawing on the crucial role being in control serves for humans and their rather limited opportunities to adjust the environment to their needs, Rothbaum et al. (1982) sought to expand the meaning of control by describing it in terms of two rather than one process. The initial conceptualization of control as consisting of individuals' ability to intentionally alter the environment to their benefit has been entitled *primary control*. The second process pertaining to individuals' inclination to intentionally fit in with existing circumstances has been labeled *secondary control*.

The epistemic value of the secondary control construct has been attested by numerous studies and various psychological research areas. Nonetheless, its conceptualization varies, and some of it recently disputed (Skinner, 2007). One major approach (Heckhausen & Schulz, 1995) interprets secondary control as maintaining individuals' sense of control by attempting to affect the self (rather than the environment). Another conceptualization (Morling & Evered, 2006, 2007) has been prompted by revisiting Rothbaum et al. (1982) conceptualization of secondary control and questioning its coherence on grounds that it oscillates between motives: to control and to fit in with existing circumstances. To resolve it, Morling and Evered suggested that "people exert secondary control when they adjust some aspect of the self and accept circumstances as they are" (Morling & Evered, 2006, p. 272).

Our approach contends that while common to primary and secondary control is the effect individuals impress toward achieving their goals, the targets and ensuing strategies differ. In primary control the target of change is the environment and the strategy is behavioral. In secondary control the target is the self and the strategy is cognitive and involves adjustment of goals and beliefs about the self, others, and self-others relationships. In other words, the ultimate goal of person-environment fit can be achieved by having an effect on the environment (primary control) or – as also suggested by Heckhausen and Schulz and Morling and Evered –on the self (secondary control).

Although new to psychology, secondary control is as old as the Old Testament and Jewish *Mishna (Ethics of the fathers,* concluded at the end of the second century):

> He that is slow to anger is better than the mighty; and he that ruleth his spirit [is better] than he that taketh a city (Proverbs, 16, 32).
> Who is rich? He who rejoices in his portion. Who is mighty? He who subdues his passions (Ben Zoma, Ethics of the fathers).

The primacy of primary control. A basic premise of much of current research concerns the primacy of primary control, contending that the ultimate goal of human behavior to exert control over the environment is universal and shared by all people regardless of age, culture or any other contextual factor, even when temporarily – for reasons related to one or more of the contextual factors mentioned above – they find themselves in a situation that calls for the employment of secondary control strategies (Heckhausen, 1999; Heckhausen & Schulz, 1995, 1999; Rothbaum et al., 1982).

In fact, as they describe individuals' tendency to enhance personal gains by influencing existing realities as *primary* control and by accommodating to existing conditions as *secondary* control Rothbaum (Rothbaum et al., 1982) and Weisz (Weisz et al., 1984) concur with the primacy of primary control. Agriculture, the hierarchical structure of societies, and warfare are three historical and universal examples of primary control behaviors employed in all cultures at all times.

Therefore, at issue is not the universal use of primary control but rather the latitude of secondary control employment; that is, how accessible and commendable secondary control is in different cultural settings and interpersonal situations. Overall, without tuning to reality – physical and social – humans may fail to notice the conditions necessary for gaining primary control. Thus, the importance of subgoals served by secondary control orientation may not be less than that of the ultimate primary control goal.

Cultural Contexts

The cross cultural relevance of the primary and secondary control construct has been introduced in the seminal work of Weisz et al. (1984). While the "flow with the stream" as an indicator of secondary control (rather than of relinquished control) has been suggested in the original Rothbaum et al. (1982) analysis, Weisz et al. (1984) found it particularly relevant for control orientations of Japanese, and regarded it as an instance of the *value mediation hypothesis.* This hypothesis posits that whereas the individualistic activist, self-centered approach of western thinking encourages primary control, the collectivistic or interdependent orientation of non-western cultures prompts secondary control.

Much of the empirical research that examined these propositions compared Japanese and western societies such as Canada, the United States, Germany (Friedlmeier & Trommsdorff, 1998; Seginer, Trommsdorff, & Essau, 1993; Trommsdorff & Friedlmeier, 1993), and Switzerland (Nakamura & Flammer, 1998), and to a lesser extent Asian and White Americans (Lam & Zane, 2004), and Israeli Druzes and Jews (Halabi-Kheir, 1992; Seginer, 1995; Seginer et al., 1993). However, their results only partly support the *value mediation* hypothesis. Particularly, Malaysians score higher than Germans and Israeli Druzes score higher than Israeli Jews on both primary and secondary control (Seginer, 1998b; Seginer et al., 1993).

An alternative interpretation. Limiting their analyses to adolescents, Seginer et al. interpreted their findings as supporting the *multiple transitions hypothesis.* For Malaysian and Druze adolescents multiple transitions pertain to cultural and development transitions. Drawing on Rothbaum et al. (1982), the hypothesis posits that the demands created by their co-occurrence lead transition to modernity adolescents to endorse both primary and secondary control beliefs. Thus, while the value mediation interpretation may explain the basic tendency of westerners to endorse more strongly primary control orientations and non-westerners to endorse more strongly secondary control orientations, the multiple transition hypothesis addresses circumstances in which individuals expand their control beliefs repertoire to deal with both self needs and community demands.

However, their tendency to score higher than western adolescents on primary control may have yet another explanation. It draws on Heckhausen and colleagues' (Wrosch, Heckhausen, & Lachman, 2000) interpretation of older people's tendency to score higher than younger adults on primary control. Thus, the relatively high primary control orientation of Druze and Malaysian adolescents – like that of the older people in Wrosch et al.'s study – may reflect a need rather than reality. Older adults score relatively high on primary control to compensate for their dwindling objective control, and Druze and Malaysian adolescents score high on primary control to compensate for deference to family and community authority.

The interface between culture and interpersonal primary-secondary control domains. Another study (Seginer, 1998b) focused on domain specific aspects of primary and secondary control orientations applying to three interpersonal relationships: with parents, friends, and teachers. Its findings show that cross cultural differences are in fact domain specific. Thus, although relative to Jewish adolescents Druze adolescents score higher on secondary control for all three domains, they are equally high on primary control pertaining to the two adult interpersonal domains: parents and teachers. The exception is the peer relationships domain. All adolescents understand peer relationship as demanding less primary control than relationships with parents and teachers, but Druze adolescents score significantly lower than Jewish adolescents.

Obviously, the stability of these findings needs additional support and should be tested on other groups of western and non-western adolescents. However, it does support the distinction between global and domain specific aspects of control orientations, particularly emphasized by self researchers (e.g., Harter, 1999; Marsh, 1986; Rosenberg, 1979). Recently, the relationship-specific scale has been used to study Asian and White American college students. Assessing their independent and interdependent self construals and using a global rather than the three domain specific control orientations, Lam and Zane (2004) showed that the independent self construal mediated the ethnicity-primary control link and the interdependent self construal mediated the ethnicity-secondary control link. This finding may reflect the personality dynamics of Asian and white Americans or the specific attributes of the global scale and need to be further tested.

Developmental periods, and adolescence in particular, as context. Adolescents–and in recent generations also emerging adults – have been assigned the developmental task of preparing for independent adult life. This task cannot be performed without a sense of agency that leads adolescents to strive for autonomy and perceive themselves as harnessing the environment to serve their needs. As many American children have been told:

> You have brains in your head.
> You have feet in your shoes.
> You can steer yourself
> any direction you choose. (Dr. Seuss, 1990)

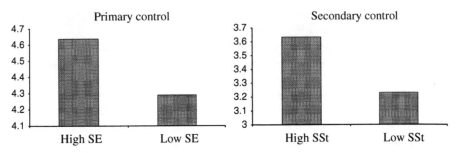

Fig. 3.6 Primary and secondary control scores for high and low Self-Esteem (SE) and Self-Stability (SSt)

This view has led researchers (Heckhausen, 1999; Trommsdorff, 1994) to suggest that adolescence is a time when primary control is high and secondary control low. A study conducted in Israel (Guter, 1995) has shown this empirically. Emerging adults (ranging in age from 19 to 21 and serving in the military) described themselves as more primary than secondary control oriented. However, individual differences have been related to self esteem and self stability: primary control is positively related to self-esteem and secondary control is negatively related to self stability (Fig. 3.6). In other words, to gain primary control individuals enlist their sense of self competence, deemed necessary for controlling the environment. To practice secondary control, on the other hand, the necessary personal quality is flexibility without which individuals are unable to accommodate themselves to environmental demands.

Primary and Secondary Control and Future Orientation

The relation between primary and secondary control and future orientation has been first indicated by Trommsdorff (1994) who pointed to the function both serve in reducing uncertainties and regulating behavior. These functions are especially relevant for three adolescents' and emerging adults' universal developmental tasks: education, work and career, and marriage and family. Their pursuit shares a common goal of changing the environment to serve such essential personal needs as status, income and relatedness.

However, the motivation prompting and the behaviors ensuing from the hopes, goals and plans related to each of these developmental domains also demand accommodation of the self to the requirements, rules, and values set by society. These considerations lead to three predictions: that future orientation is related to primary control, to secondary control, and to what Weisz et al. (1984) considered as the balance between them. However, granting the relevance of contextual factors, the effect of primary and secondary control on each future orientation domain has been examined in the context of culture and gender.

The nature of prospective life domains. The differential relations between primary and secondary control and the various future life domains draw on the nature of control orientations as pertaining to the person-environment interface and the multidimensionality of the environment, past, present, and future. As noted earlier, prospective life domains – describing individuals' projections of the self in various social roles – have been described in terms of two dimensions: their main *theme* as either instrumental (e.g., higher education, work and career) or relational (marriage and family, interpersonal relationships) and their distance from the present as near or distant (Seginer & Lilach, 2004).

Earlier work on the relations between control orientations and future orientation drew on this two-dimensional characteristic of the future orientation domains and predicted that, particularly during adolescence, instrumental domains will be affected by primary control more than by secondary control, and relational domains – where accommodating to others' needs is essential – will be affected more by secondary than by primary control (the *thematic* hypothesis). The second prediction posited that the effect of control orientations will be stronger for near than for distant life domains (the *distance* hypothesis).

Showing that primary control is positively associated with the *higher education* and *collective issues* domains, analyses of two samples of Israeli Druze and Jewish adolescents (Halabi-Kheir, 1992) supported the *distance* hypothesis but only partly supported the *thematic* hypothesis. Thus, the more individuals view themselves as able to master the environment and overcome obstacles set by it, the more salient higher education is for them. The relevance of *mastery* is further supported by the negative relation found between higher education and secondary control, meaning that not only is the salience of higher education positively related to a sense of harnessing the environment to fit one's needs but it is negatively related to any adjustment of the individual to fit to the environment's demands. The positive relation found between primary control and *collective issues* (relational domain) should be understood in light of the Israeli reality of Israeli-Arab political tension that brings to the fore sense of mastery rather than of accommodation.

Analysis of a third Israeli sample (Guter, 1995) showing stronger effect of primary control orientation on instrumental than on relational domains further supports the thematic hypothesis. The effect of secondary control is lower than the effect of primary control, and in most instances non significant. Thus, altogether our findings show that granting high value to future developmental tasks, having confidence that future hopes, goals and plans will be materialized (the motivational component of future orientation), thinking about the future (the cognitive representation component) and engaging in future oriented exploration of future options and decision making (the behavioral component) are all related to a sense of mastery of the environment rather than to an obligation (or at least an understanding of the need) to accommodate it.

Relating these findings to Trommsdorff's (1994) proposition that underlying the relation between control orientations and future orientation are functions of uncertainty reduction and self regulation, common to both orientations, our findings raise two additional considerations. The first indicates that, for adolescents, future thinking is understood as facilitating uncertainty reduction mostly by means of primary control orientation. Moreover, the finding indicating that primary control is mainly related to the instrumental and not to the relational domains suggests that adolescents understand the accommodating nature of relational domains but given their preference for primary control orientations are either reluctant or hesitant to think about them in terms of secondary control orientations. The second consideration pertains to cultural and gender factors and is discussed below.

Culture and gender effects. Israeli data also show that overall primary and secondary control orientations are more relevant to the future orientation of Druze than of Jewish adolescents. For Druze boys, prospective *work and career* is understood in terms of secondary rather than primary control, *military service* is negatively related to primary control, *but self concern* is related to both primary and secondary control orientations.

The overall picture for Druze boys is that they construe their future as requiring accommodation of self to the environment, and particularly to the values, norms and expectations of their family and community elders. For Druze girls the picture is more similar to that of Jewish girls and boys: *higher education* future orientation is associated with primary control and the *collective issues* domain is negatively associated with secondary control. However, relationships with *others* is negatively associated with primary control and positively associated with secondary control. Thus, the thematic hypothesis regarding the relation between primary and secondary control and the relational domains is supported only for Druze girls.

Primary and secondary control and future orientation: summary. Empirical analyses of the relation between primary and secondary control and future orientation show that whether future orientation is related to primary or to secondary control depends on the nature of the future orientation domain as well as on the interface between culture and gender. Israeli girls and boys of different cultural-political backgrounds consider the fulfillment of hopes, goals and plans in the *higher education* and *collective issues* domains as requiring that individuals affect the environment rather than accommodate to it. The one group more influenced by secondary control is Druze boys. Why this tendency is more prevalent among them than among Druze girls can only be conjectured.

Two reasons need to be considered here. One is that Druze boys may regard themselves as bearers of the Druze religion (whose principles can be learned only by men) which – as all other religions – emphasizes deference to God and to the community and its elders. The second is that Druze girls, like Arab girls (Seginer, 1988a,b, 2005; Seginer & Halabi-Kheir, 1998) understand the value of education and the action they have to take to fulfill hopes, goals and plans regarding higher education (Seginer & Mahajna, 2004). However, as suggested by Heckhausen and her colleagues (Wrosch et al., 2000), their endorsement of primary control may reflect a need rather than a reality.

Cognitive Abilities and Future Orientation

The relations between cognitive abilities and future orientation have been examined in only a few studies. First among them has been Greene's (1986) attempt to examine the effect of cognitive abilities on future orientation. Underlying her study has been the premise that, given the hypothetical nature of future thinking, it will be related to abstract thinking which according to Inhelder and Piaget (1958) develops during adolescence. However, Greene's findings show that among adolescents, future self-representations are unrelated to abstract thinking. Instead, they are related to age, representing adolescents' experiences and exposure to others.

Two explanations of these findings might have been the specificity of the ability measure and adolescents' cultural background, and the non-linearity of the effect of cognitive abilities on future orientation. That is, whereas by the time they reach adolescence individuals have all mastered the level of abstract thinking necessary for future self-projection, this may not be the case for younger children.

The first explanation has been tested by Nurmi and Pulliainen (1991) on a sample of Finnish adolescents (11 and 15 years old) showing that for this sample intelligence (assessed by figure analogy task) *is* positively related to the cognitive representation of the future pertaining to education. The second explanation has been tested by Gelberg (1996). He assessed the effect of school ability in reading and arithmetic on representation of the future self among 2nd, 4th and 6th graders and found only moderate correlations (ranging from r = 0.20 to 0.35, p < 0.001) between cognitive abilities and representation of future self. Thus, Gelberg's findings partly support Greene's findings for younger children in a different cultural setting (Israel) and the employment of a different cognitive ability measure. The independence of future orientation from cognitive abilities is underscored by the finding that among 2nd graders the relation between cognitive abilities and representation of the future is higher than among 4th and 6th grades.

Summary: The Effect of Self and Personality on Future Orientation

Research reviewed in this chapter indicates that future orientation is prompted by psychological well-being indicated by self-esteem, self-agency, a sense of social embeddedness, optimism, psychological empowerment, and primary control rather than by the need to compensate oneself for feeling lonely (loneliness), protect oneself against anticipated failure (defensive pessimism), and secondary control. In line with a recent study showing that in normal participants depression is related more to past than to future thinking (Eysenck & Payne, 2006), depression does not affect the relations between loneliness and defensive pessimism (respectively) and future orientation. Nonetheless, not all domains and all components are equally affected by psychological well-being. Thus, loneliness is associated with the relational (and particularly *interpersonal relationships*) but not with the instrumental domains, primary control is related to instrumental domains and particularly *higher education*, and secondary control to relational domains and particularly the *others* domain (pertaining to family, friends, and peers).

While analyses focusing on domain density (the thematic approach) indicated domain specificity, analyses focusing on the three components approach to future orientation show that regardless of the thematic focus of the domain psychological well-being indicators directly affect the motivational component and via it the cognitive representation and behavioral components, thus underscoring the pivotal role of the motivational aspects of future orientation (e.g., Nuttin & Lens, 1985; Nurmi, 1991; Raynor & Entin, 1983; Trommsdorff, 1983). In a similar vein, cultural differences are found for the thematic approach studies but not for the three-component model where the direct effect on the motivational component is found for Jewish and Arab adolescents. This issue is further discussed in Chap. 8.

Chapter 4
Future Orientation Sex Differences

As controversial as the topic of sex differences has been, researchers tend to agree that it involves more political considerations than do most other topics of psychological research (Bem, 1993; Eagly, 1995; Hyde, 1996; Scarr, 1988). For contemporary researchers, at issue are three fundamental questions: how prevalent sex differences are, which attributes are consistently susceptible to gender differences, and how dependent are they on biological, social and cultural factors and the interaction among them (Sternberg, 1993). Drawing on psychobiological research on sex hormones effects of the hormone prenatal environment (Hines, 2004) and the human body (Hampton & Moffat, 2004) and developmental studies on sex differences identified as early as infancy (McClure, 2000) and reinforced by adults (Bem, 1993) so that even sex-neutral adult roles are gender specific, it is plausible that girls and boys construct their future orientation differently. To examine these issues the present chapter opens with review of pertinent approaches to sex differences and continues with review of research on future orientation sex differences.

Sex Differences: Their Extent, Origins and Underlying Processes

The obvious physical and biological differences between girls and boys, women and men and early interest in individual differences led psychologists to assess sex differences (e.g., Anastasi, 1958) even before the distinction between "sex" as the biological aspect and "gender" as the social aspect of describing females and males was employed, and a theoretical framework for predicting such differences was formed. The impetus for the systematic study of sex and sex differences has been the work of Maccoby and Jacklin (1974) in which they summarized data accumulated over the years on sex differences.

While their analysis indicates women and men differ only in some aspects of cognitive abilities and aggression, subsequent studies are divided in their conclusions. At one end stands research prompted by evolutionary psychology and social role theory. This research indicates sex differences in areas linked to different ancestral adaptive mechanisms of males and females (evolutionary psychology) (Buss, 1994, 1995b) and to the different role occupancy and sex-typed expectations set for

R. Seginer, *Future Orientation*, The Springer Series on Human Exceptionality,   91
DOI 10.1007/978-0-387-88641-1_4, © Springer Science+Business Media, LLC 2009

women and men (social role theory) (Eagly, 1987; Eagly & Mitchell, 2004; Eagly & Wood, 1999). At the other extreme are feminist theorists (Bem, 1993; Hyde & Plant, 1995; Hyde, 2005) who, like the social role theorists, explain sex differences as the result of social and cultural mechanisms, but based on meta-analyses (Hyde, 2005) show that in fact they are few and tend to be small. The theoretical underpinnings of each of these approaches and their major findings are presented below.

Evolutionary Psychology

The evolutionary psychology approach draws on psychological interpretations of modern Darwinism (Cronin, 1991). Buss described it as focusing on "... the analysis of the human mind as a collection of evolved mechanisms, the contexts that activate those mechanisms, and the behavior generated by those mechanisms." (Buss, 2004, p. 50). What identifies a psychological mechanism as "evolutionary" is that throughout evolutionary history it has proven itself as a successful solution of a specific adaptation problem.

Sexual selection. Central to the issue of sex differences is the mechanism of sexual selection that explains sex linked behaviors among animals and humans. Applied to humans (Trivers, 1972), the basic assumption has been that, concerned with future generations, both women and men search for mating partners that will maximize fitness of their offspring, and consequently compete for access to the best mate. However, because women and men differ considerably in parental investment, the interests underlying their sexual selection and same-sex competition and the behaviors ensuing from it are guided by different considerations. Women search for a mate with good genes, resources, and parental skills and males search for women who are young (fertile) and – because of paternity uncertainty – promise sexual fidelity (Buss, 1995a, b). Meta-analysis of mate selection strategies differentially used by women and men (Feingold, 1992) confirmed Trivers' model: women more than men value socioeconomic status, ambition, character, and intelligence but not in characteristics unrelated to offspring survival such as sense of humor.

Evolutionary psychology main proposition is that to maintain sexual selection ancestral women and men were required to develop different evolutionary adaptive solutions which underlie human sex differences since. These are reflected in a wide variety of human functioning ranging from cognitive to physical abilities and interpersonal relationships. Reviewing this research, Buss (1994, 1995a, 2004) and Archer (1996) listed several sex-linked abilities, values and practices. Specifically, in the cognitive domain females have an advantage over men in spatial location memory which was essential for ancestral women's food gathering (Silverman & Eals, 1992) whereas men have an advantage over women in spatial rotation essential for hunting. Women value economic and intellectual resources more than men and men exert greater sexual control, express greater sexual jealousy, and behave more aggressively toward other men (intermale aggression) (Daly & Wilson, 1994).

Does mate selection vary by culture? To demonstrate the universality of sex differences as they are guided by the principle of sexual selection, Buss and colleagues

(Buss et al., 1990) analyzed data collected from over 9,000 adults residing in 37 societies. These societies are distributed across six continents and five islands and vary on criteria of economic development, political systems, and mating value orientations (i.e., polygyny vs monogamy, cohabiting without marriage).

Their findings showed that cross cultural differences notwithstanding, overall women more than men preferred mates that can provide financial support, possess high social status, ambition and industriousness and are of older age. However, women and men share high preferences for mates of good health and attractive physical appearance (as an indicator of good health), dependability and stability, and love and commitment. Men more than women value physical appearance, chastity (Buss & Schmitt, 1993), and young age, though age difference varies from 1 to 2 years among monogamous cultures to 6 to 7 years among polygamous cultures. where only as men grow older do they accumulate enough resources to attract multiple wives (Buss, 2004).

A recent reanalysis (Eagly & Wood, 1999) of Buss et al. data examined cultural differences with the particular purpose of showing that sex differences co-varied with the extent to which cultures endorse gender equality values. Gender equality values have been assessed by two aggregate measures: *gender empowerment measure* and *gender-related development index* (United Nations Development Program, 1995). The first measures participation of women relative to men in economic, political and decision-making roles. The second gauges women's access to resources that provide them with good health, wealth, education and literacy (*plus* points) and sex inequality on each of these capabilities (*minus* points).

Not surprisingly, these analyses show that some differences are more strongly affected by cultural values of gender equality than others. To illustrate, men's preference for mate's provision of domestic services (good housekeeper and cook) and women's preference for their mate's earning capacity decrease as gender equality increases. In a similar vein, as gender equality increases, both women's and men's preference for mate's age difference (i.e., older men for women and younger women for men) decreases. However, preference for physical attractiveness shows a more complex picture. Physical attractiveness varies with gender equality for women (who as gender equality increases value it less) but less for men (who regardless of gender equality values prefer a good looking mate) and only when absolute scores rather than the relative rank of each society (calculated only by Eagly & Wood) is considered.

Social Role Theory

The social role theory of sex differences was developed by Eagly (1987, 1995) to explain the evolvement of gender roles. While evolutionary psychology attributes the origin of differences between women and men to sexual selection, social role theory attributes them to the position of women and men in the *social structure* created by their distribution into different activities such as domestic activities for women and paid jobs for men (Eagly & Wood, 1999).

The social basis of gender role allocation. Differential role allocation gives greater power and status to men (gender hierarchy) than to women and results in two processes that contribute to the perpetuation of differences between women and men: the development of dominant behavior in men and subordinate behavior in women, and the acquisition of specific skills, beliefs and resources necessary for successfully performing these roles. Thus, although initially the distribution of women and men into different tasks and social roles may have been determined by biological factors such as women's childbearing and men's physical strength, their persistence in post industrial societies is more adequately explained by social than by biological considerations, and specifically by propositions drawing on gender role theory (Eagly & Wood, 1999).

Gender role theory. Like other role theories, gender role theory focuses on social expectations. These expectations are formed and prescribed by society and communicated to its members in the context of social interactions (Deaux & Major, 1987, 2004) anticipating that they engage in role appropriate activities. Nevertheless, gender roles differ from other social roles in several ways: they are consensual, expectations linked to them apply to much of individuals' daily life and hence they have greater scope, and they pertain to general personality attributes rather than to mere specific behaviors (Eagly, 1987). As a category, gender is more salient than other role defining dimensions (Deaux & Major, 1987) and considered socially appropriate (Eagly, 1987). Consequently, gender-related expectations affect the definition of other roles. Their power is especially significant in the world of *work and career* where:

> Interacting with a concrete other evokes primary cultural rules for making sense of self and others pushing actors to sex categorize one another in each of these situations. Sex categorization pumps gender into interactionally mediated work process by cueing gender stereotypes, including status beliefs, and by biasing the choice of comparison others. (Ridgeway, 1997, p. 231).

Gender linked personality characteristics and behavioral tendencies. The gender-linked personality characteristics and behaviors ensuing from them can be subsumed under two overarching categories: communion and agency (Bakan, 1966). In the context of gender roles, communion pertains to caring and nurturant behaviors as well as interpersonal sensitivity, and agency to such attributes as self-assertion, independence, and direct and adventurous personal style (Eagly, 1987).

Behavior consistent with gender role expectations, like behavior emanating from other social roles, is prompted both by social pressure and by intrinsic motivation. Consistent with role theory of sex differences, meta-analyses conducted by Eagly and her associates show that women are less involved than men in aggression intended to inflict physical pain and injury (Eagly & Steffen, 1984), receive more help but give less help than men (Eagly & Crowley, 1986), and in leadership roles tend to adopt more democratic and less autocratic style than do men (Eagly & Johnson, 1990).

Gender role conflict. In times of social change, when social expectations are eased and women may enter social, political and occupational roles that traditionally have been considered suitable for men, threat to gender equality continues. Slow to change societal expectations may lead to a role conflict (Eagly, Karau, & Makhijani, 1995) and internalized sex role expectations (even slower to change) may lead to an inner struggle and together deter women from seizing up the opportunity.

The Gender Similarity Approach

Employing narrative analysis (Bem, 1993) as well as quantitative meta-analyses, the gender similarities approach (Hyde & Plant, 1995; Hyde, 2005) contends that differences between women and men are few and overall small. Particularly telling is Hyde's (2005) review of 46 studies that examines sex differences by means of meta-analyses. Of the 124 effect sizes reported by those studies, 78% are small or close to zero.

The 22% showing medium and large effect sizes indicate that men score higher than women on several motor performance behaviors, masturbation, positive attitudes toward casual sex, physical aggression, and some aspects of spatial perception, and women score higher than men on smiling and agreeableness (as one of the Big Five personality measures). Of special relevance to this chapter are meta-analysis findings on the moderating effect of age on self esteem gender differences. These differences grow larger from childhood to early and middle adolescence but decline in adulthood.

Socialization of Gender Roles

Initially, research on gender role socialization – as socialization pertaining to other roles, skills, and beliefs – assumed that parents' gender-related expectations, or as Bem described it ". . .their gender-stereotyped preconceptions of what girls and boys are supposed to be like" (Bem, 1993, p. 134) are the basis for socialization of gender roles (Jacklin & Reynolds, 1993). However, at present researchers draw on both unidirectional (in which parents are the agents and children are the target of socialization) and bidirectional models (consisting of both parent and child characteristics) and focus on factors that affect the *construction* of parents' differential gender role behavior and factors that affect the *effectiveness* of gender roles socialization (Pomerantz, Fei-Yin Ng, & Wang, 2004).

Mother-child interaction as a gender role socialization context. An early analysis of the gender role socialization considering both mother and child characteristics has been Chodorow's (1978) analysis that focused on the gender specific mother-child interaction in infancy and early childhood. Drawing her analysis on object relations theory, Chodrow contended that Western society social arrangements, by which women are the sole caregiver of young children, lead to sex differences in mother-child relationships. Girls' identity develops in response to similarity and attachment to their mother whereas boys' identity develops in the context of differences which generate sense of separateness and independence.

These differential relationships lead to *gendered personalities* that result in women's need to have children and men's desire to participate in alienated work structures produced by advanced capitalism, and consequently reproduce social structure. Thus, Chodrow's analysis and her emphasis on the Western industrial context of mothers' exclusive responsibility for childcare complement Eagly's (1987) analysis of gender role as emanating from and reproducing Western social structure.

The peer group as a gender role socialization context. In contrast to Chodrow's emphasis on the relevance of mothers to gender role socialization, Maccoby (1990) contended that peers rather than mothers are responsible for gender role socialization. According to her view, mothers respond to children's needs and characteristics rather than to their gender whereas the peer group anticipates gender specific behavior. In support of her thesis, Maccoby reported findings showing that children prefer interaction with a same-sex partner or group. These same-sex groups act as "powerful socialization environments" (Maccoby, 1990, p.516) for forging gendered behavior that both girls and boys employ as they move to cross-sex interactions during adolescence. Their preference for interacting with same-gender individuals preserves gender-specific interaction style and continues into adolescence and adulthood.

A study (Suh, Moskowitz, Fournier, & Zuroff, 2004) of the interaction styles between same- and opposite sex friends and romantic couples supports this proposition for adults. In their interaction with same-sex friends, women are more agreeable and men are more dominant. However, although scoring higher than men on trait communion, women are less agreeable with opposite-sex friends and romantic partners, and both sexes are less submissive with same-sex than with opposite sex friends or romantic partners. Thus, in the context of opposite-sex friendship and romantic relationship, the gender-role interaction style of women is not preserved, refuting also the relevance of the gender hierarchy proposition.

Summary. Although research on sex differences is not unequivocal and its data-based conclusions depend on the theoretical approach underlying it, it may be summarized by the following three points. First, gender similarities may be more prevalent than sex differences. Second, although women and men differ in their trait scores so that women score higher on communion traits and men on agency, contextual factors – ranging from the dyad or group sex composition to economic opportunities and cultural orientations – increase or decrease these differences. Third, sex differences identified in young children are explained by inherent biological characteristics and socialization processes taking place in the family and the peer group.

Future Orientation Sex Differences and Gender Similarities

Prediction of future orientation sex differences depends on two considerations: the *theoretical approach* researchers use for developing their predictions and the *future orientation dimensions* they choose to study.

Theory Based Predictions

Of the three approaches discussed in this chapter, the feminist approach predicts no sex differences and the evolutionary psychology and gender role theories predict that women and men construct their future orientation differently. These predictions are detailed below.

Evolutionary psychology. This prediction is based on the *mate selection preferences* proposition that women's preferences are for men who can offer them the security of professional skills, stable job and high status, and men's preferences are for women committed to family obligations and domestic responsibilities. Attuned to these cross-sex preferences, in constructing their future orientation adolescent girls will invest more in the construction of *relational* domains like marriage and family, and adolescent boys in the construction of *instrumental* domains such as work and career.

Gender role theories. Although generated from different theoretical premises, the predictions of the social structural approach do not vary from those of evolutionary psychology. Both approaches predict sex differences and both underscore male dominance and gender hierarchy. However, the gender role theory approach attributes sex differences to structural processes by which the different distribution of roles among males and females gives greater power and status to men than to women which thus lead to *gender* differences. Consequently, two processes emerge and contribute to the perpetuation of differences between women and men: the development of dominant behavior in men and subordinate behavior in women, and the acquisition of specific skills, beliefs and resources necessary for successfully performing these roles.

Given that even in the postindustrial society – where the importance of physical strength for men and domesticity for women is less pronounced – differential gender role expectations continue to be consensual, a prediction drawing on this approach posits that women construct their future orientation by investing more in the relational prospective domains and men by investing in the instrumental prospective domains.

The feminist approach. Drawing on the feminist approach that women and men differ on only few characteristics (Hyde, 2005; Bem, 1993) the prediction is that girls and boys (or women and men) will construct similar rather than different future orientation. This will be reflected in all aspects of future orientation, particularly in the density of future orientation domains, extension into the future, and scores on the motivational, cognitive representation, and behavioral components as they apply to various future orientation domains.

Three questions on future orientation sex differences. In sum, the application of evolutionary psychology, gender role theory, and feminists' similarity hypothesis to future orientation generates three basic questions. The first is whether the future orientation constructions of women and men, and particularly of adolescent girls and boys, differ? Assuming sex differences exist, the next two questions are whether girls invest more in relational domains such as marriage and family and interpersonal relationships, and whether boys invest more in instrumental domains like

higher education, work and career, and military service (where it applies)? The rest
of this chapter examines these issues by reviewing pertinent empirical data reported
in recent years.

Gender Effects on the Themes and Extension
of Future Orientation

As indicated by the title of this section and substantiated by findings presented in
Table 4.1, the answer to the question whether girls and boys construct different or
similar future orientations is not "Yes" or "No", but rather "It varies and depends on
contextual factors" (for a similar conclusion, see also Greene & DeBacker, 2004).
The overall picture is that sex differences are primarily a function of time and place,
the latter signifying such categorical dimensions as ethnicity, social class, rural vs
urban residence, minority vs. majority, and immigrant status.

Future orientation sex differences: a recent history perspective. The first big
studies on future orientation sex differences were conducted during the 1950s, as
societies in different parts of the world were emerging from the aftermath of World
War II and not long before the women's lib movement in the United States were
formed. The studies of Douvan and Adelson (1966) in the United States, of Mönks
(1968) in the Netherlands, and of Trommsdorff and her colleagues in Germany (e.g.,
Trommsdorff, Lamm, & Schmidt, 1979) describe how girls and boys viewed their
future in that era. The extensive work of Douvan and Adelson will be described in
more detail followed by the work of Mönks and Trommsdorff and her associates,
referred to in several parts of this book.

The Douvan and Adelson (1966) study. The relevance of historical context to
future orientation is exemplified by Douvan and Adelson's (1966) study of American adolescents in the mid-1950s (1955–1956). Respondents (a representative sample consisting of 1,925 girls and 1,045 boys 14–16 years old in grades 7–12) were
interviewed on adolescent development relevant topics such as values, aspirations
and the formation of feminine identity, close relationships applying to family and
friendship, and contextual factors pertaining particularly to family structure and
what, following Bronfenbrenner (1979), we presently refer to as the macrosystem.

Douvan and Adelson's approach to future orientation sex differences has to be
understood in terms of the pivotal role they assumed future orientation plays in the
development of adolescents and their transition to the adult world:

> Separate the present of adolescence from its future in adulthood, and a hollow and super-
> ficial picture is about all one can hope to reveal. Adolescence in all cultures, especially in
> our own, is bound inextricably to adult reality. (Douvan & Adelson, 1966, p. 229).

Considering the gender-differentiated culture that characterized the United State
and Western Europe in the post World War II era – eventually bringing about the
Women's Lib movement – one can understand why Douvan and Adelson's chapter on adolescent future orientation is in fact divided into two parts: the future
orientation of boys and the future orientation of girls (in that order). Like other

Table 4.1 Studies examining future orientation gender differences

Study	Participants Background characteristics	Age/grade	Variables	Measures	Main findings
Anthis et al. (2004)	149 (55 males) young adults (mostly European-Americans)	18–25 years (mean age 21)	Identity dimensions of exploration and commitment across eight domains: occupation, religion, politics, values, family, friendship, dating, gender roles. Hoped and feared possible selves	Ego Identity Process Questionnaire (EIPQ) Possible Selves Inventory (PSI) (open-ended)	No gender differences are found for interpersonal PSI, but women generate significantly more feared interpersonal possible selves, and more balanced interpersonal possible selves
Greene (1990)	104 Caucasian students (13 males and 13 females from 4 age groups)	10th & 12th graders, College sophomores and seniors	Future expectations pertaining to achievement, relational, experiential and existential domains	Structured interviews where a semi-structured questionnaire was administered	Boys extend themselves to more distant points in the future and project future events that are more evenly distributed across life course. No gender differences in the distribution in the different prospective domains
Greene and Wheatley (1992)	82 (39 males) Caucasian working class with some college education	20 years	Psychological profile characteristics (abstract reasoning, psychological distress, self concept and self-esteem), future orientation variables	90 min semi-structured individual interview including proportional reasoning measure, brief symptom inventory (BSI), self esteem, self concept questionnaire, and	Men show greater overall spontaneous extension than women. No sex differences in number of future events, and occupational events, but women list more family

Table 4.1 (continued)

Study	Participants		Measures	Main findings
	Background characteristics	Age/grade		
				related events, and anticipated entry into full time employment, marriage and parenthood and at an earlier age than males. Men have an overall longer extension and specifically in the career domain
			orientation variables (e.g., absolute number of events, spontaneous and constrained extension)	open-ended Future orientation questionnaire
Kerpelman & Mosher (2004)	267 African American adolescents (168 girls) attending a rural high school in the South	7th–12th graders	Educational and occupational future orientation	Future orientation questionnaire assessing education and career	Girls score higher than boys on both the education and career domains
Kerpelman and Schvaneveldt (1999)	1267 (25% men and 75% women) singles (never married, no children)	18–25 years	Role identity salience regarding career, marriage, and parenthood	Pie Measure for role identity; role identity salience (LLRS) (Likert scale), personal attributes questionnaire (PAQ), identity interview with parents	Women place greater importance on the parental identity than did men, but no gender differences about value of career or marital identities. Gender differences in the anticipated timing of career and marital roles acquisition (men earlier on career, women earlier on marriage)

Table 4.1 (continued)

Study	Participants Background characteristics	Age/grade	Variables	Measures	Main findings
Knox et al. (2000)	212 (85 boys) high school students	9th–12th graders 14–19 years (mean age 16.4)	Possible selves, 14 categories (e.g., other- and self-oriented descriptors, physical appearance and health, psychological functioning, education, occupation, material & financial, relationship). Global self worth	Hoped-for and feared possible selves questionnaire. The Self-Perception Profile for Adolescents Global self-Worth Scale	Hoped for possible selves: boys list occupation, relationship and interpersonal selves, and girls list relationship and interpersonal and occupation. Feared possible selves: boys mention most frequently the categories of physical illness and death and general failure, and girls list relationship and interpersonal and physical illness & death
Lamm et al. (1976)	50 girls and 50 boys lower and middle class German adolescents	14–16 years	Density of family, occupation and personal development (personal domains), and economy, politics and environment (public domains), and extension, perceived control and optimism/pessimism for each	Hopes and fears open-ended questionnaire and Likert-type questionnaire for assessing optimism	Boys express more hopes and fears than girls, but girls express more private domain and public domain (politics, environment) hopes and fears. Lower class boys have a more extended future orientation and score higher on occupation and education than girls. Middle class boys score higher on occupation density but no extension gender differences. Boys score higher on perceived control, but not on optimism-pessimism

Table 4.1 (continued)

Study	Participants Background characteristics	Age/grade	Variables	Measures	Main findings
Malmberg & Trempala (1997)	194 (108 boys) Finnish and 158 (84 boys) Polish respondents from secondary and vocational schools in urban and semi urban areas	17 years	Subjective assessment of 3 life domains: occupation, education, family; self esteem; extension	Probability estimation for successful accomplishment of developmental tasks (Likert scale); subjective generational comparison (in comparison to parents' life); Rosenberg's self-esteem scale (Likert scale). Control over future scale	Finnish and Polish girls estimate the highest and Polish boys the lowest probability for attaining educational goals. Girls anticipate moving away from home, finding a partner and having children earlier than boys. Finnish vocational school girls estimate moving away from home the earliest while Polish boys estimate the latest to leave
Mehta et al. (1972)	High and low SES American and Indian adolescents (N = 96, 12 in each SES x Nation group)	13–15 years	Future time extension	Open ended questionnaire	No gender by SES differences are found
Mönks (1968)	627 girls and 797 boys from Dutch high, middle and low SES	14–21 years	Essays coded in term of self and personality, school and vocation, family and home, society and state, religion and church, travel, material sphere, science fiction categories	Anticipated autobiography essay	Girls list fewer statements than boys (5 vs 9), boys list twice as many school and occupational statements than girls and girls list more marriage and family statements. Boys have clearer and

Table 4.1 (continued)

Study	Participants Background characteristics	Age/grade	Variables	Measures	Main findings
					more detailed concepts regarding political and social procedures, and science fiction. Family and home are placed second for girls but fourth for boys
Nurmi (1989)	Longitudinal and cross-sectional research (N = 57 10–11 years and 14–15 years Finnish respondents)	10–11 years and 14–15 years	Future orientation was analyzed in terms of 10 categories of hopes and fears (e.g., profession and occupation, education and schooling, marriage and family, parents, others, property, leisure, collective issues (peace and war), and their complexity of plans, level of realization, and knowledge about realization	Interview, background data questionnaire, and 2 intelligence tests	Among girls but not among boys fears about war increase with age; boys' affect towards the future grows more positive with age, whereas girls' affect becomes more negative. Internal control regarding realization of fears increase for boys and decrease with age for girls. Girls list more family- and leisure-related hopes than do boys. 15 years-old boys are more optimistic than 11-year-old boys whereas the opposite is true for girls

Table 4.1 (continued)

Study	Participants Background characteristics	Age/grade	Variables	Measures	Main findings
Nurmi et al. (1993)	Australian (younger 95 boys and 104 girls and older 87 boys and 81 girls); Finnish (younger 67 boys and 86 girls and older 56 boys and 107 girls)	13–14 years and 16–17 years	Density scores and temporal extension for 13 categories (Nurmi et al., 1995)	Hopes and fears (open-ended) questionnaire	Finnish girls list more educational goals and concerns than all other groups. All girls list more occupational and family-related goals and concerns than do boys, and boys list more leisure and property-related goals than do girls. Younger adolescents' educational goals are more extended into the future, and older Finnish boys have an overall longer temporal extension than others
Nurmi et al. (1995)	120 (71 boys) Australian, 102 (36 boys) Finnish, and 46 (23 boys) Israeli adolescents	16–17 years. High school students	Density scores and temporal extension for future life domains like education, work and career, marriage/ children, leisure/ vacations, friends, parents, health, military service, property, global issues; exploration and commitment education, occupation and family	Hopes and fears questionnaire (open-ended), exploration and commitment questionnaire	Girls express more future education hopes and score higher on education-related exploration and commitment, Israeli boys express more military service hopes and fears than girls. No gender differences for the occupational and family domains. Israeli and Finnish (but not Australian) girls express more education fears than do boys, and all girls list more family-related fears

Table 4.1 (continued)

Study	Participants Background characteristics	Age/grade	Variables	Measures	Main findings
Poole and Cooney (1987)	162 (83 males) Singapore adolescents and 440 (184 males) Australian (Sydney) adolescents	Mean age 15 and 14.6, for Singapore, Australia, respectively	Personal (e.g., education, work, courtship and marriage, Leisure and sports, travel, health) and societal (e.g., environment, population, community issues, the economy, employment, political and international) categories	Life possibilities questionnaire: respondents listed 6 personal and 6 societal expected events, their time, and emotional tone (pleasant or unpleasant) for individual and for society. Acquaintance with occupations questionnaire (list all known occupations) and how realistic it was for them to work in those occupations	Australian girls and Singapore boys list more marriage events. Girls had shorter median time spans than boys. No gender difference regarding optimism. Australian boys list more environmental, psychological and lifestyle events and fewer political events then girls. For the Singapore adolescents, more girls than boys list events related to their country; no gender differences for Australians
Salmela-Aro, Vuori, and Koivisto (2007)	561 Finnish adolescents (284 girls) from two middle-sized cities	9th graders	Frequency of personal goals listed by respondents in the following categories: school, education/occupation, property, friends, family, leisure, and self	Personal Project analysis (PPA) inventory	Gender differences represent instrumental-relational division of labor: boys score higher than girls on property and educational-occupational goals; girls score higher than boys on leisure, self concerns, family, and friends related goals

Table 4.1 (continued)

Study	Participants		Age/grade	Measures	Variables	Main findings
	Background characteristics					
Seginer (1988a)	115 (61 males) Israeli Jewish and 116 (67 males) Arab adolescents		High school 12 graders	Open ended Hopes and Fears questionnaire	Salience and specificity scores for each of the school and matriculation, military service, higher education, work and career, marriage and family, self, others, collective issues domains	Jewish boys score higher on military service and work and career (hopes) and girls score higher on marriage & family (hopes and fears) and Others (fears). Arab girls score higher on higher education (fears), self concerns (fear and hope) and others (fears). No specificity gender differences among Jewish adolescents; among Arabs, girls score higher than boys on education (hopes), and work and career (fears). Boys score higher than girls on collective issues (fears)
Seginer (1988b)	112 (67 boys) Jewish and 116 (67 boys) Arab adolescents		High school 12 graders	Open-ended hopes and fears questionnaire	See Seginer (1988a)	Jewish boys score higher on military service and work and career (hopes) and girls on marriage and family (hopes and fears), and others (fears). Arab girls score higher on higher education (fears), self (hopes and fears), and others (fears). Arab boys score higher on collective issues (fears).

Table **4.1** (continued)

Study	Participants		Measures	Main findings
	Background characteristics	Age/grade		
				No specificity gender differences for Jewish adolescents; Arab girls score higher on higher specificity re education (hopes) and work and career (fears), and boys on collective issues (fears)
Seginer and Halabi-Kheir (1998)	276 (126 boys) Israeli Druze and 308 (122 boys) Jewish adolescents	9th and 12th graders	Open ended Hopes and Fears questionnaire	Druze sample: girls score higher on relational domains (marriage and family, others) and in personal development via education hopes, and boys score higher on the agentic domains (e.g., work and career) hopes, and on fears about collective issues. Jewish sample: girls score higher on the relational domains (marriage and family) and personal development via education (hope and fears), and boys score higher on agentic domains (military service)
			Density scores for each of the domains listed in Seginer (1988a)	

Variables

Table 4.1 (continued)

Study	Participants Background characteristics	Age/grade	Variables	Measures	Main findings
Seginer and Schlesinger (1998)	112 (58 boys) kibbutz adolescents and 112 (61 boys) urban adolescents (1984 sample) 101 (41 boys) kibbutz adolescents and 113 (59 boys) urban adolescents (1992 sample)	12 graders	Density scores for each of the following domains: School & matriculation, Military service, Higher education, Work and career, Marriage and family, Self, Others, and Collective issues	Open ended Hopes and Fears questionnaire	Girls score higher than boys on hopes regarding higher education, marriage and family and others. Boys score higher than girls on hopes regarding military service and work and career. Girls score higher than boys on fears concerning marriage and family and others. Boys score higher than girls on fears regarding school and work & career
Sundberg, Poole, and Tyler (1983)	50–150 boys and girls from India, Australia and the U.S.	9th graders (15 years)	Time scale, affective tone, and event content	Open-ended questionnaire on personal life possibilities	Australian girls show longer time spans than the other girls, and Indian boys show longer time spans than Indian girls, and American girls and boys. No gender differences regarding the affective tone. Indian girls mention education, work, travel, acquisitions and specific occupation more often than Indian boys. American and Australian gender differences varied, but all boys scored higher on acquisitions and girls on autonomy

Table 4.1 (continued)

Study	Participants Background characteristics	Age/grade	Variables	Measures	Main findings
Trommsdorff et al. (1979)	German 24 male and 24 female lower and middle SES secondary school students	14–16 years at time of measurement 1. Measurement 2, 2 years later	Future orientation in four different categories: personality and self actualization, physical well-being and appearance, family, and occupation: extension time, internal and external control, and optimism-pessimism measures	Open-ended hopes and fears	Girls list fewer hopes and fears in the area of physical well-being & appearance than boys (measurement 2). Boys have a more extended future orientation (measurement 2) than in measurement 1. Boys have a more extended future orientation in the occupational domain, and in measurement 2 boys have a more extended future concerns in the personality and self-actualization and the physical well being & appearance domain. Girls are more optimistic regarding their family, and boys regarding physical well-being & appearance (2nd measurement)
Yowell (2000)	38 (20 boys) Latino elementary school students. All students U.S. citizens from low SES	8th graders. Ag: M = 13.4	Five domains of possible selves: education, occupation, family, friendship, personal well-being and their temporal extension, optimism, internal control, priority, specificity and hopes-fears balance	FOQ = Future Orientation Questionnaire (interview)	No gender differences in hoped-for selves by domain. Girls prioritize educationally related hoped, and boys prioritize occupationally related hopes; girls scored lower on extension. No gender differences on optimism, feared selves, and hopes/fears balance, but boys scored higher on control

psychologists (Erikson, 1968) and sociologists (Parsons & Bales, 1955) of that era, Douvan and Adelson believed that whereas boys assume responsibility for the construction of their future identity primarily through choice of future occupation, girls' future identity is vicarious and depends on the man each will marry and the family each will raise, and is hence uncertain.

Similar to other studies of adolescent future orientation, to assess girls' and boys' future orientation and particularly their notion of adulthood Douvan and Adelson asked them about their plans and expectations for the future, particularly regarding their life plans and the domains of education and work. However, assuming future orientation also consists of a deeper less formulated and more emotional dimension, they also tapped adolescents' daydreams and adult admired models.

Their findings supported boys' tendency to construct an instrumental, coherent, and goal-directed future orientation and girls' tendency to construct a fuzzy future orientation. How could girls know who they would grow up to be if they don't know who will wish to marry them? This also explains why girls developed two separate images of the future: the realistic and the fantastic. The dependence of much of their future on an as yet unknown future husband limited the range of their plans to the time before marriage and resulted in unclear and non-coherent representations about higher education and occupational choices. Their fantasies on the other hand consisted of dreams of marriage, glamour and physical beauty. These findings correspond to findings of an exploratory study conducted among women's college sophomores who were requested to write an essay about the life they expected to live in 10 years time.

Between 46 and 48 of the total group of 50 girls included each of the following elements in their picture of future life: marriage to a successful professional man or junior executive; three or more children; home in the suburbs; daily activities including chauffeuring, shopping, and food preparation; family income of $20,000 a year or more; a station wagon car; membership in community organizations. Most telling is the reaction of 2 of the 50 participants in a post-experimental debriefing that presented them with those results. These girls claimed that the life they described was not the life they wished for but the only life they knew, and therefore the only life they could realistically wish for. By contrast, "the boy's future conceptions are all of one piece and heavily infused with the rhetoric of reality" (Douvan & Adelson, 1966, p. 52).

Douvan and Adelson's findings clearly reject the gender similarity hypothesis formulated by feminist psychologists (Bem, 1993; Hyde, 2005), and equally support explanations of sex differences as emerging from adaptation of ancestral women and men (evolutionary psychology) and from social structure processes that allocate women and men to different social positions that result in different attitudes, skills, and conceptions of their future as adults (social role theory). However, the emphasis they put on the adolescents' obligation to social demands, particularly those emanating from the goal-oriented nature of American society, suggest that, if asked, Douvan and Adelson would have endorsed the social structure explanation.

The Mönks (1968) and Trommsdorff et al. (1979–1982) studies. In a study conducted in the Netherlands 6 years later, Mönks (1968) found similar trends. Thus, whereas education and occupation (as a combined category) were ranked first in importance by both girls and boys, boys wrote down twice as many statements as did girls. In a similar vein, girls were more concerned with marriage than were boys and boys were more concerned with political and social issues. The limited future orientation Douvan and Adelson reported for American girls was also found for Dutch girls. This has been indicated by two findings that show the lesser concern girls have about the future: girls' mean number of statements concerning self and personality and the mean total number of statements listed by them were about half those listed by boys.

In a similar manner, *German* girls listed more hopes and fears than boys regarding the family domain and boys listed more hopes and fears than girls regarding the occupational domain (Lamm, Schmidt, & Trommsdorff, 1976; Trommsdorff & Lamm, 1980; Trommsdoff, Burger, & Füchsle, 1982; Trommsdorff et al., 1979).

Future Orientation Sex Differences: Recent Findings

More than 30 years after Douvan and Adelson collected their data from a representative sample of American high school students, Greene and Wheatley (1992) reiterated their findings with a much smaller sample of older adolescents (whose mean age was 20). Specifically, their findings (as well as those of Greene, 1990) show that more boys describe their future in terms of an overall longer extension into the future than do girls, and that more girls than boys anticipate marriage and parenthood, and at a younger age. The findings that girls expect to enter adulthood at an earlier age but have a shorter future extension time thus suggest that the ambiguity of girls' idea of the future reported by Douvan and Adelson (1966) persisted through the generations. Be it for reasons of time, sampling, or assessment methods, Mello's (2008) findings based on 5-wave longitudinal NELS:88 data show females and males have similar educational expectations trajectories, but females' expectations of attaining a professional occupation higher than those of males.

More recent data collected in Australia, Finland, Israel (Jewish population), Poland, and the United States show that some sex differences persist whereas others have grown smaller. Finnish and Polish girls (Malmberg & Trempala, 1997) as well as American Latino girls (Yowell, 2000) continue to anticipate earlier and more rapid transition to adulthood than boys, American girls anticipate greater likelihood of feared possible selves (Anthis, Dunkel, & Anderson, 2004; Knox, Funk, Elliott, & Bush, 2000) and referred to interpersonal relationships more frequently than did boys. As predicted, American girls (Anthis et al., 2004) as well as Australian (Nurmi, Poole, & Kalakoski, 1993; Poole & Cooney, 1987), Finnish (Nurmi et al., 1993), and Israeli Jewish (Seginer, 2001a) girls all address family domain issues more often than their boy counterparts. An exception is a recent study of Finnish comprehensive school students (Nurmi, in press) showing that, while girls scored higher than boys on educational, social (friends), and self goals and boys scored higher than girls on occupational goals, they equally endorsed family goals.

Regarding the work and career domain, only two studies carried out in the United States (Knox et al., 2000; Yowell, 2000) reported that girls refer to it less frequently than do boys. Moreover, as girls close the career gender gap they become more concerned with educational issues (Malmberg & Trempala, 1997; Nurmi et al., 1993). This is particularly true of girls growing up in societies undergoing social change such as Poland (Malmberg & Trempala, 1997), or aspiring personal and generational mobility such as American Latinos (Yowell, 2000) and Israeli Arabs (Seginer, 2001a).

In all, these findings support the *social roles* approach to gender differences and indicate the relevance of socio-cultural context. The changing times and particularly the effect of women's lib ideas are particularly evident here. In the post-World War II era, as women returned to domestic roles, the effect of gender roles on the future orientation of girls and boys was stronger than in more recent times. Eagly and Mitchell's conclusion about political attitudes and voting behavior sex differences applies also to recent findings on future orientation:

> Despite the emphasis of our analysis on sex differences, these differences may be eroding in modern societies in which the roles of women have undergone relatively rapid change. As a consequence, gender roles are under pressure to change, and such changes will likely decrease actual sex differences in the long run, thereby increasing the behavioral flexibility of both men and women. (Eagly & Mitchell, 2004, p. 201).

The Cultural Context of Sex Differences

Early future orientation studies focused on comparisons. Although gender was many times of only secondary concern for them, by reporting separately about girls and boys these studies have informed us about the relevance of sex differences across different cultural and social groups.

The future orientation of western and non-western girls and boys. One of the early studies to examine adolescents' future orientation (Sundberg et al. 1983) compared three cultural settings: Australia, India, and the United States. Focusing on cross-cultural sex differences, researchers posited that these differences will be largest in India. Given that India is an eastern traditional society that allows girls only limited freedom of choice and independence in charting their future, it was predicted that Indian girls will adhere to traditional gender roles more than their American and Australian counterparts. This will result in a shorter extension into the future by girls than by boys and in investing less in such instrumental domains as education and occupation.

These predictions have only partly been borne out. Indeed, Indian girls scored lower on extension to the future. Nonetheless, they listed issues related to future education and occupation more often than boys. The authors were not sure as to how to interpret these findings and suggested two explanations. One drew on traditional values that privilege boys over girls. Applied to schooling it suggests that school attendance is based on different selection criteria for girls and boys: only the exceptionally talented and motivated girls but a less selective group of boys secure parents' willingness to send them to school. The second explanation drew on economic necessity. In the small Indian towns where data were collected, girls are required to look for a job to help in the support of their families whereas boys can enjoy a longer period of education. In all, however, both explanations took a traditional point of view in which only the parents' but none of the girls' interests have been considered.

The Israeli studies. A third explanation for the findings described above draws on data collected from two Israeli groups: Jewish adolescents of economically under-privileged groups whose high school curriculum included a college preparation educational program (the MABAR program) and Arab adolescents. These data focus on the adolescents' point of view and underline the *meaningfulness* of higher education for girls who differed in culture and ethnicity but shared the common characteristic of growing up underprivileged. Thus, among the Jewish adolescents (Seginer, Dan, & Zeliger, 1998) as among the Arab adolescents (Seginer, 2001a), girls devoted a larger part of their prospective life space to higher education than did boys (Fig. 4.1).

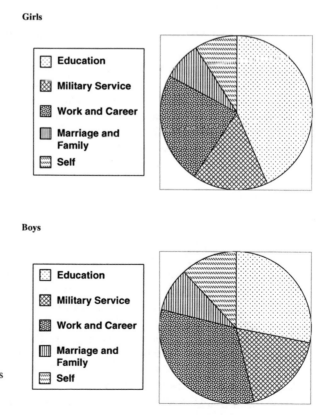

Fig. 4.1 The future life space of Israeli Jewish low-achieving adolescents (the MABAR project): hopes density score for girls and boys

These data as well as those about sex differences among Indian adolescents thus indicate that, by constructing their future orientation, adolescent girls chart an adult-hood which diverts from the adult life of their mothers and older sisters. However, so stated it differs from Douvan and Adelson's (1966) approach that investment in the future is part of the process of adaptation to existing social structure. Under-lying their contention that "adolescence in all cultures, especially in our own, is bound inextricably to adult reality" (Douvan & Adelson, 1966, p. 229) is a cultural continuity proposition by which the adolescents of today will assume adult roles and interpret them in a way similar to that of earlier generations. This assumption cannot be applied to social and cultural groups undergoing social change.

Thus, the lesson Indian and Israeli Arab and Jewish girls teach us is that in times of cultural change, particularly applying to transition to modernity, when the collec-tive adult schema does not correspond to their aspirations girls construct an alterna-tive schema for their adult life, and view education as the main means for personal change. As frequently expressed in the future orientation hopes and fears narratives of our Arab girl respondents "education is a weapon in women's hands" (Seginer & Mahajna, 2003, 2004).

The Hoped For and Feared Future of Transition to Modernity Girls: The Case of Israeli Arab and Druze Girls

One consistent finding emerging from our research on the future orientation of Israeli adolescents in the last 20 years has been the importance Arab and Druze girls attribute to higher education. Long before they viewed education as "a weapon", Arab and Druze girls expressed a greater concern for higher education than all other Israeli groups (i.e., Arab and Druze boys and Jewish girls and boys) (Seginer, 1988a, b, 2005; Seginer & Halabi-Kheir, 1998). Moreover, in some samples (Seginer, 2005) Arab girls listed fewer hopes and fears regarding marriage and family than did Arab boys and Jewish girls. This finding was not replicated for Druze girls. Relative to the Druze boys the density of their marriage and family domain is higher and the density of their work and career domain is lower in both the hoped for and feared prospective life space (Seginer & Halabi-Kheir, 1998).

Intertwining prospective adult roles. Another distinguishing feature of the hopes and fears narratives of Arab and Druze adolescent girls is their *intertwining* nature (Seginer, 2005). Across several studies conducted in recent years (e.g., Halabi-Kheir, 1992; Mahajna, 2007; Margieh, 2007; Seginer & Mahajna, 2004) it has been shown that, while the hopes and fears narratives constructed by Arab and Druze boys and Jewish adolescents each relates to one prospective life domain, Arab and Druze girls intertwine two or three domains, most commonly higher education and marriage but also career and family, and education, career and community inter-ests. Although the cultural and political affinity between Israeli Druzes and Arabs is debatable, both societies are guided by collectivistic orientations characterized by familism and male dominance (Seginer, Shoyer, Hossessi, & Tannous, 2007).

As their narratives illustrate, girls of both groups use the intertwining strategy to negotiate access to higher education.

Twelfth grade *Druze* girls (Seginer, 2001) intertwine higher education with both family and community interests:

> To be a teacher and educate the next generation, to open an educational center for illiterate women. (No. 5).
>
> To be educated and help develop our community. (No. 12).
>
> Get degrees and certificates that will prepare me to work so I can help my husband. (No. 78).
>
> To work as a simple journalist, to write bulletins about the Druze community, to be a housewife for 1 year without being employed, to be an announcer on a TV program for the Druze community, organize meetings between Israeli Druzes and Druzes from the rest of the world; to work at least once for the Monte Carlo radio station. (No. 173).
>
> To be a competent and famous social worker, to be a good and successful housewife, that our village will develop, for example by opening a women's center. (No. 174).

Narratives collected from 16- to 18-year-old Arab traditional girls (Seginer & Mahajna, 2004) show how the intertwining strategy evolves. Whereas 10th graders (age 16) express their desire for independence and defiance of traditional expectations for early marriage, for 12th graders (age 18) the future is governed by expressions of the intertwining strategy. Thus, the 16-year-olds describe their future in the following way:

> I hope to continue my studies and be a strong woman able to cope with all the difficulties and hurdles in my way. I don't want to be just a woman who gives in quickly. I want to contribute to our society and be a good and devoted housewife. (No. 29).
>
> I want to be a History teacher. I want to study because "education is a weapon in the woman's hands". Marriage is not important right now. (No. 32).
>
> I hope to be a famous lawyer. Therefore, I hope God will help me with my studies. As to getting married, I want to get married only after age 20. (No. 27).
>
> I want university education and to be an educated woman. Then I want to get married. (No.42).

An exception to 16 year defiance has been expressed by one 10th grader who understood the wisdom of intertwining earlier than her friends and wrote:

> Sometimes I sit by myself imagining I am a married teacher with wonderful husband and children. I don't want much. I want only to have a respectable job so that I can be economically independent so that my husband will not control my economic life because as a result he will also control my opinions, behavior, and ideas. I want to be recognized as an educated well-respected

woman. On the other hand, I have no objection to take care of my husband and family and serve them and be obedient to my husband as long as he does not get in the way of my aspirations, independence and self-respect. (No.77, age 16).

At age 17 (11th grade) girls are still focused on personal advancement by means of education. Their preference is clear: education first:

I hope to graduate from high school cum laude. I want to continue my education at the university and be important and contributing to my society. I hope public opinion about women and girls will change some day so that girls will not get engaged [to be married] while still in junior high school. I hope to find in my partner the attributes I am looking for: 26 years old, educated, sensitive, not religious, social, self-reliant, good natured, and a people-loving person. (No. 46).

Every girl in this world aspires for a successful future. I am like that. The first goal I have set for myself is achieving high grades on my matriculation certificate so that I can be admitted to the university. When I finish my [university] studies I will start thinking of getting married and choose a person so that we will understand each other. (No 49).

Honestly, the future is important for everyone. I myself am very busy with the future which causes me to be worried and hopeful, optimistic and interested [in various subjects] all at the same time. My hope is to be a successful student and get married but my preference is first continuing my education. (No. 67).

In 12th grade (age 18), as they approach high school graduation, family and communal pressure to get married and lead a traditional life rather than go on with university education grows stronger. Consequently, defiance is replaced by negotiations expressed by the intertwining strategy:

I hope to get a good matriculation certificate to make my father happy. And then I want to continue in some college so that I can be economically independent so that I can make all my hopes come true. (No. 4).

First of all I hope God will help me so that I can be successful in my studies and work. I hope to be a teacher, loved by both my students and my colleagues. I hope my married life will be successful and I will excel in my role as a wife and as a mother. I hope my husband will be well educated, religious, and respectful so that we can base our married life on understanding and mutual respect. (No. 223).

I hope to live quiet and happy married life, to have children and take good care of them, I hope to make my husband happy and be happy with him. As to education, I hope to go into higher education at the university or a college and be an important woman of value to our society. (No. 236).

I hope to be an important woman in our society. I hope to be an educator in the future and get married to a devoted and respectable person and together we will raise a family based on mutual respect and understanding. (No. 250, age 18).

Given that the intertwined narratives echo Arab girls' negotiation with their families and wider social circles about pursuing higher education, and used by them as a strategy for narrowing the gap between the culturally prescribed and personally desired prospective life courses for women, the intertwining strategy should be less prevalent in socio-cultural settings that endorse higher education and career development for women. This has been illustrated by data collected recently among Arab girls who attend college (Margieh, 2007).

Their narratives included three main themes: education, career, and marriage and family. However, none of the 67 female participants used the intertwining strategy. Specifically, with the exception of one girl who aspired to be "an exemplary mother", all others were not concerned with promising that pursuing a career would not interfere with fulfilling their traditional roles. Among their hopes were:

I have many hopes and aspirations, but my most important hope is to be a successful teacher at age 25, and that everyone will love and respect me. And to be an exemplary mother and have a nice family. (No. 16, age 19).

I am a married woman and pregnant. I hope I will have an easy delivery and that every thing will be OK, with God's help, and the baby will be healthy And that my relationships with my husband will be good. That I will be a good student and got high grades, and continue to graduate school and obtain MA and PhD degrees. I hope to find a job in my major [biology], and consider myself successful and develop myself in the right way and travel all over the world, no matter at what age. (No. 20, age 19).

By comparison, here are the hope protocols of 12th grade (age 18) Jewish girls who attended a college-bound prestigious high school:

To move to an apartment of my own, to live on a kibbutz, travel abroad, be a scientist, find a partner. (No. 53).

To be accepted to a dance company, boyfriend, driving license, pass successfully the matriculation exams, be in a military combat unit, study in medical school or law school, get married and have children, develop my career, develop a political career. (No. 52).

Military service, professional military service, get married, university studies, start a career, have my first child. (No. 55).

Thus, girls growing up in traditional settings, particularly Moslem and Druze girls from rural areas, aspire to higher education as a means for personal emancipation and negotiate their way to higher education by intertwining traditional family roles with modern higher education. However, considered a "hot topic"

(Montemayor, 1983), much of this negotiation never gets voiced in parent-adolescent face-to-face interactions, and many of the high ability achievement oriented girls settle for lesser education in a close-by college. Yet, as will be shown in Chap. 7 (Future Orientation Outcomes), higher education future orientation affects their investment in school work and results in high academic achievement.

Future Orientation Motivational and Behavioral Components Gender Differences

As the future orientation conceptualization has expanded from uni-dimensional cognitive to three-component models (Nurmi, 1991; Seginer, 1995, 2005), findings about sex differences encompass the motivational and behavioral components as well.

Future orientation gender differences: 14 Israeli studies. Of the 14 studies carried out in Israel in the last decade (Table 4.2), five were carried out with Jewish adolescents (10th to 12th graders), two with former Soviet Russia new immigrants, one with kibbutz adolescents and one with Jewish emerging adults. Four studies were performed with Arab adolescents (11th graders), and one with Druze adolescents (11th graders). Of the four Arab groups, one lived in a big mixed city and three in smaller all-Arab towns. The Druze adolescents attended a Druze high school serving two neighboring villages adjacent to the big mixed city.

The emerging adult groups consisted of single women and men (mean age 24) who completed their military service and made a decision to take up university education, although for various reasons as high school students they did not complete requirements for matriculation certificate (one of the two university admission requirements). This certificate is awarded in Israel to high school graduates who pass state examinations held by the Ministry of Education and administered to high school juniors and seniors.

The overall picture is one of relatively few gender differences. More meaningful, however, is the direction of these gender differences. Almost without exception, girls score higher than boys. Across different ethnicities, cultural background, living conditions and age, girls emerge as the group who grants higher value to higher education, work and career, and marriage and family, some of them have a greater sense of internal control over their hopes, goals, and plans for the future, invest more in exploring different options and have made up their mind concerning higher education, career, and marriage and family. As they think (cognitive representation) about each of these prospective domains, they list more hopes as well as more fears than do their counterpart boys.

Future orientation gender differences: international studies. Only few international studies included motivational and behavioral variables (Table 4.1) and those included show a diversified picture. When the future pertains to educational hopes, goals and plans, girls score higher than boys. These tendencies are particularly evident in girls' tendency to have higher confidence in attaining educational goals

Table 4.2 Future orientation gender differences in 14 Israeli samples

	Jewish									Arab				Druze
Future orientation variables	1	2	3	4	5	6	7a	8a	9b	10	11	12	13	14
Higher education/work and career														
Value		F>M		*F>M*						F>M	F>M	*F>M*	*F>M*	F>M
Expectance		F>M								F>M	F>M			F>M
Control			F>M		*F>M*		F>M		*F>M*	F>M	F>M			F>M
Hopes			F>M		*F>M*					F>M	F>M			
Fears			F>M		*F>M*									
Exploration							F>M		*F>M*	F>M	F>M			
Commitment						F>M			*F>M*					
Marriage and Family														
Value		F>M		F>M	F>M	F>M	F>M			F>M	F>M		F>M	
Expectance					F>M						F>M			
Control				F>M					F>M					
Hopes					F>M								F>M	
Fears			F>M											
Exploration		F>M	F>M	F>M	F>M		F>M		F>M	F>M			F>M	F>M
Commitment		F>M	F>M	F>M	F>M				F>M			F>M		

1 Seginer and Schlesinger (1998), 2 Lilach (1996), 3 Melzer (2000), 4 Seginer, Vermulst and Shoyer (2004), 5 Shoyer (2006), 6 Seginer and Shoyer (2005), 7 Toren-Kaplan (1995), 8 Nakash (2000), 9 Noyman (1998), 10 Seginer (2001), 11 Seginer (2001), 12 Sleiman (2001), 13 Margieh (2007), 14 Seginer (2001). *Italics* indicate that findings pertain to the Work and Career domain

a New-immigrants from former USSR

b Emerging adults

(expectance) (Malmberg & Trempala, 1997) and being more involved in exploration of and commitment to educational issues and plans (Nurmi et al., 1995). While these findings may indicate girls' negotiations for equality of opportunities via education, they also show that to date these negotiations are age-specific. As females face adulthood they tend to accept traditional roles. Thus, emerging adults maintain the sex role division and women attribute higher value to parenting than do emerging adult men (Kerpelman & Schvaneveldt, 1999).

More telling are Nurmi's (1989) findings that as girls enter middle adolescence their view of the future becomes bleaker. Thus, while as boys grow up from age 11 to 15 they become more optimistic about the future and have a greater sense of control over it, for girls the reverse is true: as they grow up their view of the future becomes less optimistic and their sense of control decreases. Whether these differences emerge in response to viewing adult women and men around them or reflect the experience of being 15 for girls and boys, girls anticipate a less encouraging future than do boys. Eighteen years later (Salmela-Aro et al., 2007), 15-year-old Finnish girls (growing up in a social system where over 40% of parliament members are women) list more family, friend, leisure, and self-related goals, and boys list more property and education-occupation related goals. Data collected in the 1970s show that German girls and boys did not differ in how optimistic they were about the future but boys felt more control over it than did girls (Lamm et al., 1976).

Although these findings are sparse and based on data collected in different times and places, the overall impression they give is that girls more than boys treat the future with an approach-avoidance attitude and equality of the sexes may not begin in adolescence.

Gender differences in social context. Our finding that with few exceptions, across different ethnicities, living conditions and developmental periods, girls invest more in constructing future orientation raises the question Why? The answer is not clear, not the same for all groups, and relates both to personal characteristics and social context of girls and boys. Nonetheless, all explanations relate to social structural gender inequality and women's aspirations to overcome the traditional division of labor by pursuing a career while at the same time preserving their commitment to raising a family. As indicated by the Arab and Druze girls' narratives, relatively early in life they realize that to strive for academic excellence, they must also prove commitment to traditional women's roles, and devotion to their family and community.

Gender differences among children. As reported in Chap. 2, as early as 2nd grade, the future orientation protocols of girls contain fewer existential (i.e., global and not goal-directed) hope narratives than the protocols of boys (Gelberg, 1996). When the *density* scores of girls and boys narratives are summed over for 2nd, 4th and 6th graders, the results are even clearer: a larger share of their prospective life space (indexed by the total number of hopes and fears, respectively) is devoted to the education and marriage and family domains and a smaller share to the non-specific non-goal oriented self concerns domain. Boys devote a larger share of their prospective life space to work and career and do not differ from girls in the relative weight of the military service domain (Fig. 4.2).

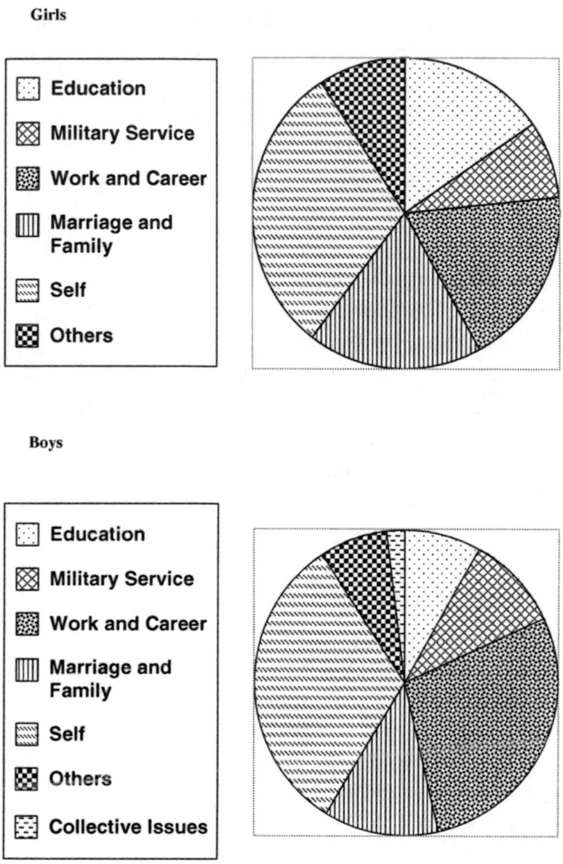

Girls

Boys

Fig. 4.2 The future life space of Israeli Jewish elementary school children: hopes density score for girls and boys

Gender differences and gendered distribution of roles. One explanation of gender differences reported above, relevant to all cultural groups, draws directly on the gendered distribution of social roles: the world is more open and offers greater opportunities to men than to women. Thus, to find their place in the world of work and career women must be more intentional, goal oriented and altogether invest more in thinking and planning the future than men. In addition, considering the biological clock and the social timetable constructed for women and men, girls are expected to make their transition to adulthood and particularly assume their family roles earlier than boys who may train themselves, experiment, and take time off from the social normative developmental track for longer periods. Thus, boys are less rushed to enter adulthood than are girls. This is clearly reflected in the average age of marriage which is several years younger for women than for men.

Gender differences among Arab adolescents. Explanation of the differences in the future orientation of Arab adolescents rests on two additional considerations.

One is the differential status of women and men in Arab families. Boys, like adult men, are the privileged sex in Arab society. Applied to the family setting, since childhood they – like adult men – are exempted of any domestic chores and responsibility for younger children, have authority over their sisters regardless of their age, and are served by family women. This sex-related differential pattern of socialization also has its negative consequences because it raises boys to be more dependent and less mature than girls.

In the realm of academic achievement, this reliance on others is reflected in parental involvement. While girls' academic achievement is treated by surveillance so that the higher their grades the lower their parents' demandingness, boys' academic achievement is treated by encouragement so that the higher their achievement the more they are pampered, encouraged and rewarded (Seginer & Vermulst, 2002). Thus while Arab girls have to prove their worthiness by helping with domestic chores (Seginer, 1992b) and working hard at school, Arab boys earn their privileges by belonging to the dominant sex, and doing well at school gets them extra rewards. Altogether, their social milieu gives boys a greater sense of security about the future and consequently fewer challenges and concerns than it gives girls.

The second consideration specific to Arab and Druze adolescents pertains to girls and boys sex role beliefs. Studies of these beliefs among Arab and Jewish girls and boys (Mar'i, 1983; Seginer, Karayanni, & Mar'i, 1990) show that Arab girls hold more liberal sex role beliefs than do Arab boys. In our recent studies this greater liberalism is voiced in the girls' narratives cited above. Moreover, these beliefs have a direct effect on Arab adolescent girls' future orientation as it applies to the motivational component of their prospective educational domain and their optimism about fulfilling hopes and goals pertaining to prospective marriage and family domain (Seginer & Mahajna, 2004).

While this explanation is concerned more with the condition and characteristics of Arab girls, conditions specific to Arab boys should also be considered. Of particular relevance to boys is the protracted Jewish-Arab conflict which has led to compulsory military service for Jewish adolescents (two years for girls and three for boys) and Druze boys but excludes Arab adolescent boys. Consequently, whereas for Israeli Jewish adolescents and Druze boys military service is part of their normative future path, it is not for Arab boys and may thus incite a sense of powerlessness.

Summary

Guided by the main current approaches to sex differences this chapter has examined two hypotheses about future orientation sex differences. Based on feminist theories of gender similarities, the hypothesis has been that girls and boys will construct similar future orientations. Based on *evolutionary psychology* and *gender role theory* the prediction has been that for different underlying processes, in developing their future orientation adolescent girls will invest more in the construction of *relational* domains like marriage and family, and adolescent boys will invest more in the construction of *instrumental* domains such as work and career.

However, findings presented in this chapter show the contextual nature of future orientation gender differences. Data collected in the late 1950s in the United States confirmed the gender differences hypothesis, indicating that because they regarded their future life as depending on the man they would marry, girls' future orientation extended less into the future than boys' future orientation and their protocols included fewer narratives about the work and career domain and more narratives about the marriage and family domain.

Data collected since the 1980s in the United States, Europe (Belgium, Finland, Germany, Holland, and Poland), Australia, Singapore and Israel only partly replicated those earlier findings. While in some European studies girls outline a shorter future time perspective than boys and are concerned more with marriage and family and less with work and career issues than boys, other studies reported no differences and thus supported the *gender similarity hypothesis* or showed that where gender differences are found girls score higher than boys. This finding applies particularly to girls from transition to modernity societies (such as India, Israeli Arabs and Druzes, and Singapore) but also from western societies (such as Israeli Jews). Its explanation, however, should take into consideration factors affecting both girls and boys. For girls it is aspirations for personal progress whereas for boys the narrowing gender differences emanate from several contextual factors that curb or possibly delay their concern about the future.

Altogether, at the present time, girls' future orientation is less gendered than it had been in the mid-twentieth century when early future orientation research was conducted. Nonetheless, particularly for girls growing up in traditional and transition to modernity societies, the world is still more gendered than they would hope it to be. This is illustrated in the hopes and fears narratives of Israeli Arab girls; as they approach adulthood their images of the future become more aligned with traditional reality than are those of younger adolescent girls.

Chapter 5
The Effect of Parenting on Future Orientation

Until recently, research on adolescents' future orientation was mainly concerned with macrosystemic effects. Researchers contrasted the future orientation of Singapore and Australian, Indian and American, Israeli Arab and Jewish adolescents, working class and middle class adolescents, native-born and new immigrants, kibbutz and urban raised youth. Underlying this research interest has been an assumption that macrosystemic forces consisting of cultural beliefs, attitudes, values, and adult role expectations serve as building blocks for the construction of adolescent future orientation and thus make socio-cultural settings a viable issue in the study of future orientation.

Missing from this research have been issues related to adolescents' proximal environment pertaining particularly to relationships and pertinent beliefs. Thus, whereas in other areas of developmental psychology interest in the effect of family environment preceded consideration of cultural settings, social class and other aspects of the macrosystem, in future orientation research analysis of the effect of distal context indicators preceded the study of the effect of the proximal context as it relates to parents, siblings, peers, friends and other interpersonal relationships.

Consequently, the purpose of this chapter and the one following it is to examine future orientation in the context of parent-adolescent (this chapter), sibling and peer relationships (next chapter) and their culture specificity. This chapter consists of four sections that examine the effect on future orientation of *relationships* with parents and parents' pertinent *beliefs* in their *cultural contexts*. The effect of adolescent-parent relationship is discussed in two sections. The first summarizes early research on the effect of family atmosphere and parenting on future orientation and the second presents recent studies that examine the *positive parenting* model of future orientation. The third section addresses the effect of parental beliefs on future orientation and the fourth examines the intergenerational transmission of future orientation.

In accordance with much of current conceptualization of adolescent parenting and for reasons drawing on theoretical, methodological and policy-making considerations, research discussed in this chapter is directional and focuses on the effect of parents on their children. However, this by no means refutes the viability of parent-child reciprocity and the relevance of child factors to parenting and parental beliefs.

R. Seginer, *Future Orientation*, The Springer Series on Human Exceptionality,
DOI 10.1007/978-0-387-88641-1_5, © Springer Science+Business Media, LLC 2009

Family Atmosphere, Parenting and Future Orientation

This section starts with a review of three studies that laid grounds for contemporary research on parenting effects and proceeds with studies that focus on the effect of positive parenting – as the construct often used in adolescent parenting research – on various indices of adolescents' future orientation.

Early Studies on the Effect of Parenting on Adolescent Future Orientation

Parental support. The earliest study on the effect of parent-adolescent relationship on future orientation was carried out by Trommsdorff and her associates. Drawing on social learning theory they predicted that in adolescence parental support and encouragement prompt two personality inclinations that lead to positive attitudes toward the future and willingness to pursue future goals: sense of *internal control* and *optimism* about the outcomes of one's behavior. These hypotheses have been confirmed; adolescents who perceive their parents as supportive and encouraging express greater optimism toward the future and construct more extended and differentiated future orientation (Trommsdorff, 1983; Trommsdorff, Burger, & Füchsle, 1982). Summarizing this work (originally published in German) Trommsdorff wrote:

> ...we assumed that the experience of parental acceptance would foster a positive, self-assured future orientation in the child. As a matter of fact, we were able to show for adolescents from different age groups that persons who perceived their parents as loving and supporting had a more trusting, hopeful, and positive future orientation, believed more in personal control of their future... (Trommsdorff, 1986, p.125).

Family atmosphere. Prompted by these findings, Nurmi (1989; Nurmi & Pulliainen, 1991) and Pulkkinen (1990) continued the study of family effects on future orientation. The three studies focus on family atmosphere but ask different questions and use different methods. Pulkkinen's study is retrospective. It focuses on emerging adults' (age 20) memories of parents' child rearing practices and time spent together in childhood and shows that positive memories are associated with emerging adults' optimism regarding the future, and memory of time spent together with parents is positively related to all aspects of future orientation assessed by the study.

Although memories are constantly changing and liable to manipulation (Loftus, 2003) they do reflect parental behavior as *experienced* by the emerging adults and are therefore considered a valid indicator of home atmosphere. Particularly relevant is *time spent together*. Seldom included in research designs, its importance draws on the logic that as adolescents and parents spend more time, particularly as a dyad, they have more opportunities to exchange ideas and sentiments. As elaborated in a subsequent section, time spent together may also explain why the effect of mothers' parenting on adolescents' future orientation is greater than that of fathers.

Like Trommsdorff and her associates, Nurmi and Pulliainen (1991) examined the effect of parental affect. However, contending that along with closeness, support and encouragement, parents also vary in the extent to which they control, supervise, and exert authority over their children (Schaefer, 1965), Nurmi and Pulliainen also assessed parental control. Their hypothesis has been that the effect of these dimensions on future orientation is age-dependent. Affect (indexed by family discussions) has a greater effect on older adolescents' (age 14–15) future orientation and parental control on the future orientation of preadolescents' (age 10–11).

The importance of including both dimensions of parent-adolescent relationships has been indicated by their effect on future orientation. Parental discussions prompt adolescents' interest in future marriage and family domain and parental control hinders their interest in future education. Moreover, for the 14- to 15-year-olds, optimism about the future is prompted by family discussions whereas, for the 10- to 11-year-olds, optimism is related to low level of parental control. As noted by Nurmi and Pulliainen, the relation between family discussions and interest in the marriage and family domain may be explained by the positive family model families having frequent discussions set for their adolescent children. Thus, in addition to the positive effect of parental warmth and support reported by Trommsdorff and by Pulkkinen, Nurmi and Pulliainen's findings show the hindering effect of parental control and the domain specific relevance of parental practices and behaviors for adolescents' future orientation.

Positive Parenting and Future Orientation

Although adolescent-parent *relationship* is only one aspect of parenting, its examination has become so prevalent (Collins & Laursen, 2004; Steinberg & Silk, 2002) that often when researchers refer to parenting they in fact describe adolescent-parent relationships and use *positive parenting* as an umbrella term subsuming constructs like authoritative, autonomous-accepting, enabling (vs restrictive), child centered parenting, and individuation and connectedness facilitating parenting. The observation that behavior indicating positive parenting changes with age of child (Maccoby, 1992a) suggests that parenting is affected not only by parents' personality, values, beliefs and cultural practices but also by children's age-dependent characteristics and behavior and by parents' appraisal of those characteristics and behavior as normative.

Positive parenting and future orientation: the rationale. The proposition about the effect of positive parenting on various aspects of adolescents' future orientation draws on both general and future orientation specific considerations. The general consideration relates to the extensive research on the influence of adolescent-parent relationships on adolescent adjustment indicated by psychological well-being, interpersonal and close relationships, school achievement and law-abiding behavior (Collins & Laursen, 2004; Steinberg & Silk, 2002).

Doubts about the effect of positive parenting on children and adolescents' adjustment (Maccoby, 1992a) notwithstanding, these findings can be explained in terms of the generalized complementary value of parental acceptance, autonomy and authority (limit setting). Parental support, warmth and acceptance, and autonomy granting engender a sense of security and self competence essential for the pursuit of developmental tasks, and parental authority serves as an external reminder of responsibilities and priorities and a safeguard against peer pressure or failed judgment. Empirical evidence for the relevance of limit setting for adolescent adjustment has been presented by the findings of Beyers and Goossens (1999) on the negative effect of low limit setting on school performance and its positive effect on deviant behavior.

The future orientation specific consideration relates to the relevance of parental support, warmth and acceptance for prompting a positive outlook and the relevance of parental autonomy granting for the motivation to explore future options and develop exploration skills. Underlying the latter is application to future orientation of the cognitive-motivational principle of *least necessary expenditure* stating that individuals will not exert maximal effort "... on easier tasks or on tasks that overtax one's ability" (Heckhausen, 1977, p. 314).

Specific to the effect of positive parenting on future orientation it suggests that adolescents will invest in the construction of the future to the extent they appraise their families as supporting (rather than hampering) an independent search of a future course. In this context, the role of parental limit setting is to contain exploration and experimentation by reiterating age-appropriate Dos and Don'ts and setting external limits against what adults regard as unsafe risky adventures.

Positive parenting and future orientation: empirical findings. Research conducted among German adolescents showed that child centered parenting (Kracke, 2002; Kracke & Schmitt-Rodermund, 2001) is related to adolescents' career exploration and to its intensification across time. Studies carried out among Israeli Jewish and Arab adolescents examined the effect of two aspects of fathers' and mothers' positive parenting on the motivational, cognitive and behavioral components of future orientation: parenting style and parenting behavior.

Despite cultural differences, the greater difficulties Arab adolescents will encounter in reaching a successful career and the overall lower concern of Arab adolescents about prospective life course domains (Seginer, 2005), the pattern of relations between parenting style and future orientation is similar for Jewish and Arab adolescents. In both groups *authoritative* parenting facilitates future orientation thinking to a greater extent than indulgent, neglectful or authoritarian parenting. Assessment of parenting *behavior* shows that for both Arab (Suleiman, 2000) and Jewish (Melzer, 2000) adolescents, perceived parents' autonomy granting and parental acceptance predict optimism and a sense of self efficacy about the future. However, whereas for Arab adolescents granted autonomy is a better predictor than parental acceptance, for Jewish adolescents parental acceptance is a better predictor than parents' granted autonomy.

Thus, while the cultural specificity of parenting effects (Chao, 2001) applies to the comparison between Arab and Jewish adolescents, its nature too is culture specific. However, positive parenting is relevant to the future orientation of both Arab and Jewish adolescents, albeit expressed by different indicators.

Positive parenting and future orientation: summary. Findings of research conducted in two western cultural settings (Germany, Jewish Israel) and one transition to modernity cultural setting (Arabic Israel) suggest both across-culture similarities and differences. When analysis focuses on an overall authoritative style, the effect of authoritative parenting on future orientation applies to all three cultural settings. However, when analysis is carried out at the level of perceived parental behavior, the effects are culture specific so that parental acceptance is more relevant for the construction of future orientation among modern adolescents and granted autonomy for the construction of future orientation among transition to modernity adolescents. Recent analyses (Mahajna, 2007), described below in more detail, show similar tendency for Israeli Arab girls.

However, a more significant finding pertains to the weak (though consistent across several cultural groups) direct relations between parenting and future orientation. One way to interpret it is to concur in doubting the effect of parenting on children's development. The other is to suggest that, particularly during adolescence, the effect of parenting on future orientation is indirect. The processes that link parenting and adolescent future orientation are examined in a multiple step model discussed below.

The Positive Parenting Multiple Step Model

Underlying the development of this model has been the pivotal role of the self in mediating social environment and individuals' behavior, discussed in Chap. 3. In addition, two assumptions guide the multiple step approach and the model describing it. The first – discussed earlier in this chapter – pertains to the unidirectional vs reciprocal nature of parent-adolescent relationships, and the second pertains to the relevance of experienced parenting and discussed in the next section.

Experienced parenting. Shared source variance concerns notwithstanding, the conceptualization of parenting as perceived by adolescents has become a common approach in research on adolescents' parenting (e.g., Chao, 2001; Gray & Steinberg, 1999; Silk, Morris, Kanaya, & Steinberg, 2003). The endorsement of this approach weighs the *methodological assumption* that shared source variance inflates observed relationships between variables against the *psychological premise* on the meaning of experienced environment underlying self theory, social learning approach (Bandura, 1986) as well as early and more recent research on child development (e.g., Bronfenbrenner, 1979; Thomas, 1928), personality (e.g., Kelly, 1955; Rotter, 1981) and social psychology (Lewin, 1936).

Particularly relevant to this approach are Murray's (1938) distinction between *alpha* press and *beta* press corresponding to the objective and subjectively experienced environments, respectively, and attribution researchers' (e.g., Jones & Nisbett, 1971; Kelley, 1967) distinction between realities as experienced by the actor and appraised by the observer. Consequently, the parenting model presented here focuses on experienced parenting, as reported by adolescents. As its empirical estimates show, the model applies to girls and boys across various cultural settings.

The Five-Step Model of Future Orientation Parenting

The initial model (Seginer, 2005; Seginer et al., 2004) consists of five steps: perceived positive parenting (in some studies indexed as autonomous-accepting and in others as authoritative parenting), self-evaluation, and the motivational, cognitive representation, and behavioral components of future orientation. The model (Fig. 5.1) depicts a process through which perceived positive parenting is directly linked to self-evaluation, and via it to the motivational, cognitive, and behavioral components of future orientation. As described in Chap. 1, the motivational component of future orientation is directly linked to the cognitive representation and behavioral components, and indirectly – via cognitive representation – to the behavioral component. The rationale underlying the relations between parenting, self-evaluation and future orientation is described in the following sections.

Positive parenting. Positive parenting, described in terms of autonomous-accepting parenting or authoritative parenting, subsumes parental involvement/acceptance, strictness/supervision, limit setting, and autonomy granting (Chao, 2001; Gray & Steinberg, 1989; Steinberg, Lamborn, Dornbusch, & Darling, 1992). Across the years researchers have conceptualized it in two ways: as *enacted* by parents and observed in quasi-experimental settings (Allen, Hauser, Bell, & O'Connor, 1994; Grotevant & Cooper, 1985, 1986, 1998) and as *perceived* and reported by adolescents (e.g., Gray & Steinberg, 1999). Both approaches show that adolescents' self-esteem and ego development (Allen et al., 1994), psychosocial development (Gray & Steinberg, 1999), and identity exploration (Grotevant & Cooper, 1985, 1986, 1998) are positively linked to positive parenting.

The indirect relations between positive parenting and future orientation. The proposition that positive parenting (PoPa) is indirectly related to future orientation draws on two sets of relations that are theoretically sound and empirically substantiated. The first is between positive parenting and adolescents' self as individuals learn to know it through interaction with their subjectively constructed social environment. Parents' primacy in shaping children's conception of self draws on their continuous and stable relationships and has been empirically supported by findings showing that both observed (Allen et al., 1994; Grotevant & Cooper, 1985, 1986, 1998) and perceived (Gray & Steinberg, 1999) positive parenting are related to several indicators of adolescent competence, including self-esteem (Allen et al., 1994). The effect of various indices of perceived positive parenting on self-evaluation

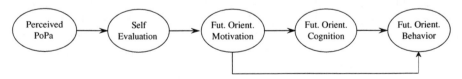

Fig. 5.1 The perceived positive parenting (PoPa) future orientation model

has been also substantiated by recent studies conducted in different cultural settings (Farruggia, Chen, Greenberger, Dmitrieva, & Macek, 2004; Laible, Carlo, & Roesch, 2004; Laursen, Furman, & Mooney, 2006; Shek, 2007).

The relation between the self and future orientation has been extensively discussed in Chap. 3. As noted there, conceptually this relation draws on the premise that self-evaluation is one of several indicators of emotional health (Grotevant, 1998) and the empirically supported conjecture (Melges, 1982; Nuttin & Lens, 1985; Seginer, 2003) that individuals' ability to engage concomitantly in present demands emanating from their social roles, interpersonal relationships and cognitive activity and think, plan, hope and be concerned about the future requires a fair amount of emotional health.

As discussed earlier in Chap. 3, the relevance of self-evaluation draws on the observation that evaluation is central to human thinking (James, 1890; Harter, 1999; Osgood, Suci, & Tannenbaum, 1971) and that the tendency to evaluate other individuals, experiences and objects in context extends also to oneself. Engaged in this process individuals use the same good-bad, positive-negative or beautiful-ugly criteria they employ for evaluating other individuals and objects. This process becomes especially relevant in adolescence when behavior is guided by self-evaluation rather than – as in childhood – by parental behavior (Harter, 1999; Higgins, 1991). However, the effect of parents, peers and other closely related people does not disappear altogether. Instead it becomes indirect: interaction with these figures continues to shape adolescents' self-evaluation (e.g., Harter, 1999) which in turn affects future orientation thinking.

Links between self-evaluation and future orientation. The relations between the various aspects of the self and future orientation are presented in Chap. 3. Underlying are the generalized effect that self-evaluation has on individuals' functioning and specific considerations particularly related to the motivational component of future orientation. However, as discussed in detail in Chap. 3, self evaluation has multiple expressions. Shoyer (2001, 2006) has identified the relevance of two of them to future orientation: self-esteem and self-agency (Harter, 1999; Stern, 1985).

Self-agency is especially relevant to adolescents and underscores their specific need for assuming responsibility and developing a sense of self-reliance and independence. Thus conceptualized self agency is akin to Fromm's (1941) sense of *freedom to* (rather than the less mature *freedom from*) and to Grotevant and Cooper's (1986, 1998) process of individuality and connectedness.

Consequently, the value individuals attribute themselves – as expressed in self-esteem and self-agency – extends to the value they give to instrumental (work and career) and relational (marriage and family) adult roles, to the confidence that hopes, goals, and plans related to these prospective roles will materialize and to a sense of internal control over behavior outcomes. Our data have shown that self evaluation also affects instrumental emerging adulthood future domains such as higher education for Israeli Arab girls (Mahajna, 2007 described below; Seginer & Mahajna, 2003, 2004) and military service for Israeli Jewish adolescents (Ablin, 2006).

Empirical Estimates of the Model

This model has been empirically estimated by several studies; in each, the fit of the data to the model is tested by structural equation modeling (SEM) on data pertaining to two future life domains: higher education or work and career (instrumental domain), and marriage and family (relational domain). Common to the three studies described below is that latent (theoretical) variables are each linked to two or three manifest (empirical) variables with sufficiently high loadings. For space and clarity reasons and to avoid redundancy here as well as in Chaps. 6 and 7, only a selection of the empirical estimates figures is presented.

Study I: Israeli Jewish girls and boys. The first study (Seginer et al., 2004; Shoyer, 2001) to estimate this model was carried out among 458 Israeli Jewish high school students (224 girls and 234 boys) who grew up in small, educated, urban middle class families. At time of data collection respondents were all 11th graders in a matriculation-track (college-bound) program in two urban high schools serving middle class residential areas and expected to do their compulsory military service upon graduating from high school. That meant postponing entry into higher education by at least 2 years for girls and 3 years for boys.

Empirical estimates were carried out on work and career (instrumental domain) and marriage and family (relational domain) separately for girls and boys showing that, as predicted, for all four empirical models self-evaluation is positively related to the motivational component but not to the cognitive and behavioral components. Testing an alternative model in which self-evaluation is omitted and positive parenting is directly linked to the three future orientation components resulted in nonsignificant paths between positive parenting and the future orientation components. Thus, positive parenting affects future orientation only indirectly via adolescents' self evaluation. In addition, the across time changes in gender differences (Chap. 4) are also reflected in the findings of this study. Overall, the empirically estimated models of girls and boys do not differ, except for one link: the effect of mothers' positive parenting on boys' self-evaluation and via it on the motivational component of future orientation is stronger for boys than for girls.

Study II: Israeli Jewish Adolescents. In a second study that tested this model, data were collected from matriculation-track (college-bound) adolescents (N = 358, 215 girls) who described future orientation pertaining to the two life domains of work and career, and marriage and family, and positive parenting as defined by three empirical variables: autonomy, acceptance, and limit setting. Like in the Seginer et al. (2004) study, the proposition has been that positive parenting is indirectly linked to future orientation via two aspects of the self: self esteem and self agency (Shoyer, 2001, 2006). The analysis – carried out separately for mothers and fathers – shows a good fit of the empirical models and indicates that positive parenting is linked to the motivational component of future orientation via both self esteem and self agency (Fig. 5.2, for fathers' results only).

These findings reiterate the effect of perceived positive parenting on self evaluation and via it on future orientation. Adolescents holding high self-evaluation also value more highly the two adult roles of work and career and marriage and family,

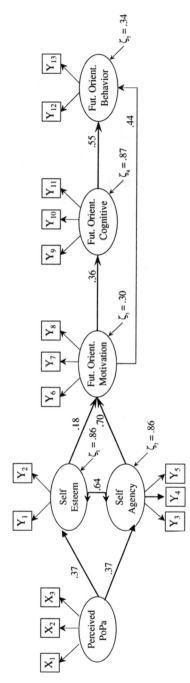

Fig. 5.2 Empirical estimate for a model of perceived positive parenting (PoPa) (father) and work and career future orientation: Jewish adolescents. X_1 = perceived positive parenting/acceptance; X_2 = perceived positive parenting/granted autonomy; X_3 = perceived positive parenting/limit setting re peers relations; Y_1 = self esteem/positive; Y_2 = self esteem/negative; Y_3 = self agency/independence; Y_4 = self agency/self reliance; Y_5 = self agency/self assurance; Y_6 = value; Y_7 = expectance; Y_8 = internal control; Y_9 = my future occupation; Y_{10} = my future professional career; Y_{11} = my future workplace; Y_{12} = exploration; Y_3 = commitment. Factors loadings (lambdas) range from .36 to .94; N = 358; χ^2 (97) = 246.11; p <.000; RMSEA = .07; CFI = .93

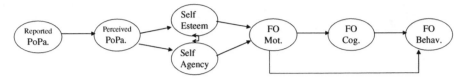

Fig. 5.3 The parent reported and adolescent perceived positive parenting (PoPa) future orientation model. Reported PoPa = positive parenting as reported by parents; perceived PoPa = positive parenting as perceived and reported by adolescents

feel more confident that their hopes, goals and plans in each of these domains will materialize and consider themselves responsible for fulfilling these hopes, goals and plans. Indirectly the two aspects of the self also prompt thinking about each of these domains (the cognitive component) and involvement in exploring future options and making a decision regarding each domain (the behavioral component).

Study III: Israeli Jewish adolescents and their parents. Shoyer (2006) extended the study of the effect of perceived positive parenting on future orientation by asking about the effect of positive parenting as reported by parents. This led her to construct a six-step model in which parenting as reported by parents preceded the adolescents' perceived positive parenting variable (Fig. 5.3).

Its empirical estimate shows that the effect of parents' reported parenting on future orientation for both the work and career and the marriage and family domains is *indirect* and linked to self esteem and self-agency and consequently to the three future orientation components only via adolescents' perceived parenting. Thus, whereas adolescent perceived parenting is indirectly linked to future orientation via the two self-evaluation variables (self-esteem and self-agency), parents' reported parenting is indirectly linked to future orientation via adolescent perceived parenting and the two self evaluation variables.

However, when reported parenting is included, mothers' perceived parenting is also *directly* linked to the motivational component for both the work and career and the marriage and family domains. The differential relationship between mothers and fathers and their adolescent children – reported in several studies (e.g., Youniss & Smollar, 1985) – is reiterated in these findings and indicates its validity outside the United States and one generation later. It also underscores the greater meaning relationship with mothers than with fathers have for these adolescents as they construct their future. In light of Larson, Moneta, Richards, Holmbeck, and Duckett (1996) findings that adolescents spend twice as much time with mother than with father, it may also reiterate Pulkkinen's (1990) findings that time spent with parents have a positive effect on several aspects of future orientation.

Future Orientation Multi-Step Model in Cultural Context

Our next question has been whether the multi-step model initially constructed to describe parenting effect on the future orientation of western adolescents also fits nonwestern adolescents, in particular traditional and transition to modernity groups.

This question has been examined on three samples of Israeli Arab adolescents and emerging adults: the first consisted of over 200 Arab (mostly belonging to Arab Christian communities) emerging adult women and men (Margieh, 2007), the second of over 700 Moslem Arab girls (Mahajna, 2007), and the third of 891 Moslem Arab girls and boys (Seginer, Shoyer, & Mahajna, 2008). Recently, the model has also been tested on a sample of 819 ultra-orthodox Jewish girls who belong to the chabad community and attend its all-girl high schools (Dekel, 2009).

Study I: Arab emerging adults. Margieh's analysis replicated the Israeli Jewish adolescents' empirical model, showing that perceived positive parenting affects adolescents' future orientation via adolescents' self evaluation (indexed as self esteem) for both the higher education and the marriage and family domains.

Study II: Moslem Arab adolescent girls. Mahajna's (2007) study took a different point of departure and consequently presented a more complex picture. Aware of the cultural uniqueness and diversity of the Israeli Moslem society, he designed his research to examine two additional issues. One addressed within-cultural differences of the effect of parenting on future orientation. Assuming the relevance of empowerment to the reality of Moslem girls, the second issue addressed self evaluation in terms of *psychological empowerment.*

By assessing parents' education, mother employment and sib size, Mahajna identified three social settings: traditional (low level of mother and father education, mother does not hold a paid job, and large sib size), transition-to-modernity (mother and father have higher level of education than traditional parents, mother does not hold a paid job, smaller sib size) and modern (mother and father have higher education, mother holds a paid job as a teacher or secretary, and a small sib size).

However, possibly because of generations of Moslem tradition influence and the recentness of higher education and women employment, these demographic characteristics did not result in differences in the effect of parenting on future orientation, and the future orientation parenting model is empirically estimated for all three social settings. Differences are found however between the domains: psychological empowerment links parenting and future orientation pertaining to higher education but not to marriage and family.

The relevance of this finding is underscored by analyses of Israeli Arab girls' hopes and fears narratives. As they spontaneously defended their desire for higher education the phrase "education is a weapon in women's hands" repeated itself across several cohorts (Mahajna, 2007; Seginer & Mahajna, 2003, 2004), thus indicating their awareness of the pertinence of psychological empowerment to prospective higher education.

Study III: Moslem Arab adolescent girls and boys. Our third study (Seginer et al., 2008) examines the future orientation multiple step model also for Israeli Arab boys. In this model the self is indicated by two theoretical variables: self esteem and psychological empowerment. Its empirical estimates show two findings worth noting: that the theoretical model is estimated for girls and boys and for both life domains (higher education, and marriage and family), and that psychological empowerment – initially introduced to the study of future orientation of Israeli Arab girls by Mahajna (Mahajna, 2000, 2007; Seginer & Mahajna, 2003, 2004) is

a. Girls

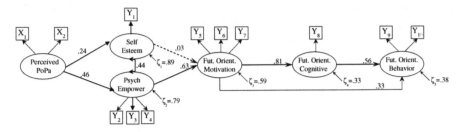

b. Boys

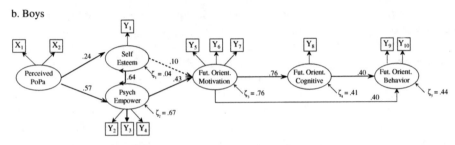

Fig. 5.4 Empirical estimate for a model of perceived positive parenting (PoPa) (parents) and higher education future orientation: Arab adolescents. X_1 = perceived positive parenting/acceptance; X_2 = perceived positive parenting/granted autonomy; Y_1 = self esteem; Y_2 = psychological empower/intrapersonal; Y_3 = psychological empower/interpersonal; Y_4 = psychological empower/behavioral; Y_5 = value; Y_6 = expectance; Y_7 = internal control; Y_8 = cognitive representation; Y_9 = exploration; Y_{10} = commitment. Factors loadings (lambdas) range from .48 to .96; **a.** N = 585; χ^2 (48) = 181.25; p < .001; RMSEA = .07; CFI = .95; **b.** N = 306; χ^2 (48) = 136.61; p < .001; RMSEA = .08; CFI = .94

particularly relevant for girls (Figs. 5.4). This is indicated by the stronger links for girls than for boys between psychological empowerment and between psychological empowerment and the motivational component.

Study IV: Israeli Jewish chabad adolescent girls. Chabad youth grow up in a social setting where individuals and families are guided by strict observance of religious law and Rabbinical authority. Girls and boys attend separate schools; as they reach adolescence boys attend the *Yeshiva* and girls an all-girls high school that offers both religious and general college-bound curriculum. Although the nature of their traditional reality is considerably different from that of the Moslem girls, empirical estimates of the future orientation model with data collected from them similarly show the greater relevance of psychological empowerment than of self esteem for future orientation. Specifically, while perceived positive parenting affects both self esteem and psychological empowerment, only psychological empowerment is positively linked to the motivational component of future orientation for both the work and career and marriage and family domains (Dekel, 2009).

a. Girls

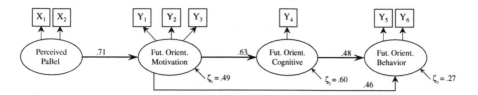

b. Boys

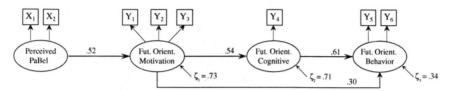

Fig. 5.5 Empirical estimate for a model of perceived parental beliefs (PaBe) and higher education future orientation: Arab adolescents. X_1 = mothers' beliefs; X_2 = fathers' beliefs; Y_1 = value; Y_2 = expectance; Y_3 = internal control; Y_4 = cognitive representation; Y_5 = exploration; Y_6 = commitment. Factors loadings (lambdas) range from .40 to .97; **a.** N = 585; χ^2 (17) = 45.87; p < .001; RMSEA = .05; CFI = .98; **b.** N = 306; χ^2 (17) = 44.20; p < .001; RMSEA = .07; CFI = .97

Summary. The validity of the multiple parenting and future orientation model has been supported by analyses of data collected from several (altogether nine) groups of Israeli Arab and Jewish adolescents. While the model depicting the indirect effect of parenting on future orientation via the self is satisfactorily estimated for all groups, cultural differences can be identified, particularly regarding gender differences (more prevalent among Arab than among Jewish adolescents) and the role of psychological empowerment for Arab and ultra-orthodox Jewish girls, and of self agency for Jewish adolescents.

Parents' Beliefs and Adolescents' Future Orientation

Beliefs pertain to the ideas and subjective knowledge individuals hold about a specific issue. Their effectiveness comes from their nature; as described by Goodnow and Collins:

> ...[they] are often marked by a touch of myth, are linked to action, have a possible "executive" function, are suffused with affect, and are often accompanied by a sense of attachment and ownership on the part of the believers. (Goodnow & Collins, 1990, p. 12).

Underlying a wide variety of conceptual approaches to beliefs has been a core definition that refers to their origin, evolvement, and structure. Beliefs are based on personal and cultural knowledge, their construction occurs in an ongoing process of exchange with other individuals and societal institutions, and their stability is maintained by assimilating new experiences into current beliefs. So conceptualized, beliefs have a dual function: they organize *individuals'* thinking and guide their behavior, and consequently also affect *socio-cultural* stability.

Parental beliefs. Parental beliefs consist of the ideas, expectations, and subjective knowledge individuals hold about issues relevant to their role as parents (McGillicuddy-De Lisi & Sigel, 1995). However, although researchers examine the direct effect of parental beliefs on children's and adolescents' outcomes, this effect is at least in part indirect and occurs as a result of parents' belief-prompted behaviors (Seginer, 1986b). These behaviors affect child outcomes either directly or – as suggested by Goodnow and Collins (1990) – by creating conditions that instigate child outcomes. In all, the parents' beliefs-child behavior relations draw their strength from the multiple paths – some direct and other indirect – between them.

Parents' beliefs consist of four broad categories: beliefs about *social issues* relevant to children's development, *parenting* and *child rearing*, *children* as a social category, and beliefs about each individual *child*. Each of these belief categories is affected by parents' personal knowledge, developmental folk theories and cultural values, and child characteristics. Although research on the effect of parental beliefs on adolescents' future orientation may address all four categories, to date much of it has been carried out on the effect of parents' beliefs about women's roles and hence applies particularly to girls.

At an earlier stage (Seginer & Mahajna, 2004) this research was guided by two premises. The first is that the effect of parents' beliefs on adolescent future orientation is mediated by adolescents' beliefs. The second is that while girls' beliefs about women's roles are relevant to all three future orientation components regarding both instrumental (higher education, work and career) and relational (marriage and family) domains, these effects differs in two major ways. First, girls' beliefs are directly related only to the motivational component of future orientation and via it to the cognitive representation and behavioral components. Second, traditional beliefs are negatively (inversely) linked to instrumental domains' future orientation and positively linked to marriage and family future orientation.

Empirical Studies

The effect of parents' beliefs about women's roles on future orientation has been examined in two studies of Israeli Arab girls (Mahajna, 2007; Seginer & Mahajna, 2004, Seginer et al., 2008) and one study of Israeli Jewish ultra-orthodox girls (Dekel, 2009). In the Arab studies parental beliefs pertain to girls' two competing trajectories: higher education and early marriage. The relevance of these beliefs to Arab girls' future orientation regarding higher education and work and career drew on the tension between women's traditional roles as wives and mothers and the girls' pursuit of equal opportunities for education and career (Buhrke, 1988; Spence

& Hahn, 1997). In the Jewish study beliefs pertained to women's roles. The effect of these beliefs on Arab and Jewish girls' future orientation is described below.

Arab girls Study I (Seginer & Mahajna, 2004). In this study respondents are high school students (age 16–18) from rural traditional families characterized by high devotion to Islam (high religiosity), parents' low level of education and occupation and large sib size. The patriarchal nature of the Israeli Arab society (e.g., Barakat, 1993; Haj-Yahia, 2002) – indicated by fathers' acting as authority figures and chief decision makers within their families, especially pronounced in traditional families – led us to focus in this study on fathers' beliefs as perceived by their adolescent daughters.

Guided by findings that across different cultural settings and age groups women express more liberal beliefs than men and endorse women's rights for equality of opportunities (e.g., McHugh & Frieze, 1997; Tashakkori & Thompson, 1991) the prediction has been that girls will perceive their fathers' beliefs regarding women's roles as relatively conservative. Nonetheless, perceived fathers' beliefs will have a direct effect on girls' beliefs and via it on future orientation.

The postulated link between perceived fathers' and girls' beliefs about women's roles drew on two culture-specific considerations. The first has been that as their daughters approach age 17 (Israeli minimum marriage age for women) the beliefs of traditional Arab fathers about women's roles – as they apply to the choice between higher education and early marriage – become particularly salient and known to their daughters. The second consideration has been that in traditional settings the relation between parents' and children's beliefs is inadvertently supported by the endorsement of these beliefs by other social settings as well.

Although empirical estimates show a good fit of the estimates to the model, perceived parental beliefs are *not* related to girls' beliefs. Instead, they are directly related to girls' academic achievement (see also Chap. 7 on future orientation outcomes). Our explanation for these results rests on a cultural perspective and draws on Cashmore and Goodnow's (1985) study on the beliefs of parents and adolescents from Anglo-Australian and Italian-Australian groups.

Their findings show that, compared to girls of Anglo-Australians background (parents born in Australia), girls of Italian-Australian background (parents emigrated from southern Italy to Australia as adults) have low actual and perceived agreement with their parents' beliefs. Thus, Cashmore and Goodnow's as well as our results suggest that in both settings girls adapted to social change faster than did parents. Consequently, standing at the crossroad of traditionality and social change, rural Arab girls distance themselves from fathers' perceived beliefs. Nonetheless, although girls' thinking (indexed by beliefs and future orientation) is not affected by fathers' perceived beliefs, their behavior (indexed by academic achievement) did.

Arab girls Study II (Mahajna, 2007; Seginer et al., 2008). Like in Study I, this analysis focuses on Israeli Arab adolescent girls (age 16–18, N = 617) but differs from it in two major ways: participants' demographic characteristics and the definition of parental beliefs. In Study I respondents all lived in rural traditional families and parental beliefs have been defined in terms of fathers' beliefs as perceived by girls. In Study II respondents represent a wider range of socioeconomic characteristics extending from traditional to transition to modernity and modern families (low religiosity, parents' level of education above high school, both mothers and fathers hold white collar or professional jobs, and small sib size), and parental beliefs are defined in terms of mothers' and fathers' beliefs as both reported by them and perceived by girls. Consequently, the path through which parents' beliefs affect girls' future orientation can also be examined for parents' *reported* beliefs.

Analyses carried out for the higher education and marriage and family future orientation domains show that parents' *reported* beliefs are linked to the motivational component of future orientation both directly and indirectly via girls' perceived parental beliefs (Seginer et al., 2008). However, generational disparity is particularly indicated for the higher education domain. Although parents' reported beliefs are linked to girls' perceived beliefs and to the motivational component, both links are *negative*, indicating that parents least endorsing higher education prompt their daughters to perceive parents as providing high support for higher education, to develop high value for higher education and believe that their chances to materialize higher education hopes, goals, and plans are high and under own control (motivational component).

The time elapsed between data collection in Studies I and II and socioeconomic differences may explain why in Study II (but not in Study I) *perceived* as well as *reported* parental beliefs are directly related to the motivational component of future orientation for both domains (as well as to academic achievement). Nonetheless, the negative links between parents' reported beliefs, girls' perceived beliefs and the motivational component found in Study II indicate that the tension between parents and adolescent girls has not subsided but rather changed its markers.

Jewish ultra-orthodox girls (Dekel, 2009). This study was conducted among ultra-orthodox 10th to 12th grade (age 16–18) high school girls (N = 819). As noted earlier, these girls grow up in a social setting governed by strict observance of religious law and Rabbinical authority and attend all-girls schools. Like the traditional Arab girls in Study I they describe their own and their parents' beliefs about women's roles, and like in Study I the hypothesis has been that perceived parental beliefs affect adolescent girls' future orientation. Dekel's findings show that the model is estimated for both the work and career and marriage and family domains, but the links between beliefs and the motivational component of future orientation are domain specific.

For the work and career domain, perceived parental beliefs are linked to the motivational component only indirectly via girls' beliefs, whereas for the marriage and family domain, perceived parental beliefs are directly linked to girls' beliefs and to the motivational component, and were the sole link to it. In other words, for these Jewish ultra-orthodox girls the value of marriage and family, and the subjective probability of and control over materializing hopes, goals, and plans regarding it are affected by how girls perceived their parents' beliefs about women's roles and not by how they construct their own beliefs.

Arab girls and boys (Seginer et al., 2008). Although the pressure on Israeli Arab girls to marry early is stronger than on boys, both are expected to abide by traditional familistic values. Therefore, recently Seginer et al. (2008) have extended their analysis of the effect of parental beliefs on future orientation to boys. With one exception pertaining to a significantly stronger link between parental beliefs endorsing higher education and the motivational component of future orientation higher education (girls higher than boys), the empirical estimates of the parental beliefs model (Fig. 5.5) is similar for girls and boys.

However, predictions that the effect of parental beliefs endorsing higher education will be *negatively* related to the motivational component of marriage and family future orientation, and will be higher for girls than for boys, have not been corroborated. Instead, the model cannot be estimated for girls; for boys the model is empirically estimated and the *positive* link between parental beliefs and the motivational component is sustained. Thus, while for boys parental beliefs endorsing higher education are an asset relevant for marriage and family as for higher education, for this cohort of girls, parental beliefs endorsing higher education are found to be irrelevant for their future orientation about marriage and family.

Parents' Beliefs and Adolescents' Future Orientation: Summary

At this point, our knowledge about the effect of parental beliefs on adolescents' future orientation draws mainly (but not solely) on studies that examined girls from two distinct socio-cultural settings: Israeli Arab and Jewish ultra-orthodox. Their nature as undergoing social change (Israeli Arab community) and holding to religious faith and lifestyle in the midst of secular society (Jewish ultra-orthodox community) made parental beliefs about women's roles particularly pertinent antecedents of future orientation about instrumental (higher education, work and career) domains and to a lesser extent also of the relational (marriage and family) domain. Our studies show that parental beliefs about women's roles, be they reported by parents or perceived by their daughters, affect future orientation. Nevertheless, the nature of the links between beliefs and future orientation is domain and cohort specific.

In the Israeli Arab society, in transition from traditionality to modernity and challenged by issues of national identity, parents' *reported* beliefs affect girls' future orientation only indirectly via girls' *perceived* beliefs. For the Jewish ultra-orthodox girls, parents' perceived beliefs affect future orientation for both domains but the structure of the effect is domain-specific. Motivation to engage in future orientation about work and career is affected by perceived parental beliefs indirectly via girls' beliefs and motivation to engage in future orientation about marriage and family is directly affected by perceived parental beliefs but not by girls' beliefs.

The applicability of the perceived parental beliefs model to Arab boys has been tested recently, showing its relevance for the motivational component of both higher education and marriage and family domains. However, given that the effect of parental beliefs is stronger in collectivistic societies where beliefs are commonly shared by the community, the effect of parental beliefs on adolescent future orientation must be examined in other social settings as well.

Intergenerational Transmission of Future Orientation

While socialization or family context research asks how family processes affect child outcomes, intergenerational transmission research focuses on child outcomes and asks whether children's attitudes, beliefs, or behavior are congruent with those of parents. In other words, the question is whether serving as a social learning setting, families, and particularly parents, facilitate the conservation of those aspects of cultural orientations and behavior patterns endorsed by them. Applied to future orientation this research is based on two assumptions. The first is that out of concern for their adolescent children parents are involved in future thinking about them which relates to the three future orientation components, and the second is that in the process of family interaction, parents communicate their views about adolescents' future orientation and consequently influence adolescents' future orientation constructions.

The extent to which adolescents' future orientation is congruent with the future orientation parents constructed for them has been examined in six studies carried out in five different cultural settings.

The German Setting

The first study to examine parent-adolescent congruence was conducted by Trommsdorff (1983). Comparing the responses of adolescents (15–17 years old) and their mothers to future orientation questionnaires (in which mothers related to their daughters' or sons' future orientation), Trommsdorff found that mothers and adolescents constructed different future orientation images. Particularly, mothers anticipated earlier timing of future events (both hoped for and feared of) than did adolescents and were overall more optimistic than adolescents about the distant future. However, mothers' optimism was also affected by their child's gender. Regarding both the near and the distant future, mothers were more optimistic about their sons' than about their daughters' futures.

The Italian Setting

The relation between parents' and adolescents' future orientation in the Italian setting must be understood in the context of Italian ideas about parents' responsibilities toward their adolescent and emerging adulthood children. As emphasized by Scabini "parents bear the fundamental task of guiding young people with respect to future choices and providing direction to their child's growth" (Scabini, Marta, & Lanz, 2006, p. 90).

Analysis of the future orientation of Italian adolescents and their parents (Lanz, Rosnati, Marta, & Scabini, 2001; Scabini et al., 2006) resulted in three important findings. First, higher congruence in listing hopes (only 22–27% of the domains listed by parents and adolescents were dissimilar) than in listing fears (62–65%

of the domains listed by parents and adolescents were dissimilar). Second, parents and adolescents agree on the three core domains (education, work and career, and marriage and family) but while parents focus mainly on these three, the future orientation of adolescents is more elaborate and includes more domains such as social relationships and sex, as well as more narratives. Third, in contrast to Trommsdorff's (1983) findings about German mothers, Italian parents expected their children (both girls and boys) to assume transition to adulthood (higher education) and adulthood (work and career, marriage and family) roles at an *older* age than did adolescents. In addition, Italian parents had less confidence in their children's internal control over future education and career but were more optimistic than their children regarding goal realization.

The Finnish Setting

Employing the global (rather than domain-specific) approach to future orientation, Malmberg, Ehrman, and Lithen (2005) examined intergenerational transmission by relating to two aspects of adolescent future orientation as reported by adolescents and their parents: the importance of adolescents' future goals and the probability of attaining them. Intergenerational transmission is indexed by similarity and associations. Specifically, the researchers assessed the extent to which adolescents and parents similarly scored on the importance of goals and probability of attainment, and the relations between all four indices.

Overall their findings concur with those found for all other cultural groups: in certain aspects, but not all, the future orientation of adolescents and their parents are similar and interrelated. However, these researchers go one step further by specifying how parents affect adolescents' future orientation. Thus, the effect of parents' estimate of goal fulfillment on adolescents' goals is both direct and mediated by adolescent-parent relationships, and adolescent-parent relationships also affect adolescents' estimate of goal fulfillment.

The Israeli Setting

In the Israeli setting the analysis of future orientation transmission was examined in two ways. Following the work of Trommsdorff and Scabini et al., the first approach focused on the similarity between parents' and adolescents' future orientation scores and assessed adolescent-parent congruence. The second approach focused on the three component model and examined the relations between adolescents' and parents' scores and correspondence between adolescents and parents empirical models.

The congruence approach. Given the pivotal role of the motivational component in linking between both family and intrapersonal variables and future orientation, the congruence approach focused on the three variables subsumed under it: value, expectance, and control. By examining congruence between adolescents' (Jewish, 11th graders) and parents' endorsement of the motivational variables for four domains – military service, higher education, work and career, and marriage and family – Schlesinger's (2001) study highlighted the multiple aspects of future orientation congruence. Considering domains, *higher education* was the domain on which *in*congruence was most pronounced and *military service* the domain on which parents and adolescents were most congruent. Addressing variables, *expectance* (indexing subjective probability of materializing hopes, goals, and plans) was the variable on which parents and adolescents were incongruent in all four domains. However, regardless of domain or variable, parents consistently scored higher than their adolescent children.

Mahajna's (2007) study of Israeli Arab high school girls and their parents focused on parents-adolescents' congruence on only one domain: higher education. His results show that congruence is variable dependent. Parents attribute lower value to higher education than do their daughters. Like Israeli Jewish, German and Italian parents, they are more optimistic about the materialization of their daughters' hopes, goals, and plans, but like their Jewish counterparts (Schlesinger, 2001) appraise internal control as high as do their daughters.

Summary

While in some specific aspects parents and adolescents similarly construct adolescents' future orientation, overall adolescents do not draw on their parents' future orientation. Thus, although parents are concerned with their children's future and are able to translate this concern into motivational, cognitive, and behavioral aspects of future orientation in various prospective domains, these constructions are only partly associated with their adolescent children's future orientation. Underlying these findings are two psychological processes. The first is described by *social learning* theory contending that recurrent family interaction leads adolescents to model their future orientation after that constructed for them by parents. The second is described by *attribution theory* and its analysis of actors-observers differences (Jones & Nisbett, 1971). Applied to adolescents and parents, while some of the relevant information underlying the construction of future orientation is commonly shared by adolescents and their parents, other information is unique to each.

Thus, regardless of the nature of parent-adolescent relationships, parents' knowledge of their children's experiences and feelings is limited. Moreover, as underlined by Jones and Nisbett, even when actor (adolescent) and observer (parent) hold similar information, they differ in the *salience* of various aspects of that information. Consequently, adolescents and parents process the information differently and altogether approach the construction of future orientation from different perspectives.

The Three-Component Model: Parent-Adolescent Correspondence

Asking parents about the future orientation they wished for their children, Shoyer (2006) examined the correspondence to adolescents' future orientation in two domains: work and career (instrumental) and marriage and family (relational). Her findings showed that parents' wished-for future orientation affected adolescents' future orientation in two ways. The first relates to the *model structure*, showing that it holds for both parents and adolescents. Specifically, the motivational component is directly linked to the cognitive and behavioral components and the cognitive component is directly related to the behavioral component when the model is estimated for both. The one exception is the model for fathers' wished-for *career* future orientation which consists of only two components: motivational and cognitive.

The second parents-adolescents relation pertains to each of the components. This analysis shows that such relations exist for mothers but not for fathers. Specifically, mothers' *cognitive* component is directly related to adolescents' cognitive component for both work and career and the marriage and family domains. For the work and career domain (but not for the marriage and family domain) mothers' *behavioral* component (pertaining to the exploration and commitment acts mothers think need to be carried out) is directly linked to adolescents' work and career behavioral component.

These findings suggest three conclusions. First, mothers' but not fathers' wished-for future orientation components are congruent and possibly affect adolescents' future orientation. Second, the effect of mothers' wished-for future orientation on adolescents' future orientation is maintained only for the cognitive and behavioral components. Third, adolescents' motivational component is (indirectly) affected by positive parenting and not by mothers' wished-for future orientation motivational component.

Drawing on Trommsdorff's (1983) question whether adolescent-parent relationships affect similarity between their future orientation, Shoyer (2006) compared the effect of mothers' on adolescents' future orientation for adolescents who described adolescent-parent relationships as high vs low. Her findings show that, for the work and career domain, the effect of mothers' cognitive component (how often she thinks and talks about career issues) is positive only for adolescents who experienced high parent-adolescent relationships.

For the marriage and family domain, however, a positive effect of mothers' on adolescents' motivational component is found for the *low* adolescent-parent relationships but not for the high adolescent-parent relationships group. This finding suggests at least two interpretations. One pertains to the multiple faces of adolescent-parent relationships. Adolescents who do not view their relationships with mother as positive nevertheless keep their relationships with them by sharing values, expectancy and sense of control regarding marriage and family (the motivational component).

The second interpretation relates to adolescent-mother relationship as facilitating similarity between the motivational component of marriage and family. It suggests that while under high positive parent-adolescent relationships adolescents feel free to endorse values and appraise expectance and control over the materialization of hopes and plans regardless of those developed by mothers, under less positive parent-adolescent relationships adolescents feel more obliged to follow their mothers. Alternatively, they may be less confident to develop their own views.

Parents as Models

Although future orientation research does not address modeling, data collected from 11th grade Arab adolescents (Suleiman, 2000) is relevant here. These data show that in response to an open question about career options, girls (n = 129) spontaneously mentioned the following occupations: teacher, sports teacher, English teacher, social worker, medical doctor, pediatrician, dentist, pharmacist, psychologist, journalist and TV announcer, engineer, travel agent, lawyer. By comparison, boys (n = 75) mentioned medical doctor, lawyer, engineer, computer engineer, and accountant. Given that of these adolescents less than one third grew up in families where one or both parents had above high school education, and considering the low prevalence of these professions at present in the Israeli Arab population in general and among women in particular, it is plausible that the majority did not use their parents as models of career.

Thus, as a group, Arab adolescents and especially girls develop an educational and career future orientation that is different from that of their parents' generation. For them, as for other adolescents in the majority world (Kagitcibasi, 1996), future orientation is not an act of intergenerational continuity but rather of bridging multiple worlds (Cooper, in press).

The Meaning of Parent-Child Congruence

Although parent-child congruence has been considered an indicator of intergenerational transmission, it is liable to alternative interpretations (Seginer & Vermulst, 2001). One pertains to confounding which may occur under two conditions: as a result of genetic inheritance or across-cohort value stability (Van IJzendoorn, 1992). The other relates to similarity between values endorsed by the family and societal institutions such as the educational and the political systems. Super and Harkness' (2002) analysis of the developmental niche described it as *across-system regularities*.

To control for their confounding effect when assessing congruence, a statistical procedure has been developed (Lanz, Scabini, Vermulst, & Gerris, 2001; Vermulst, Van Leeuwe, and Lanz, 2003) that compares the mean of the observed congruence score of related dyads (e.g., parent-adolescent) with the mean of expected congruence score of unrelated 'artificial dyads' (e.g., parent of one family and adolescent of another family). Analyses showing significant congruence scores for the parent-child dyad would indicate an intergenerational transmission while analyses showing significant congruence scores for the artificial dyads would indicate a cultural rather than intergenerational transmission.

Statistical analysis cannot inform us about the *process* through which the parent-child dyad has reached its congruence. However, relational psychoanalysis (Gordon, Aron, Mitchell, & Davies, 1998), and educational and developmental research suggest that interpersonal situations as diversified as the psychoanalytic process

(Bromberg, 2006), kindergarten classrooms (Leseman, Rollenberg, & Rispens, 2001), or mother-child interaction (Gini, Oppenheim, & Sagi-Schwartz, 2007) result in the *coconstruction* of meanings. Drawing on this approach, parent-adolescent congruence – to the extent it exists – may indicate a process of *coconstruction* rather than or together with intergenerational transmission of adolescents' future orientation.

Summary: How Parents Facilitate the Construction of Future Orientation

Based on a rich body of knowledge on family socialization and parent-child relationship as facilitating the development of children and adolescents, this chapter focuses on three issues considered pertinent to how adolescent construct future orientation. The first two – pertaining to parent-adolescent relationship and parental beliefs – focused on *conditions* for the construction of future orientation. Studies drawing on this approach have been mainly interested in parents' behavior as experienced by adolescents. However, their results indicate that, given the interactive nature of the family, the extent to which parent-adolescent relationship facilitates the construction of future orientation relates not only to this relationship but also to adolescents' self representation.

Specifically, the effect of parent-adolescent relationship on future orientation is indirect and linked via the adolescents' self. However, the specific aspect of the self linking parenting and future orientation is culture specific: *self esteem* and self agency for Israeli Jewish adolescents who grow up in middle class families and attend the secular school system, and *psychological empowerment* for Moslem high school girls growing up in a society undergoing social change as well as for Jewish ultra-orthodox girls. Conversely, the effect of parental beliefs as reported by parents (Arab participants) and perceived by girls (Arab participants, Jewish participants) has a direct effect on future orientation.

The third issue pertains to the congruence between adolescent future orientation as viewed by parents and constructed by adolescents. Underlying it are two assumptions. One is that parents' future thinking also relates to their children, and the second is that parents communicate their adolescents' future orientation views. Five studies carried out in four cultural settings show that overall parent-adolescent congruence has been limited. Although the pattern of parent-adolescent differences is culture specific, one difference has been found in all studies: compared to their children, parents are more optimistic about their children's future. This may explain why, despite limited similarity, in the one study that examined it, mothers' future orientation for adolescents is positively related to adolescents' future orientation. Finally, the interpretation of congruence as indicating transmission of future orientation from parents to adolescents needs to be expanded and the effects of culture on both and parent-adolescent coconstruction further explored.

Chapter 6
The Effect of Contemporaries: Siblings and Peers

This chapter builds on two observations of wide agreement: that the majority of contemporary children grow up with siblings and that, as children enter school, time spent with peers gradually increases and so does their influence. Obviously then in wishing to understand the effect of the social environment on adolescents' future orientation siblings and peers must be included and their influence relative to each other and to parents must be tested.

Consequently, the chapter is guided by three main questions. The first focuses on the effect of sibling and peer relationships and asks whether each adds to the effect of parents on adolescents' future orientation. The second question concerns the effect of sibling and peer relationship in the context of the other, specifically asking whether each adds to the influence of the other on adolescents' future orientation or alternatively substitutes for it. However, a recent cross-cultural study on of the effect of interpersonal relationships on self-esteem and perceived social support (Seginer, Shoyer, Hossessi; & Tannous, 2007) highlights the cultural relevance of this issue. The study shows that the relative effect of sibling and peer relationship varies across cultures so that the self esteem and social support of adolescents growing up in traditional societies (Israeli Arab and Druze in this case) are affected by sibling more than by peer relationship whereas the self esteem and social support of western (Israeli Jewish) adolescents are affected more by peer than by sibling relationship.

The third question relates to the *joint* effect of parenting, sibling and peer relationships. At issue is whether by sharing similar experiences and facing comparable problems, siblings and peers have greater influence than parents on adolescents' future orientation, or conversely that in spite of developmental changes in adolescents' interpersonal relationships and reduced time spent with parents (Larson et al., 1996), parents remain the most significant figures in adolescents' lives (Collins & Laursen, 2004) and thus relationship with them continue to influence adolescents' future orientation.

Although this chapter focuses on the effect of interpersonal relationships, two other channels through which siblings and peers affect adolescents' future orientation are pertinent: *beliefs* held by them, and direct adolescent-siblings and face-to-face peer interaction. Before setting out to examine how they affect future orientation the significance of sibling and peer relationships to adolescent development is reviewed.

R. Seginer, *Future Orientation*, The Springer Series on Human Exceptionality,
DOI 10.1007/978-0-387-88641-1_6, © Springer Science+Business Media, LLC 2009

Adolescent Sibling Relationship

Although the majority of children and adolescents grow up with siblings, early and middle childhood children spend more time with siblings than with parents (McHale & Crouter, 1996), and relations with siblings last longer than with parents (Lamb & Sutton-Smith, 1982), until 1990 research on sibling relationship has been sparse (Dunn, 2005) particularly relative to research on parent-adolescent relationship (Collins & Laursen, 2004). Underlying it are several reasons.

One is early human development theories that viewed childhood as a socialization opportunity aimed at training youths to be well-socialized adults and parents as the adults in charge of this training (Maccoby, 1994). A second draws on findings indicating adolescents' tendency to spend more time with peers (Larsen et al., 1996). Finally, a methodological consideration pertaining to the multivariate nature of family composition is also relevant here. Children may grow up in small, middle size or large families, in an all-girl, all-boy or mixed gender constellation, be firstborn or youngest, and belong to intact, single-parent or step-parent families. Nonetheless, research that has been carried out focused on two main issues: sibling interaction and the quality of their relationship in the context of age differences, parent-child relationship, and parents' differential treatment.

Sibling interaction. From early age on, sibling relationship is characterized by *complimentarity* (Dunn, 1983) emanating from older siblings' greater competence, power and status. However, although complimentarity remains stable throughout adolescence, its specific nature varies with age and gender. Thus, in early and middle childhood, older siblings and particularly older sisters serve as caretakers and teachers of their younger siblings (e.g., Azmitia & Hesser, 1993; Lamb, 1978); as they reach adolescence, caretaking and teaching are substituted by provision of information and advice about present tasks (Seginer, 1992b, 1998a) and future plans (Tucker, Barber, & Eccles, 1997).

The quality of sibling relationship. Research on the quality of sibling relationship ranging from positive (warmth, support, admiration) to negative (rivalry, jealousy, negative affect) focuses on two main issues: the factors affecting sibling relationship quality and its behavioral and developmental outcomes. Not surprising, positive sibling relationship is associated with positive developmental outcomes particularly reflected in competent peer relationship (Brody, 1998; Yeh & Lempers, 2004) and extreme negative sibling relationship is associated with negative peer relations (Bank, Patterson, & Reid, 1996).

Although some studies indicate the effect of early friendship (Kramer & Kowal, 2005) and peer relationship (Yeh & Lempers, 2004) on adolescent sibling relationship, much of the research has focused on the effect of parent-child relationship (parenting), as described below.

The effect of parenting on sibling relationship. These studies focus on two questions: how parents' differential treatment and parent-child relationship affect sibling relationship?

The overall conclusion has been that differential treatment (i.e., perceiving parents as being warmer or less demanding toward one's siblings) leads to poor sibling relations only when considered unfair (Kowal & Kramer, 1997) and that in child-hood (Brody & Stoneman, 1995; Dunn, 1992) and adolescence (Seginer, 1998a) sib-ling relationship are similar to parent-adolescent relationship. Explanation (Brody, 1998) for these findings (as well as for findings on peer relationship reported below) comes from three psychological approaches: attachment theory (Bowlby, 1973) con-tending that children reconstruct parent-child relationship in other close relation-ships (Sroufe & Fleener, 1986), social learning theory (Bandura, 1977) positing that parent-child relationship serves as a model for other interpersonal relationships, and personality theory proposing that personality characteristics such as child's temperament (Brody, Stoneman, & Burke, 1987) similarly affect all interpersonal relationships.

However, under specific stressful conditions – not always identified in commu-nity samples (Seginer, 1998a) – siblings and especially older siblings may *compen-sate* for relational deficits with others. Such relational deficits may evolve under stressful life events and family relationships (Bank & Kahn, 1982; Bryant, 1992; Dunn, Slomkowski, & Beardsall, 1994; Gass, Jenkins, & Dunn, 2007; Jenkins, 1992), parental stress (Cummings & Smith, 1993), cultural transitions as the case is among Israeli Arabs (Seginer, 1992b), and children's social isolation (East & Rook, 1992).

Overall, as research on sibling relationship has developed, its complex nature, the relevance of parenting, and the processes that moderate and mediate its effect on adolescent outcomes become clearer. As noted in the next section, these issues are particularly relevant to our understanding of the effect of sibling relationship on future orientation.

The Effect of Sibling Relationship on Adolescents' Future Orientation

Given that sibling relationship is one of several family subsystems and that parent-adolescent relationship is relevant to future orientation, two questions are pertinent here: whether the model describing the effect of sibling relationship resembles the model describing the effect of parent-adolescent relationship on future orientation, and whether in a model including both adolescent-parent and adolescent-sibling relationship, sibling relationship affects adolescents' future orientation above and beyond the effect of parent-adolescent relationship (Fig. 6.1)? Two issues should be underscored here. First, following the rationale presented in Chap. 5, the effect

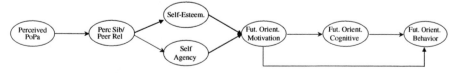

Fig. 6.1 The interpersonal relationships future orientation model

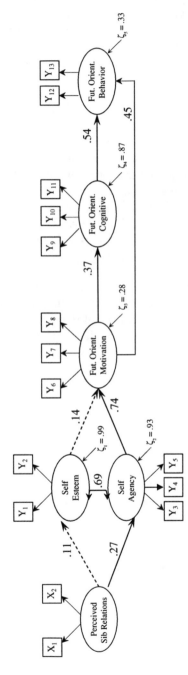

Fig. 6.2 Empirical estimate for a model of perceived sibling relationship, self and work and career future orientation: Jewish adolescents. X_1 = perceived sibling relationship/support; X_2 = perceived sibling relationship/future related; Y_1 = self esteem/future related; Y_1 = self esteem/ positive; Y_2 = self esteem/ negative; Y_3 = self agency/independence; Y_4 = self agency/self reliance; Y_5 = self agency/self assurance; Y_6 = value; Y_7 = expectance; Y_8 = internal control; Y_9 = my future occupation; Y_{10} = my future professional career; Y_{11} = my future workplace; Y_{12} = exploration; Y_{13} = commitment. Factors loadings (lambdas) from .36 to .94; N = 358; χ^2 (82) = 232.21; p < .001; RMSEA = .07; CFI = .92

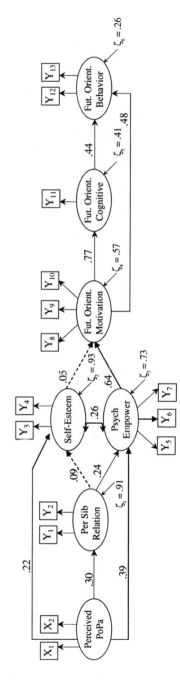

Fig. 6.3 Empirical estimate for a model of perceived positive parenting (PoPa), perceived sibling relationship, self and higher education future orientation: Arab adolescent girls. X_1 = perceived positive parenting/acceptance; X_2 = perceived positive parenting/granted autonomy; Y_1 = perceived sibling relationship/positive; Y_2 = perceived sibling relationship/future related; Y_3 = self esteem/positive; Y_4 = self esteem/positive; Y_5 = psychological empower/intrapersonal; Y_6 = psychological empower/interpersonal; Y_7 = psychological empower/behavioral; Y_8 = value; Y_9 = expectance; Y_{10} = internal control; Y_{11} = my future education; Y_{12} = exploration; Y_{13} = commitment Factors loadings (lambdas) from .37 to .98; N = 585; χ^2 (68) = 203.43; p < .001; RMSEA = .06; CFI = .96

of all interpersonal relationships (i.e., parent-adolescent, sibling and peer relationships) are conceptualized and assessed as experienced and perceived by adolescents. Second, although the two subsystems are interrelated, in the model examined in our research perceived parenting precedes perceived sibling relationship and directly affects it.

Empirical estimates of the effect of sibling relationship. Our analysis (Fig. 6.2) shows that the effect of perceived sibling relationship – like the effect of perceived parenting on future orientation – is indirect and linked via the self. Moreover, the indirect effect of sibling relationship on future orientation is not an artifact of family atmosphere but rather has an added net effect (Fig. 6.3). Thus, as in the case of academic achievement (Seginer & Golan, 2007) "the rich get richer" and adolescents experiencing positive parenting also enjoy positive sibling relationship that in turn have a positive effect on future orientation.

However, while perceived parenting is linked to future orientation via both self esteem and self agency, sibling relationship is linked only via self agency, attesting to the broader effect parenting – relative to sibling relationship – has on adolescents' self and to the different self paths through which family relationships affect future orientation.

Adolescent Peer Relations

Siblings and peer relationships differ on two main dimensions: choice (Kandel, 1978, 1986) and permanence. The short-lived nature of peer relationship (Brown, 2004) has been a major reason why our research on peer relationship (Seginer, 1998a; Seginer, Shoyer, Hossessi; & Tannous, 2007) has focused on the quality of peer relations rather than on the number of close friends, sociometric nominations or peer characteristics. Moreover, peer selection is limited by geographical, socio-economic, educational and personal interests factors, and relationships within the peer group vary.

Like parents and siblings, peers may serve two main functions: as a source of warmth and support and as offering socialization opportunities. Particularly, peers may provide necessary information (Stanton-Salazar & Dornbusch, 1995; Stanton-Salazar & Spina, 2000), prompt the development of cognitive skills (Azmitia, 1988; Azmitia, Montgomery, & Cruz, 1993; Rogoff, 1990) and ideas, help children and adolescents to evaluate one's attitudes and beliefs (Piaget, 1926, 1932), and sharpen their social understanding and social skills (Hartup, 1992, 1996).

Parenting and peer relationship. The relations found between parenting and sibling relationship have also been found for peer relationship: positive parenting prompts positive peer relationship among children (Clark & Ladd, 2000) and adolescents (Cooper & Cooper, 1992; Engels, Dekovic, & Meeus, 2002), and negative parenting (indicated by parental neglect, anger, harsh discipline, or excluding children from pertinent decisions) results in associating with peers engaged in antisocial behavior (Dekovic & Meeus, 1997) and noncompliant behavior, aggression toward peers, and school misconduct (externalizing behavior).

Moreover, depending on their nature, peer groups may either exacerbate (Goldstein, Davis-Kean, & Eccles, 2005; Kim, Hetherington, & Reiss, 1999; Lansford, Criss, Pettit, Dodge, & Bates, 2003) or reduce (Lansford, Criss, Pettit, Dodge, & Bates, 2003) the negative effect of negative parenting. As indicated by a study reporting on similar effects among Chinese children (Chen, Chang, He, & Liu, 2005), the power of peer groups to curb the influence of negative parenting on young adolescents' adjustment is also found in non-western settings.

Peer relationship in cultural context. Underlying the cultural question are two issues: familism and parental knowledge. Given that familistic orientations are more prevalent in non-western societies, one obvious prediction has been that in these societies parents will have stronger effect and peers will have a weaker effect on adolescents' behavior, attitudes and beliefs than in western societies. As mentioned earlier, this prediction has been supported by recent analyses of the effect of parenting, sibling, and peer relations on the self-esteem and perceived social support of Israeli Arab, Druze (non-western) and Jewish adolescents (Seginer, Shoyer, Hossessi; & Tannous, 2007). Drawing on these findings it is expected that among Arab adolescents the effect of peers on future orientation will be weaker than among Jewish adolescents.

However, in non-western societies *undergoing social change*, adolescents view their parents as representing the world of yesterday rather than the world of tomorrow to which adolescents aspire and their knowledge of relevant issues as undated. Consequently, advice given by contemporaries may be of greater value than advice given by parents. This, as shown by earlier findings (Seginer, 1992b; Seginer & Mahajna, 2003, 2004), is particularly applicable to Israeli Arab girls growing up in traditional Moslem families where parents push their daughters to early marriage and girls aspire for higher education as means for greater personal emancipation. Lacking parental support they may turn to friends who share similar parental pressure and undergo the same generational conflict. Consequently, familism notwithstanding, non-western peers may have a stronger effect than western peers on adolescents' future orientation. The extent to which parents and peers affect the future orientation of Israeli Arab (non-western) and Jewish (western) adolescents is presented below.

The Effect of Peer Relationship on Adolescent Future Orientation

Peer relationship and future orientation. Assuming siblings and peers have a parallel socializing role, the *self mediating model* constructed for the effect of sibling relationship on adolescent future orientation is repeated for peer relationship. The comparability of the two models is demonstrated in the empirical estimate of the peer relationship model (Fig. 6.4). However, while the indirect sibling relationship-motivational component path is linked only via self-agency, peer relationship – like parenting – is linked via both self esteem and self-agency.

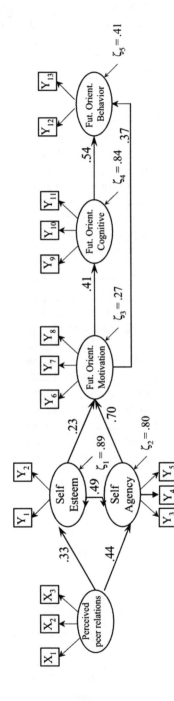

Fig. 6.4 Empirical estimate for a model of peer relations, self and work and career future orientation: Jewish adolescents. X_1 = perceived peer relationship/companionship; X_2 = perceived peer relationship/support; X_3 = perceived peer relationship/negative; Y_1 = self esteem/positive; Y_2 = self esteem/negative; Y_3 = self agency/independence; Y_4 = self agency/self reliance; Y_5 = self agency/self assurance; Y_6 = value; Y_7 = expectance; Y_8 = internal control; Y_9 = my future occupation; Y_{10} = my future professional career; Y_{11} = my future workplace; Y_{12} = exploration; Y_{13} = commitments. Factors loadings (lambdas) from .36 to .96; N = 358; χ^2 (111) = 245.65; p < .001; RMSEA = .06; CFI = .92

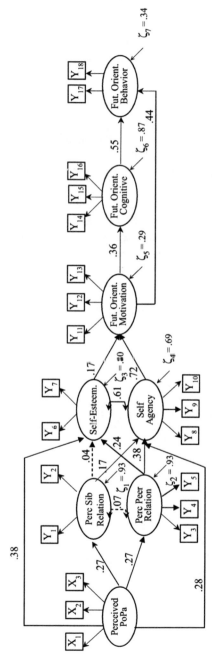

Fig. 6.5 Empirical estimate for a model of perceived parenting, perceived sibling relationship, perceived peer relations, self and work and career future orientation: Jewish adolescents. X_1 = perceived positive parenting/acceptance; X_2 = perceived positive parenting/granted autonomy; X_3 = perceived positive parenting/limit setting re peers relations; Y_1 = perceived sibling relationship/positive; Y_2 = perceived sibling relationship/future related; Y_3 = perceived peer relationship/support Y_4 = perceived peer relationship/ companionship; Y_5 = perceived peer relationship/negative; Y_6 = self esteem/ positive; Y_7 = self esteem/ negative; Y_8 = self agency/independence; Y_9 = self agency/self reliance; Y_{10} = self agency/self assurance; Y_{11} = value; Y_{12} = expectance; Y_{13} = internal control; Y_{14} = my future occupation; Y_{15} = my future professional career; Y_{16} = my future workplace; Y_{17} = exploration; Y_{18} = commitment. Factors loadings (lambdas) range from .36 to .94; N = 358; χ^2 (219) = 452.27; p < .001; RMSEA = .06; CFI = .91

Parenting and peer relationship. When parenting and peer relationship are included in the same model, like in the case of the parenting and sibling relationship (Fig. 6.3), both self esteem and self agency affect peer relationship. However, while sibling relationship is indirectly linked to the motivational component only via self agency, peer relationship is linked to the motivational component via both self esteem and self agency. Thus, the divide is not between family and non-family or between generations but rather between more and less meaningful relationships, and reiterates the growing meaningfulness of adolescent peer relations. Possibly guided by adolescents' need for individuation, relationship with siblings is linked to future orientation via self agency that indicated by self reliance, independence, and personal strength represents the interpersonal aspect of the self.

Parenting, sibling and peer relations. In light of its similar effect on future orientation, the inevitable question is whether, when added to parent-adolescent and sibling relationship, peer relationship still maintains its effect on future orientation? Figure 6.5 shows it does. Moreover, analysis of the joint effect of parent, sibling and peer relationships reiterates the effect of parenting on relationships with contemporaries and the different paths through which parenting and peer relationship on the one hand and sibling relationship on the other hand affect future orientation. Analysis carried out on Israeli Arab adolescents (Fig. 6.6) shows that despite cultural differences, the structure of the joint effects of the three interpersonal relationships on future orientation is similar.

The Future Orientation of Classmates

Underlying the decision to study this issue is a basic premise about the significance of interaction with classmates for the formation of adolescents' future orientation. Undoubtedly, classmates do not overlap with one's peer group: some classmates are not counted as belonging to the peer group and some of their peers may not be attending the same class. This is particularly characteristic of Arab adolescents whose peer group includes siblings and cousins (Booth, 2002).

However, whereas in American high schools classroom composition varies with school subject, in other parts of the world including Israel, assignment of students to their classrooms is stable across the school year and in some cases across all high school years, and based on academic and administrative considerations rather than on students preferences. Consequently, the classroom is a significant social unit and researchers' concern (e.g., Brown, 2004) that the effect of peer relationship is confounded with their selective nature does not apply.

Thus, three questions about the effect of classmates on future orientation are relevant: do classmates affect adolescents' future orientation? Does culture matter? Do peer effects vary by age?

The relations between classmates' and adolescents' future orientation. Those observing adolescents' activities during school breaks notice that much of the time between classes is devoted to talking. While group composition may change,

a. Girls

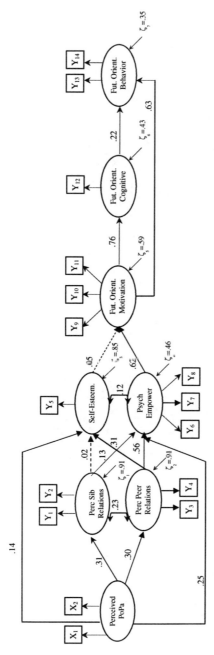

Fig. 6.6 Empirical estimate for a model of perceived parenting, perceived sibling relationship, perceived peer relations, self and higher education future orientation: Arab adolescents. X_1 = perceived positive parenting/acceptance; X_2 = perceived positive parenting/granted autonomy; Y_1 = perceived Sibling Relationship/positive; Y_2 = Perceived Sibling Relationship/future related; Y_3 = perceived peer relationship/ positive; Y_4 = perceived peer relationship/future related; Y_5 = self esteem; Y_6 = psychological empower/intrapersonal; Y_7 = psychological empower/interpersonal; Y_8 = psychological empower/behavior; Y_9 = value; Y_{10} = expectance; Y_{11} = internal control; Y_{12} = my future education; Y_{13} = exploration; Y_{14} = commitment. Factors loadings (lambdas) for girls from .33 to .97, and for boys from .48 to .97; **a.** N = 585; χ^2 (91) = 282.21; p < .001; RMSEA = .06; CFI = .95; **b.** N = 358; χ^2 (91) = 216.41; p < .001; RMSEA = .07; CFI = .94

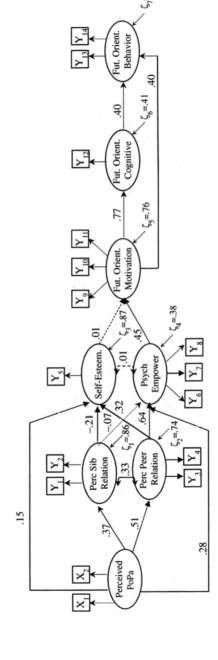

Fig. 6.6 (continued)

conversation with same-gender peers tends to be the norm. Therefore and despite the similarity between the prospective trajectory of girls and boys in many western societies, the analysis presented here is based on same-gender comparisons (Table 6.1).

This analysis shows that the relations between adolescents' and classmates' future orientation scores are of relatively low magnitude but consistent across the different variables, prospective life domains, gender, and cultural settings, specifically pertaining to Arabs and Jews. Thus, the rationale presented earlier that Arab girls may be influenced either more (because they cannot consult their families) or less (because they grow up in a familistic society) than western adolescents and the rival hypotheses deduced from them have not been supported. In a similar vein, no differences were found for gender and age comparisons. Instead, the effect of classmates is moderate but consistent across diverse conditions and future orientation domains.

Peer Influence: What Adolescents Do and Report

Group interaction effects. As in several other areas of future orientation research, Trommsdorff (1982) has been a pioneer. Along with her interest in the effect of home atmosphere on adolescents' future orientation (Chap. 5), she also studied how university students in a group setting affect each other's future orientation. Drawing on social psychology of groups theories Trommsdorff and her colleagues ran several experiments on the effect of group discussion on subjective probabilities of a person's future success (or failure) of materialization of goals among German university students.

While we would expect group discussion to prompt positive thinking and raise one's success probabilities, the results of those experiments were to the contrary. Trommsdorff's explanation of those counterintuitive results rest on the assumption that optimism regarding one's success would be regarded by the group as unduly and arrogant thus leading group members to public reduction of their positive outlook toward the future. This interpretation can be viewed in the wider perspective of cultural effects. As noted by Goodnow in relation to planning, "The nature of the general social environment gives rise. . .to variations in the extent to which planning meets with approval or disapproval and in the content areas for which planning is seen as appropriate" (Goodnow, 1997, p. 340). Correspondingly, the social setting of those students considered expressions of optimism about the future as undesirable. Nonetheless, the extent to which participants distinguished between public appearance and private beliefs, the duration of the effect of group pressure, as well as the effect of real life groups were beyond the scope of those experiments and thus were not reported.

This question has been tested in a study (Young et al., 1999) that examined the effect of conversation on the formation of future career goals among Canadian high school students (13–19 years old) who led conversations about future career issues with a self-selected partner. As researchers were observing the process the dyad

Table 6.1 The relation between adolescents' and classmates' future orientation scores

	Jewish adolescents						Arab adolescent girls			
	9th graders		11th graders				11th graders			
	Girls (n = 87)	Boys (n = 81)	Girls (n = 188)		Boys (n = 170)		Traditional (n = 225)		Transition to modernity (n = 208)	
	Higher Education		Career	Family	Career	Family	Hi Educ	Family	Hi Educ	Family
Value	0.22*	0.27**	0.28***	0.30***	0.24***	0.22**	0.14*	0.21***	0.35***	0.36***
Expectance	0.34***	0.22	0.33***	0.37***	0.29***	0.23***	0.24***	0.24***	0.27***	0.27***
Control	0.28**	0.28**	0.20**	0.25***	0.19**	0.23***	0.20**	0.17**	0.29***	0.30***
Cogn Rep Hopes	0.39***	0.48***	0.36***	0.32***	0.35***	0.29***	0.29***	0.32***	0.33***	0.23***
Cogn Rep Fears	0.15	0.54***	0.28***	0.37***	0.32***	0.26***	–	–	–	–
Exploration	0.24*	0.20	0.25***	0.37***	0.31***	0.33***	0.24***	0.34***	0.34***	0.24***
Commitment	0.22*	0.14	0.32***	0.31***	0.34***	0.28***	0.14*	0.23***	0.22**	0.30***

*p < .05
**p < .01
***p < .001

underwent in discussing career issues, they identified several steps through which conversation partners facilitated each other in reaching a better understanding ("self-refining") of their future career goals.

Common to both studies has been the effect of others on one's future orientation. However, be it the result of time and place (German university during the 1970s vs Canadian high school in the late 1990s), group composition (group consisting of several members vs dyad), self-selected vs experimentally contrived groups, or research questions and instructions given to participants, the nature of the peer effects and hence the investigators' conclusions point in opposite directions. Age (high school vs university students) is another relevant variable on which the two groups differed. Its pertinence has been attested in a study (Steinberg & Monahan, 2007) showing the greater resistance of younger (high school students) than older adolescents to group pressure. Nonetheless, these studies set the stage for further research on the effect of interpersonal interaction on the formation of future orientation.

Adolescents self reports. When asked to whom they turn when considering future oriented issues, more American adolescents reported they consult parents than peers (Brittain, 1963; Sebald, 1986). However, to understand its meaning, this tendency should be viewed in light of two other findings. One is that those adolescents followed the principle of "division of labor": they consulted their peers on peer relevant issues such as social activities (dating, clothing, music) and parents on financial, educational and future career issues that call for adult experience and expertise. The second pertains to the relevance of the social-historical context showing that as political atmosphere changed from conservatism (in the early 1960s) to liberalism (mid-1970s), the pendulum swung and adolescents reported that on future oriented issues they relied on peers' advice more than on that of parents.

Summary

At present our knowledge regarding the effect of siblings and peers on the construction of adolescent future orientation is rather limited. Nonetheless, current research provides preliminary answers to several questions. The first relates to the effect of sibling and peer relationships showing that each has positive effect above and beyond the effect of parenting on future orientation. However, while parenting and peer relationship affect future orientation via two aspects of the self – self-evaluation and self-agency for Jewish adolescents and psychological empowerment for Arab adolescents – sibling relationship affects it only via the interpersonal aspect of the self pertaining to self agency or psychological empowerment.

The extent to which peer interaction and the processes underlying it facilitate future orientation thinking and behavior has been studied even less. Results differ in the direction of the effect – that is, whether interaction with peers encourages or discourages the construction of positive plans for the future – but agree about the power of peer interaction on future thinking and adds to the overall conclusion on the relevance of contemporaries to the construction of adolescent future orientation.

Chapter 7
Future Orientation Outcomes

As previous chapters described the development of future orientation and its indicators in infancy, childhood, and adolescence, its personality correlates, gender differences, and how interpersonal relationships affect it, this chapter is about the 'What for' of future orientation? What behavioral and developmental purposes does future orientation serve? Why do individuals "need" an orientation to the future and consequently why should researchers have an interest in studying it? Answers vary from the global to the specific.

Taking a motivational approach, for Nuttin and Lens (1985) the future is the temporal zone where the objects of hopes, goals and plans are localized, while for Raynor and Entin (1982) future orientation is particularly relevant to achievement motivation. Focusing on developmental considerations, the global rationale was first suggested by Douvan and Adelson who contended that "...adolescent adaptation directly depends on the ability to integrate the future to their present life and current self concept." (Douvan & Adelson, 1966, p. 229). The specific grounds relate to future orientation as facilitating various developmental tasks adolescents and emergent adults tackle, especially as they cope with major life transitions.

However, as theoretical approaches are translated into empirical studies, all questions become specific. Consequently, this chapter looks at the effect of future orientation on five developmental outcomes relevant to adolescents, emerging adults, and midlife adults. The five outcomes are: academic achievement for adolescents, identity, intimacy, and adjustment to transition (military service) for emerging adults, and midlife men (early retirement). The conceptual framework guiding the study of each issue is outcome specific.

Future Orientation and Academic Achievement

While achievement is by no means restricted to the academic realm, with very few exceptions such as achievement in sports (Vansteenkiste, Simons, Soenens, & Lens, 2004), research has been mainly devoted to the effect of future orientation on academic achievement. Therefore, discussion of this issue opens with the conceptualization and data-based illustrations of *perceived instrumentality* as the psychological process underlying the future orientation-academic achievement link and continues with examining the structure of this link and its covariation with cultural settings, age, and future orientation domains.

The Underlying Rationale: Perceived Instrumentality

The notion of perceived instrumentality and its relevance to future orientation was first introduced by Nuttin. "...[individuals] lacking future time perspective" he wrote in his introduction to *Future time perspective and motivation* "are unable to perceive the instrumental link between their present studies and a far-distant career..." (Nuttin & Lens, 1985, pp. 9–10). In other words, without the capability for and the activation of future thinking, individuals are unable to comprehend the relevance – or *instrumentality* (Husman & Lens, 1999) – of present behavior for future goal attainment.

Concerned that perceived instrumentality signifies extrinsic motivation, Husman and Lens further contended that students, particularly high achieving students, employ instrumentality for achieving intrinsic goals which thus facilitates rather than interferes with their achievement. This has been empirically supported by studies showing the stronger effect of intrinsic (rather than extrinsic) future goals on the academic achievement of high school students (Vansteenkiste, Simons, Lens, Soenens, & Matos, 2005) from diverse cultural settings (Andriessen, Phalet, & Lens, 2006).

Perceived instrumentality and academic achievement. The development of perceived instrumentality measures (Husman & Shell, 2008; Miller, DeBacker, & Greene, 1999) made it possible to assess its effect on college students' academic self regulation and achievement. Drawing on different research questions and employing different measures of perceived instrumentality they reached seemingly different conclusions. Thus, while Malka and Covington's (2005) findings show the net effect of perceived instrumentality on academic achievement after controlling once for future orientation and once for achievement goals, Shell and Husman's (2008) findings show that, in a design including control beliefs as well as goal orientations and affect, perceived instrumentality is not significantly related to academic strategic self regulation. Together, their findings indicate the contextualization of perceived instrumentality and their outcome specificity.

The subjective meaning of perceived instrumentality. Given the importance of present behavior-future goal links, the question is whether individuals are aware of it and deliberately invest in present behavior as means for attaining their goals? Our findings show that the answer varies by gender and cultural setting. The hopes narratives of Israeli Arab adolescent girls (Seginer & Mahajna, 2004) clearly voice their understanding of this link. As demonstrated by the narratives quoted below, as they list their hopes and fears of the future these girls spontaneously explain their motivation to do well at school and gain high academic achievement in terms of their awareness that high academic achievement is a necessary – though not sufficient – condition for materializing their hopes, goals, and plans for higher education and careers:

> I would like to be a famous lawyer. That is why I hope God will help me with getting high grades. (No. 27, age 16).
> I hope to graduate from high school cum laude because I want to have university education and be an important and contributing [person] to my society. (No. 46, age 16).
> All depends on God. I hope God will help me get high grades above 100 so that I can be admitted to a university program. I want to study medicine at Hebrew University in Jerusalem. (No. 60, age 17).
> I hope to graduate from high school cum laude and get a high grade on the psychometric exam and be accepted to the University of Haifa and study psychology. (No. 61, age 17).
> Every person thinks about his future [and about his] hopes and dreams. I hope for a productive and promising future. First of all I hope to continue my education at the university and [therefore I need to] get high grades on my matriculation exams. (No. 68, age 17).
> Before anything else I hope to get good matriculation certificate and I'll do everything to get the best grades. I hope all will continue as it is now and I will continue my [university] education because education is a weapon in girls' hands. (No. 95, age 17).
> I hope to pass the matriculation exams with high grades so I can be accepted to the school of social work or medical school. (No. 198, age 18).
> I have many hopes. First of all higher education is the foundation of my life. Therefore presently I am so busy with my school work. (No. 207, age 18).

These narratives all draw from the same data set. However, while data collected from other groups of Israeli Arab girls (Mahajna, 2007; Seginer & Mahajna, 2003, 2004; Seginer, Mahajna, & Shoyer, 2007; Seginer, Shoyer, & Mahajna, 2008) all include narratives that acknowledge the importance of education and emphasize the instrumentality of working hard and achieving high grades in high school, these themes only seldom appear in *narrative* data collected from other groups such as Israeli Arab boys (Seginer et al., 2008; Suleiman, 2000) and Israeli Jewish adolescents (girls and boys) (Seginer, 2005; Seginer et al., 2004).

Underlying these differences are three factors: the different socio-cultural developmental settings of Arab and Jewish adolescents in Israel, the stronger pressure on Israeli Arab girls (than on boys) for early marriage, and their belief that higher education is their only negotiable means for breaking off the traditional path destined for Arab women. Thus, although their academic motivation is extrinsic and their perceived instrumentality emphasizes achievement rather than learning (Malka & Covington, 2005; Miller et al., 1999) as shown below, for Arab girls as well as for other adolescent groups higher education future orientation is positively related to academic achievement.

Considered in more general terms, the conclusion suggested here is that as determined goal-oriented individuals identify obstacles interfering with the achievement of their hopes, goals and plans, they become more concerned about possessing means for achieving them. Conversely, under supportive conditions, individuals and particularly adolescents develop confidence about the feasibility of goal achievement, and therefore are not concerned about – but not necessarily unaware of – means for its implementation.

Future Orientation and Academic Achievement Links: Empirical Analyses

Our next question has been whether, regardless of their awareness of and concern about means for achieving future goals, adolescents' future orientation is linked to academic achievement? Given that our research employs a multiple component and multiple domain conceptualization of future orientation in different cultural settings, answers vary. However, not to the extent cultural and cross-cultural psychology approaches may predict. To indicate commonalities and differences, the empirical findings about future orientation-academic achievement links are grouped under three headings: cultural settings, future life domains, and age.

Cultural settings. Analysis of the effect of the motivational, cognitive, and behavioral components of each of the two future orientation instrumental domains (higher education or work and career) shows that the effect of future orientation on academic achievement *does not* vary by culture. Thus, though growing up in different political-cultural settings, guided by different beliefs and value orientations, and expected to follow different life trajectories, the academic achievement of Israeli Arab Moslem girls (Mahajna, 2007), Israeli Arab girls and boys (Seginer & Mahajna, 2008), Israeli Jewish adolescents (girls and boys), and Israeli Jewish ultra-orthodox girls (Dekel, 2009) is directly affected by the behavioral component of future orientation and indirectly by the motivational and cognitive components. These links apply to the work and career domain for Jewish adolescents and to the higher education domain for Arab adolescents (Fig. 7.1a–c).

Differences in their expected life trajectories are especially pertinent here. Whereas Arab and Jewish ultra-orthodox girls are guided each by the dos and don't of their religion and their path into adulthood is determined by their parents, Israeli Arab boys follow parental advice and seek admission to an institute of higher education or enter the world of work, while Israeli Jewish girls and boys take a different path. Following high school graduation they all go through mandatory military service (2 years for girls and 3 years for boys), the majority then obtains university education, leave home as it fits with their other plans, and marry at a later age.

Yet, in one of our samples, separate analyses for Jewish girls and boys (Shoyer, 2006) show that, among boys, the cognitive component has a direct and negative effect on academic achievement so that it is *not* being too much concerned with their prospective work and career thoughts but rather being engaged in "doing" (by exploring work and career options and reaching a decision) that prompts investment

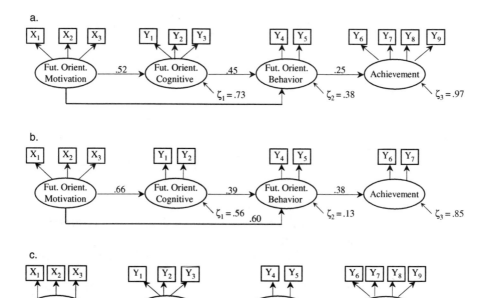

Fig. 7.1 Empirical estimates for model of higher education/work and career future orientation and academic achievement for three samples. **a.** Work and career for Jewish adolescents N = 358, χ^2 (72) = 107.61, p = 0.004, RMSEA = 0.04, CFI = 0.96. **b.** Higher education for Moslem girls N = 295, χ^2 (12) = 38.80, p = 0.001, RMSEA = 0.07, CFI = 0.94. **c.** Work and career for ultra orthodox girls N = 819, χ^2 (61) = 326.81, p = 0.001, RMSEA = 0.07, CFI = 0.90. X_1 = value; X_2 = expectance; X_3 = internal control; Y_1 = my future major/occupation; Y_2 = my future studies/professional career; Y_3 = my future workplace; Y_4 = exploration; Y_5 = commitment; Y_6 = English; Y_7 = mathematics; Y_8 = Hebrew grammar; Y_9 = literature. Factors loadings (lambdas) range from 0.40 to 0.96

in schoolwork and its resultant academic achievement. Viewed from perceived instrumentality perspective, academic achievement is prompted by exploration and commitment activities pertaining to their future hopes, goals, and plans in the domain of higher education or work and career, and specifically for Jewish boys *curbed* by being frequently concerned with prospective work and career.

In fact, exploration and commitment have a dual function: they help adolescents reach a decision about future education or career and hone their understanding that fulfillment of future hopes and plans is contingent on pertinent present behavior. A hypothetical example would be a girl who, after gathering information about a career in computer engineering, realizes that her career path starts with being a top student at school.

Domain specificity. While the structure of the relations among the three future orientation components and the effect of interpersonal relationships on future orientation (described in Chapts. 5 and 6) are consistent for the different

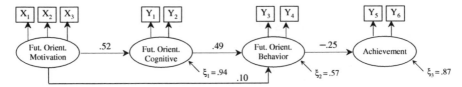

Fig. 7.2 Empirical estimate for a model of marriage and family future orientation and academic achievement: traditional Moslem girls. X_1 = value; X_2 = expectance; X_3 = internal control; Y_1 = my future partner; Y_2 = my future family; Y_3 = exploration; Y_4 = commitment; Y_5 = English; Y_6 = math. Factors loadings (lambdas) from 0.40 to 0.92; N = 617; χ^2 (86) = 253.59; p = 0.001; RMSEA = 0.05; CFI = 0.96

future orientation domains, the effect of future orientation on academic achievement is domain-specific. The stable effect of the two *instrumental* domains (higher education and work and career) on academic achievement does not repeat itself for the *marriage and family* domain. For Jewish girls and boys, ultra-orthodox Jewish girls and Arab boys prospective *marriage and family* is unrelated to academic achievement. This finding has one exception: for Israeli Arab girls the link between the behavioral component and academic achievement is negative (Fig. 7.2; Mahajna, 2007). For these girls, exploration of marriage and family options and abiding by the decision to get married early reduces interest in schoolwork and academic achievement. Moreover, concerned that such behavior will interfere with their schoolwork, high achievers purposely avoid it:

> [My hope is] to get high grades on my matriculation and psychometric exam. Therefore the most important thing now is to get the highest grades possible. Regarding marriage, the truth is that I avoid thinking about it because I think it will interfere with my schoolwork. (No. 39, age 16).
> ...And when I complete my studies, then I may start thinking about getting married. (No. 49, age 17).
> All my hopes are condensed into one: continuing my education. This is the only goal I am striving for. My education will drive me to other achievements. After I complete my studies I will start thinking about other matters like a fiancé that I hope will encourage me to continue my education. (No. 55, age 17).
> Regarding marriage, I don't think about it now because I want to complete my education first. (No. 69, age 17).

Noticeably, these narratives are expressed by the 16- and 17-year-olds and not by the 18-year-olds. As girls of this age group approach high school graduation, family and community pressure for early marriage goes up and the actuality of hopes for pursuing the higher education trajectory goes down.

The effect of age. Given that much of the work on future orientation focused on high school students, our interest in the relevance of age to the future orientation-academic achievement link resulted in studying young adolescent participants. Cognizant of an unavoidable confounding of age and distance to materialization of future hopes, we specifically asked whether the link found between future orientation and academic achievement among high school students can be identified among junior high school adolescents who will attend higher education at least 6 or 7 years later.

Our respondents were Israeli Jewish 9th graders, whom we judged capable of considering all three future orientation components. Their responses show that while the relation between academic achievement and higher education future orientation is sustained, it indicates a different meaning. Specifically, the behavioral component found linked to academic achievement among 11th graders interfere with 9th graders academic achievement.

Instead, academic achievement is directly prompted by the *motivational* component (Fig. 7.3). Viewed from the perceived instrumentality perspective, for 9th graders academic achievement is supported by the high value of higher education, confidence in materializing higher education hopes and plans, and belief in their ability to control it (empirically indicating the motivational component) and not by exploration of higher education options and commitment to one of them. Thus, underlying the perceived instrumentality of young adolescents are intrinsic motives (Husman & Lens, 1999) whose effect on the academic achievement of older adolescents is only indirect and mediated by the behavioral component.

Moreover, while for Jewish 11th graders future orientation explains only 3% of academic achievement variance, for 9th graders it explains 14% of the variance. These, together with findings about the explained variance of academic achievement for Israeli Arab girls and boys and for Jewish ultra-orthodox girls (13–15% each), suggest that cultural diversity is not the only factor underlying the differential effect of future orientation on academic achievement. Instead, future orientation is particularly facilitating adolescents facing educational challenges (S. Shoyer, personal communication, June 19, 2008).

For Jewish adolescents, 9th grade is last year of junior high school and their educational future (i.e., admission to college-bound or other high school program) is of paramount concern, for them as well as for their families. Conversely, the academic

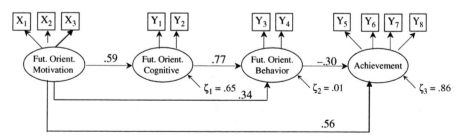

Fig. 7.3 Empirical estimate for a model of future orientation higher education and academic achievement: 9th grade Jewish adolescents. X_1 = value; X_2 = expectance; X_3 = internal control; Y_1 = my future education; Y_2 = my future major; Y_3 = exploration; Y_4 = commitments; Y_5 = English; Y_6 = math; Y_7 = literature; Y_8 = grammar. Factors loadings (lambdas) from 0.40 to 0.92; N = 168; χ^2 (39) = 77.49; p < 0.001, RMSEA = 0.07; CFI = 0.90

standing and hence the educational trajectory of the Jewish 11th grade respondents is clear. They attend one of several college-bound programs and the majority expects to enter a higher education program upon concluding military service. For 11th grade Arab adolescents reality is considerably different. Uncertainty about the feasibility of higher education in general and admission to preferred university programs in particular for girls and boys alike and family pressure exerted on girls make 11th grade a challenging year. Under these circumstances, future orientation and the perceived instrumentality it facilitates prompts academic achievement, resulting in a higher percentage of explained variance of academic achievement by instrumental (higher education or work and career) future orientation.

Summary. Findings reviewed in this section show that the effect of future orientation on academic achievement is consistent across cultural settings but varies with prospective domains and age. Specifically, the effect of each of the instrumental domains (i.e., higher education, work and career) on academic achievement is maintained for Israeli Jewish and Arab girls and boys, and for Israeli ultra-orthodox girls. However, whereas for high school adolescents (mostly 11th graders) only exploration of future options and commitment to one (the behavioral component) is directly linked to academic achievement, for junior high school students (9th graders) who are further away from higher education academic achievement is affected by the motivational component subsuming the value of higher education, confidence in materialization of hopes, goals and plans, and one's ability to control it.

For all cultural groups, except one, the marriage and family domain is unrelated to academic achievement. Exception are Israeli Arab girls for whom the behavioral component is *negatively* linked to academic achievement. Thus, while girls who accept early marriage are relatively uninterested in academic achievement, to avoid its interference with academic achievement, others who view early marriage as an obstacle to higher education avoid marriage and family exploration and commitment.

Drawing on the conceptualization developed by Lens and his research group, the link between each of the instrumental domains and academic achievement is explained by the inclination to perceive the instrumentality of academic achievement for the pursuit of higher education goals located in the future. However, for reasons related to the conflicting life trajectories that Israeli Arab adolescent girls and their parents chart for these girls, only they explicitly and richly express the instrumentality of academic achievement for future higher education. Altogether, our findings support earlier research on perceived instrumentality (e.g., Simons et al., 2000) and elucidate the process through which future orientation (pertaining to higher education) affect present behavior (academic achievement).

However, these findings highlight two additional issues. One concerns the meaningfulness of future orientation for the academic achievement of various groups and suggests future orientation pertaining to higher education and work and career is particularly relevant to groups challenged by prospective higher education, such as junior high school Jewish students, Israeli Arab 11th graders (girls and boys) and Israeli Jewish ultra-orthodox girls. The second relates to cases in which future orientation does not facilitate academic achievement but is instead *counter-*instrumental. Data presented in this chapter pertains to two instances: for Israeli Arab girls marriage and family future orientation has a negative effect on academic achievement, for Israeli 9th graders the behavioral component of higher education and for Israeli Jewish boys the cognitive component of work and career have a similar effect.

Future Orientation and Two Developmental Tasks: Identity and Intimacy

Developmental psychologists agree that future orientation, identity, and intimacy are *interrelated* adolescent developmental tasks that continue to be relevant in emergent adulthood. Developmentalists do differ, however, in their propositions about the direction of the links among the three developmental tasks. Whereas some researchers interpret Erikson's (1968) and Marcia's (1993) ego identity conceptualizations as indicating that future orientation is one aspect of ego identity, others consider future orientation as an outcome of identity formation (e.g., Dunkel, 2000; Dunkel & Anthis, 2001; Kerpelman & Mosher, 2004).

No doubt, Erikson's writings can support both positions as well as a third one contending that future orientation *precedes* identity formation and indeed sets the stage for processes underlying the formation of ego identity. This view has also been expressed in Marcia's (1983) discussion of identity development in early adolescence, and guides the approach presented in this chapter. Specifically it is here contended that, although for emerging adults the three developmental tasks function concurrently, conceptually and chronologically future orientation develops earlier and precedes the formation of identity and the ability for intimacy. To explain it, this section starts with a short review of identity and intimacy as developmental tasks.

Identity

Although the impact of Erikson's identity analysis on subsequent research has resulted in the identity statuses paradigm (Marcia, 1993) as a leading approach, the richness of Erikson's analysis lends itself to multiple conceptualizations (Waterman, 1999). Drawing on Erikson's writings, these conceptualizations describe identity as a self-produced personality organization achieved by integrating the self in time and social settings. Integration in time pertains to complementary relations between representation of the self in the past, present, and future, and integration of self and social settings pertains to the negotiation and resultant acceptance of family and peers' expectations and their community's social values, norms, and role definitions.

This integration results in a sense of sameness and continuity, in securing a subjective sense of acceptance by one's significant others, and of finding one's unique niche in society (Erikson, 1968). Consequently it guides individuals' behavior and supports their pursuit of personal meaning. While identity processes are at work across the life span, they are more intensely engaged in during adolescence and emerging adulthood.

The identity status approach (e.g., Archer, 1989; Berzonsky, 2003, 2005; Berzonsky & Adams, 1999; Marcia, 1993; Waterman, 1982, 1999) yielded a large body of research describing identity formation and its' correlates. It also led to research on processes of identity construction that specifically focused on identity styles (Berzonsky, 1989), and on the exploration processes involved in the construction of identity formation (Flum & Blustein, 2000; Grotevant, 1987) and the commitment consolidating it (Bosma & Kunnen, 2001; Meeus, Iedema, Helsen, & Vollebergh, 1999).

The Relations Between Future Orientation and Identity

For Erikson (Erikson, 1963, 1968; Berzonsky & Adams, 1999), time perspective in general and orientation to the future in particular are strongly related to identity formation. When specifically addressing the future, Erikson (1968) contended that optimal sense of identity is associated with a sense of direction and investment in the future (Erikson 1968). However, orientation to the future has also been considered by him as a developmental *precursor* of identity:

> . . .it [identity crisis] occurs in a period of the life cycle when each youth must forge for himself some central perspective and direction, some working unity, *out of* the effective remnants of his childhood and the hopes of *his anticipated adulthood. (Italics added*, Erikson, 1958, p. 14).

Marcia's approach to the relation between orientation to the future and ego identity has been age dependent. Based on earlier developmental findings, Marcia (1983) posited that, for early adolescents, self-reflection about the future serves as a precursor of identity formation. However, as is clearly reflected in the identity status interviews (Archer & Waterman, 1993; Marcia & Archer, 1993), during late adolescence and adulthood orientation to the future functions as a core aspect of identity statuses (Marcia, 1993).

Earlier research. Empirical analyses of the relations between identity and future orientation have been examined by earlier studies (Kerpelman & Mosher, 2004; Pulkkinen & Rönkä, 1994; Rappaport, Enrich, & Wilson, 1985). Although each took a different conceptual perspective, all show that identity and future orientation are positively related, albeit in different ways. Rappaport et al. showed the relation holds across time, Pulkkinen and Rönkä showed positive relations between future orientation and identity commitment, and Kerpelman and Mosher report relations between future orientation and both identity exploration and commitment.

The present approach. A basic premise of our research (Ablin, 2006; Seginer & Noyman, 2005) has been that the processes assumed by Erikson and Marcia as relevant to adolescents are also applicable to emerging adults, but the nature of the future orientation-identity relations evolve as a three phase process. In the earliest, children and young adolescents are able to think about the future but lack the experience and psychological maturity necessary for engaging in identity work. In the second phase (toward the end of mid-adolescence), as individuals are capable of it, the work of identity builds on their future orientation. Finally, in the third phase, for emerging adults and adults, both processes are at work; however, the motivation to engage in future thinking and behavior and the resultant thinking and behavioral acts prompt the work of identity. This process is reflected in positive relations between future orientation and identity formation.

Conceptually, future orientation is relevant to the time and social setting aspects of the integration of the self that according to Erikson (1968) take part in the process of identity formation. Integration of self representations in the past, present and future relates to the *temporal* aspect of future orientation whose construction draws on individuals' past and present experiences. Integration of the self and social settings (proximal and distal) draws on the *thematic* aspect of future orientation and particularly on the prospective life course domains that signify the developmental trajectory from adolescence to adulthood: higher education, work and career, and marriage and family.

Future Orientation and Identity Links: Empirical Evidence

As readers are no doubt aware, the social and economic changes most countries have experienced since Erikson (1950) first published his ideas about adolescent development and the critical role identity serves in it have resulted in the extension of the adolescence period and postponed entrance to adulthood. Consequently, researchers introduced a new intermediate developmental period describing individuals that are no more adolescents and not yet adults. Arnett (2000) described the age range 18–25 as *emerging adulthood*, Keniston (1970) as *youth*, and relating to the 17–22 age range, Levinson (1978) described it as *transition to adulthood*. This section draws from two studies of Israeli Jewish emerging adults.

The first (Seginer & Noyman, 2005) studied a group of young persons (women and men, mean age 24.1, SD = 1.9) who as high school students did not complete Israeli matriculation requirements and upon concluding military service opted to attend a college preparatory program (which under certain conditions is equivalent to fulfillment of the matriculation requirements).

The second study (Ablin, 2006) is a short-term longitudinal study conducted with two groups of boys who at time of data collection were doing military service. Group I consisted of individuals at the beginning of their military service (mean age 18.5, SD = 0.80). For them, transition from home and school to the hierarchical and non-voluntary setting characterizing military life, the initially unfamiliar peers and the physical and psychological challenges of military training and military barracks were a drastic change from home, school and peer group. Group II consisted of emerging adults who, 18 months after they were first conscripted, were half way through their military service (mean age 19.7, SD = 1.35). Both studies examine the effect of future orientation as a three-component construct on identity formation. However, each had an overall different rationale and employed different identity measures.

Study I: college preparatory students (Seginer & Noyman, 2005). This study examines the effect of future orientation on identity by focusing on the motivational and behavioral components of future life domains pertaining to adult roles: work and career and marriage and family.

The postulated relation between the *motivational* aspects of future orientation and identity emanates from the nature of each of the motivational variables, as applied to career and family. Specifically, attributing high *value* to these two consensual adult tasks and having a sense of *internal control* and confidence in the materialization of pertinent hopes and plans (*expectance*) contribute to one's identity, particularly as reflected in a sense of direction and recognition from others.

We further contended that engagement in *exploration* of each of these life domains results in a growing knowledge of self-in-context that facilitates identity consolidation. Specifically, exploration affects each of the three main aspects included in Erikson's (1968) depiction of identity as having a sense of direction, coming to terms with one's body, and anticipating recognition by significant others (a sense of connectedness). Given that *commitment* is a decision to pursue a meaningful future course, reaching it affects one's sense of identity particularly as it affirms a person's sense of direction and of connectedness.

The global (rather than domain-specific) approach to *identity* (Constantinople, 1969; Ochse & Plug, 1986; Reis & Youniss, 2004; Rosenthal, Gurney, & Moore, 1981) employed here resembles Blasi and Glodis' (1995) analysis of a sense of identity and Marcia's (1993) analysis of the subjective experience of identity as sources of meaning to one's life. Moreover, this meaning of identity more than other conceptualizations derived from Erikson's writings has been described by him in operational terms. Specifically, "...most obvious concomitants are a feeling of being at home in one's body, a 'sense of knowing where one is going', and an inner assuredness of anticipated recognition from those who count." (Erikson, 1968, p. 165). Thus, individuals' awareness of developing a sense of identity is related to three important aspects of the self: physical self, agency, and relatedness, particularly pertaining to a subjective sense of support ("recognition") from significant others.

However, findings show that not all variables subsumed under the motivational and behavioral components are linked to experienced identity. What we did find is that, for both life domains, identity is affected by *expectance* and not by control and by *commitment* but not by exploration. The effect of one variable is domain specific: the *value* of career but not that of family has a direct effect on identity. Altogether, the motivational and behavioral components of *work and career* future orientation explain almost a third (32%) of the variance of identity and the motivational and behavioral components of *marriage and family* future orientation explain slightly over a quarter (27%) of the variance of identity.

Our explanations draw on the meaning of expectance, value, and commitment particularly for emerging adults. Accordingly, the effect of *expectance* on identity indicates the relevance of one's confidence in the materialization of hopes, plans, and goals for experienced identity. Underlying it are two processes; one is pertinent to all conditions and developmental periods and the other is particularly relevant for the emerging adulthood period.

The universal process pertains to confidence in goal attainability as a necessary pre-requisite for action, particularly relevant to the agentic quality of identity. Analyses focusing on optimism (Carver & Scheier, 2001) emphasize the significance of confidence in goal attainability in *simulated scenarios*, because such make-believe scenarios (as future orientation is) offer better progress than the one currently experienced. Thus, experienced identity thrives not only on one's accomplishments but rather on what one *expects* to achieve. This is particularly important for participants of this study who – because they are still preparing themselves to be admitted to the university and are in the process of choosing a major – experience transition more intensely than other emerging adults.

The process particularly relevant to emerging adults pertains to *commitment*. Defined as a decision to pursue a future course, commitment is an act of self-definition whose relevance draws from the emerging adulthood normative expectations and the personal satisfaction of reaching decisions, particularly so when applied to career and family as major adult roles. Although commitment may be transient during high school years and therefore not as important for identity development during that period (Grotevant & Cooper, 1998), its relevance for emerging adults draws on its greater stability at this developmental period.

In summary, as indicated by the percentage of explained variance, the effect of the motivational and behavioral future orientation variables on experienced identity underscores the agentic nature of experienced identity as defined by Erikson and several other identity researchers. However, others (Josselson, 1987) criticized it, indicating the narrowness of an identity construct that focuses only on agency and the need to redefine it by emphasizing both its agentic and relational aspects.

Study II: Emerging adults in military service. In this study (Ablin, 2006) future orientation is assessed by its motivational, cognitive, and behavioral components and identity by the identity status measure EOM-EIS (Grotevant & Adams, 1984) that pertains to *ideological* (subsuming occupation, religion, politics, and life-style) and *interpersonal* (friendship, dating, sex roles, and recreation) identity. The effect of the motivational, cognitive and behavioral components (each a composite score) on achieved identity is examined both cross-sectionally and longitudinally. However, because earlier analyses (Ablin, 2006) showed similar effects for the two groups (i.e., beginning to mid-term and mid-term to end of military service), they were combined.

The cross-sectional analyses show that the specific nature of the effect of future orientation on achieved identity co-varies with future orientation domain and component, and ideological vs interpersonal identity. Nonetheless, with few exceptions, Time 1 and Time 2 results are similar. Given their conceptual affinity, achieved identity is consistently affected by the relevant behavioral component. *Ideological* achieved identity is affected by the behavioral component of the three instrumental domains (military service, higher education, and work and career), and *interpersonal* achieved identity by the behavioral component of the relational (marriage and family) domain (βs range from 0.30 to 0.70, $p < 0.001$). Achieved identity is also affected by the extent to which individuals think about the relevant future domain. However, ideological identity is *negatively* affected by the cognitive component of military service and work and career (β $= - 0.20$ to $- 0.22, p < 0.05$) and interpersonal identity is *positively* affected by the marriage and family cognitive component (β $= 0.16, p < 0.05$).

The *longitudinal* analyses show similar effects but only for the ideological achieved identity. The behavioral component of each of the three Time 1 instrumental domains (military service, higher education, work and career) has a positive effect (βs ranging from 0.33 to 0.42, $p < 0.001$) while the cognitive component of military service has a *negative* effect (β $= -0.28, p < 0.01$) on ideological achieved identity at Time 2. In other words, the effect of exploration of and commitment to each of the instrumental domains on ideological achieved identity is maintained across-time. In addition, however, across-time achieved identity is also affected by *not* being preoccupied with thinking about military service.

The operational definition closeness between the future orientation behavioral component and achieved identity no doubt confounds the effects of this component on achieved identity. However, the negative effect of the cognitive component of military service and work and career on the ideological achieved identity speaks for the validity of the future orientation-achieved identity links, yet also calls for taking this analysis one step further by examining the future orientation *profiles* of individuals with different achieved identity scores. As described in the next section, this has been carried out by using cluster analysis.

Future orientation and achieved identity: cluster analysis. Although an exploratory statistical procedure, the a priori selection of variables and number of clusters has a conceptual underpinning. Relevant to the effect of future orientation on achieved identity and adjustment (discussed in a subsequent section) is the conceptualization of future orientation as a multiple-component multiple-domain construct. For purposes of the present analysis two distinctions are pertinent. One is between military service and the civil domains, and the other between instrumental and relational domains. Consequently, two separate cluster analyses were run. One consists of *instrumental* (higher education-work and career composite variables) and military service domains, and the other of the *relational* (marriage and family) and military service domains. As demonstrated in Fig. 7.4, each has a three cluster solution.

When examined contemporaneously (by using the General Linear Model procedure) the findings for *ideological* achieved identity show that, grouped according to their scores on the instrumental and military future orientation three components, the *positive balanced* group scores higher on achieved identity than do the *military negative* and *all negative groups*; however, the *military negative* scores higher than the *all negative group*.

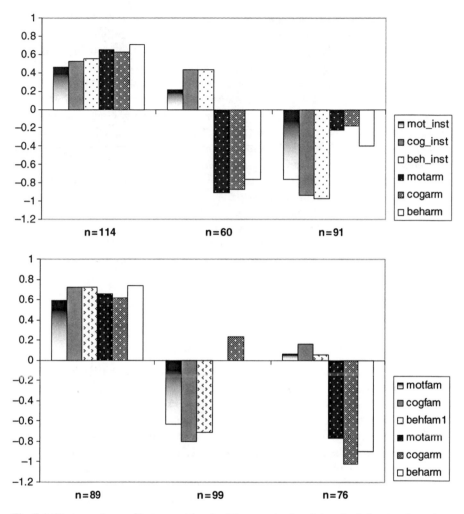

Fig. 7.4 Cluster analyses of instrumental and military service (arm) domains (*above*) and marriage and family and military service (arm) domains (*below*)

The effect of this clustering on the *interpersonal* achieved identity is similar but less differentiating: the *positive balanced* group has a stronger sense of achieved identity than the two other groups. This is also reflected in the percent of explained variance (15% of the ideological and 6% of the interpersonal achieved identity). Thus, for clusters based on the instrumental and military future orientation, it is the emotional tone (i.e., being positive vs negative toward the future) rather than domain that affects ideological and interpersonal achieved identity.

The clustering based on the family-military domains is similar to the instrumental-military clustering. The *positive balanced* group has a stronger sense of ideological and interpersonal achieved identity than the two other groups, and the *military negative* had a stronger ideological sense of achieved identity than the *family negative* group. However, longitudinally (18 months later) only the effect of the instrumental-military clusters on ideological achieved identity is maintained. The sense of achieved identity is lower for the *all negative* than for the two other groups, but the extent to which it explains achieved identity variance is similar (13%).

Altogether, these findings show the relevance of future orientation clusters (or grouping, or profiles) to individuals' sense of achieved identity contemporaneously and longitudinally. However, the longitudinal effects are maintained particularly for groups based on the instrumental-military domains.

Summary. The study of the effect of future orientation on identity formation among emerging adults has been guided by the assumption that as individuals move from adolescence to emerging adulthood future orientation does not lose its developmental significance, and one of its effects is on the formation of identity. Analyses of hypotheses derived from this assumption supported particularly the effect of the behavioral and to a lesser degree of the cognitive component. However, grouping our respondents across future orientation domains and components (by means of cluster analysis) shows the integrated effect of all three components on achieved identity.

Intimacy

Although empirical research tends to equate intimacy with self disclosure and close relationships, Erikson's writings present a more complex conceptualization of intimacy that emphasizes two abilities: to make *commitments* to intimate relationships and to develop the *ethical strength* necessary for maintaining them even at the cost of personal sacrifices (Erikson, 1963). Although the importance of the ability for intimacy is periodically reiterated, this aspect is still seldom included in the conceptualization of intimacy (Adams & Archer, 1994; Fischer, Munsch, & Greene, 1996) even by researchers drawing on Erikson's writings. Overall, researchers continue to conceptualize and assess intimacy in terms of relationships with same- or opposite-sex persons (Craig-Bray & Adams, 1986; Orlofsky, 1993; Orlofsky, Marcia, & Lesser, 1973).

Identity and intimacy. The contingent nature of the epigenetic model's stages has been especially pertinent to the dependence of intimacy on identity. For Erikson, "[It] is only when identity formation is well on its way that true intimacy – which is really a counterpointing as well as a fusing of identities – is possible" (Erikson, 1968, p. 135). In other words, the inherent difference between processes of constructing one's self definition (identity) and those of forming a union between two persons (intimacy) notwithstanding, intimacy can take place only after individuals have worked out a sense of self and reached an achieved identity.

Nonetheless, each process shares some elements with the other: although identity's main theme is the self, it contains relational aspects, and although intimacy's main theme is close relationship, it contains self aspects. Altogether both contain elements of individuality and connectedness (Dyk & Adams, 1987;

Grotevant & Cooper, 1986). Studies that assess the relation between identity and intimacy either contemporaneously or longitudinally (Adams & Archer, 1994; Dyk & Adams, 1990) support the link between them but not Erikson's (1968) contention that the identity-intimacy link is gender-related, and particularly relevant to women.

Future Orientation and Intimacy Links: Empirical Evidence

The relationship between future orientation and intimacy has not been studied before. Two considerations led Seginer and Noyman (2005) to propose it. The first emanated from similarity between meanings and processes underlying future orientation and intimacy. The key issues have been the conceptualization of intimacy as an ability for commitment to long-term relationships and of possessing personal ethical strength (Erikson, 1963), and the notion that possessing future oriented motivational forces and engaging in future oriented behaviors indicate a sense of personal strength and willingness to assume responsibility for long-term tasks, respectively.

Moreover, *willingness to assume responsibility* (which involves exploration and commitment) is facilitated by a *sense of personal strength* (expressed in the value attributed, the confidence in and a sense of inner control over the materialization of hopes and plans). This directional relation fits the three-component model of future orientation by which the motivational component affects the behavioral component, and gives it a particular meaning. Applied to the effect of future orientation on intimacy, the hypothesis has been that the motivational component variables have a direct net effect on intimacy (i.e., after the effect of the behavioral component variables is allowed for).

The second consideration regarding the future orientation-intimacy links drew on Erikson's (1964) contention that the development of the ethical strength underlying the ability for intimacy is contingent on a sense of identity and its concomitant virtue of fidelity. This has led us (Seginer & Noyman, 2005) to examine the effect of future orientation on intimacy both directly and via the effect of future orientation on experienced identity (discussed above).

These analyses, carried out on data collected from emerging adults who participated in the college preparatory program described earlier, show that overall the effect of the future orientation motivational and behavioral variables on intimacy is weaker than their effect on identity, particularly for the work and career domain (12% and 22% of the variance of intimacy is explained by the work and career and marriage and family domains, respectively). This effect grows stronger when identity is allowed to mediate the future orientation-intimacy link (percentage of explained variance goes up to 34% and 39% for the work and career and marriage and family domains, respectively). Moreover, while in this analysis identity is affected by commitment to both work and career and marriage and family, intimacy is affected by *exploration*. The effect of the motivational variables is domain specific: intimacy is affected by work and career expectance and by marriage and family sense of control.

Overall, the exploration-intimacy relation suggests that underlying intimacy as denoting interpersonal openness, warmth, friendliness and commitment to long-lasting relationship is an element of searching of the self, others and the relationships between them that continues after commitment has been made (Meeus et al., 1999). Given that emerging adults are engaged in exploration of future options (Arnett, 2000) and that participants in the Seginer and Noyman study were not married or cohabiting, the exploration-intimacy relation is especially relevant for them and others sharing their characteristics.

The net effect of the motivational variables is not as strong as expected and may thus indicate that personal strength (indexed by the future orientation motivational variables) affects intimacy indirectly via exploration. Adding this to the finding that explained variance increases when identity is added to the analysis, the picture emerging is that the ability for intimacy is affected by future oriented behavior focusing on exploration of work and career and marriage and family options and less by the motivation to engage in future orientation, and that future orientation affects the ability for intimacy both directly and indirectly via experienced identity. Although these findings represent the first analysis of the relations between future orientation and intimacy, their validity is supported by two findings: future orientation-intimacy links only partly resemble the future orientation-identity links, and the exploration-intimacy links are maintained when identity is included in the analysis.

Summary

Although all three are considered developmental tasks relevant to the emerging adulthood period, three considerations led Seginer and Noyman (2005) to predict that future orientation affects identity and intimacy. The first relates to historical changes in the Western world during the second half of the twentieth century that resulted in postponed entrance to adulthood and consequently to belated engagement in identity formation and the development of the ability for intimacy. Given that engagement in future orientation thinking is less dependent on accrued experiences and personal maturity, and as discussed in Chap. 2 has its initial indications in infancy and early childhood, middle adolescence is a suitable developmental period for expanding it. As individuals reach emerging adulthood their continued investment in future orientation serves as a basis for the work of identity formation.

The second and the third considerations are conceptual and concern the relations between future orientation and identity and between identity and intimacy. Drawing especially on ego identity approaches, these relations are founded on three theoretical contentions: that identity develops out of adolescents' anticipated adulthood (i.e., future orientation) (Erikson, 1958), that in adolescence future thinking is self-reflective (Marcia, 1983), and that the development of ability for intimacy is contingent on achieved identity (Erikson, 1968).

Analyses of two groups of emerging adults show the effects of future orientation components on experienced and ego identity and analysis of one of the groups also shows the direct and identity-linked relations between future orientation and intimacy, thus indicating that the sequence by which the construction of future orientation precedes the development of identity formation and the capacity for intimacy can be supported in cross-sectional analyses of emerging adults. However, longitudinally, the three developmental tasks are no doubt interrelated. This is particularly plausible under the assumption that the process of identity formation does not come to an end as the achieved identity status is reached but rather continues to be worked on and explored (Bosma & Kunnen, 2001; Meeus et al., 1999; Luyckx, Goossens, Soenens, & Beyers, 2006), and attested by a recent study of the relations between future orientation and identity formation indicated by exploration and commitment (Goossens, Luyckx, Lens, & Smits, 2008). Using a short-term longitudinal design, the authors have examined three rival models: future orientation (future time perspective) main effect (on identity), identity formation main effect, and a reciprocal model which indicated that across time future orientation and identity formation affect each other.

A final comment relates to cultural context. The two studies reported in this section describe the inter-relations between future orientation, identity, and intimacy among Israeli Jewish emerging adults who, in addition to having led their lives in a western setting, have also gone through several unique experiences, among them military service. Postulating that traditional cultural setting and earlier age of marriage affect the development of these three developmental tasks and the relations between them calls for continuing this research in traditional and transition to modernity cultural settings.

Future Orientation and Adjustment to Developmental Transitions

This section focuses on two developmental transitions and extends its developmental scope into middle adulthood. Specifically, it addresses the transition into and out of military service for two male groups that differ from each other in age, social background and military tasks. The first group consists of emerging adulthood conscripts and the second of non-commissioned officers who go into early retirement after 25 years of military service.

Emerging Adults' Adjustment to Military Service

Much of the developmental research on emerging adults' transitions has been devoted to transition from home to college as a common first step in the path to adulthood for youth growing up in western middle class settings. In non-western countries, the vast majority leaves home to establish their own families and are therefore unfamiliar with the experiences and opportunities characterizing this transition period. Obviously, for western youth, college is not the only transition opportunity. Americans may join the Peace Corps as well as other similar volunteer programs and, as mentioned earlier, Israeli Jewish adolescents and Druze boys serve in the military for at least 2 (girls) to 3 years (boys).

For several reasons the transitional qualities of Israeli colleges and universities are less unequivocal. Jewish male and female and Druze male emerging adults start their higher education after completing military service and often spend additional time earning money, traveling, and establishing a family. Those not married may opt to attend a university close to their parents' home (not the least for economic reasons). Finally, especially Arab and Druze girls are required to continue living at home until marriage and therefore attend a higher education institute close to home.

Drawing on research carried out in Israel, the discussion on the effect of future orientation on transitional outcomes for emerging adults focuses only on adjustment to military service of Israeli Jewish conscripts.

Entering compulsory military service. Although military service is a formative experience for Israeli Jewish girls and boys, published research on the experiences and consequences of military service is sparse. Nonetheless, its review identifies four relevant issues: motivation for military service, personal growth and transition to adulthood, relationships outside the military framework and particularly with parents, and the processes underlying adjustment to military service.

The *motivation* of potential conscripts to serve in the Israeli army (e.g., Gal, 1986; Ezrahi & Gal, 1995) has been undergoing some fluctuations but overall the majority of conscripts are motivated and view it as fulfillment of a personal obligation. As noted by Gal, military service has become "...an integral phase in the life of any Israeli youth" (Gal, 1986, p. 59). Although Gal's observations were made over 20 years earlier, they are still valid and should be understood in terms of the cultural heritage of voluntary participation in self defense organizations since the beginning of Jewish immigration to Palestine at the turn of the twentieth century (Scginer, 1999). Under these conditions, dissidence is a moral issue (Linn, 1996). Although it involves a relatively small number of reservists and even fewer mandatory service women and men, conscientious objection – like abstention from military service for any other reason – is considered gravely by the military as well as large sections of the general public.

Developmental studies of recruits show an overall positive effect of military service on individuals' sense of *personal growth* and expansion of personal boundaries (Lieblich & Perlow, 1988), an increased sense of independence, self-confidence, social sensitivity and ability for intimate relationships (Dar & Kimhi, 2001), and improved *adolescent-parent relationships* (Mayseless & Hai, 1998) which in turn has a positive effect on adjustment to military service (Mayseless, Scharf, & Sholt, 2003; Scharf, Mayseless, & Kivenson-Baron, 2004). Thus, despite the vast difference between their high school years and life under military regime that may involve physical hardships and incidents of military harshness, for the majority of young soldiers entering the military is experienced with a sense of control and coping.

Future orientation and adjustment to military service. Ablin's (2006) longitudinal design enabled her to examine several questions pertinent to adjustment to military service. These questions pertain to the effect of future orientation on adjustment as evaluated by the soldiers (self report) and their commanders cross-sectionally and longitudinally. Moreover, the psychological well-being of these emerging adults – which no doubt underlies their adjustment – can also be indicated by their future orientation endorsement after 18 months of military service. In the next sections findings and their interpretation regarding each of these issues are described.

Future orientation across time. Drawing on the relation between psychological well-being and future orientation (Melges, 1982), endorsement of future orientation is treated as an indicator of emotional health. Ablin's (2006) findings show that, similar to earlier findings on personal growth opportunities during military service (Lieblich & Perlow, 1988), as young soldiers spend more time in military service their future orientation scores for both the civil (higher education, work and career, and marriage and family) and the military service domains grow higher (Fig. 7.5). Obviously, like other longitudinal analyses, this finding confounds time in military service and age; nevertheless, it shows that despite military life restrictions, discipline, physical hardships, and limited control over one's daily routine, across time future orientation regarding both military service and civil domains is not curbed but rather promoted.

Future orientation and adjustment: contemporaneous effects. Cross-sectional multiple regression analyses of the effect of the motivational, cognitive, and behavioral components of each life domain on experienced adjustment (assessed by an adaptation of Folkman & Lazarus, 1980 emotion- and problem-focused coping questionnaire) and adjustment problems (IDF, 1983) show that the most consistent effect on both experienced adjustment and adjustment problems is that of the motivational component (with βs ranging from –0.53 on adjustment problems to 0.39 on adjustment, $p < 0.05$ to $p < 0.001$) and highest for military service.

For all domains the effect is positive for adjustment and *negative* for adjustment problems. In addition, engaging in the exploration of and reaching decisions about

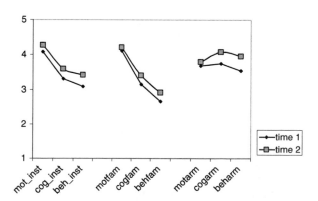

Fig. 7.5 Time 1 and Time 2 future orientation scores for instrumental, military service (arm), and marriage and family domains

military service options is associated with adjustment (i.e., a positive effect of the behavioral component on adjustment) and frequently thinking about each of the four domains is associated with higher adjustment problems (i.e., positive effect of the cognitive component on adjustment problems).

Future orientation and adjustment: longitudinal effects. Across-time, the effects on experienced adjustment are domain specific: similar to the cross-sectional analysis, both the motivational and the behavioral components of military service and the motivational component of higher education and work and career have a positive effect (βs ranging from 0.17 to 0.27, $p < 0.05$ to $p < 0.01$). However, the marriage and family components do not maintain their across-time effect. Moreover, the analyses of experienced *adjustment problems* emphasize the different role the civil and military service domains play for them.

Specifically, the cognitive (how often individuals think about domain-related hopes) component of all three civil domains has a *positive* effect (βs ranging from 0.20 to 0.39, $p < 0.05$ to $p < 0.001$) and the motivational component of all instrumental domains (i.e., military service, higher education, and work and career) has a *negative* effect on it (βs $= -0.17$ to -0.53, $p < 0.05$ to $p < 0.001$). Thus, like in the cross-sectional analysis, future orientation components vary in the extent they are associated with emerging adults' inclination to overcome military service adjustment problems. Particularly, frequently thinking about life after completing military service (be it higher education, work and career, or marriage and family) and low motivation regarding military service, higher education, and work and career enhances adjustment problems in military service.

In sum, all three components pertaining to civil and military service domains affect both experienced adjustment and adjustment problems, albeit differently. The motivational and behavioral components have a positive effect on experienced adjustment and negative effect on adjustment problems and the cognitive component has an opposite effect: it is negatively related to experienced adjustment and positively to adjustment problems. These findings prompted the pursuit of the *person approach* that focuses on future orientation profiles, created by cluster analysis of domains and components, as described next.

Future orientation profiles and adjustment: cluster analysis. The effect of future orientation clusters on adjustment and adjustment problems used the clusters initially created for examining the effect of future orientation on achieved identity.

Both cluster sets (the instrumental and military service and the marriage and family and military service clusters) predict adjustment better than adjustment problems. This is especially clear for the instrumental-military service set whose three cluster groups score differently on adjustment but not on adjustment problems. The cluster groups of the marriage and family-military service set score differently on both adjustment and adjustment problems but explain less of their variance (9% for the adjustment and 3% for adjustment problems) than the instrumental-military service set (15% for the adjustment and 3% for adjustment problems).

Moreover, the *positive balanced* group (scoring high on all three components of the instrumental and military service domains) is better adjusted than the two other groups, but the *negative military service* group (moderate instrumental and negative military service scores) does not differ from the *all negative* (scoring negatively on all components, but only moderately low on the military components) group.

The lower adjustment problems scores of the *positive balanced* group than of the two other groups thus confirm the protective potential of developing a *positive balanced* future orientation. Like the instrumental-military service, the marriage and family-military service *positive balanced* group is better adjusted than the two other groups, but unlike the instrumental-military service of the two other groups, the family negative is less well adjusted than the military negative.

In sum, the person-centered approach using cluster analysis enriches our understanding of the relation between future orientation and adjustment by showing the following findings. First, these clusters are better predictors of experienced adjustment than of adjustment problems. Second, while the *positive balanced* profile enhances adjustment low military service future orientation reduces adjustment, and is not counterbalanced by higher scores (i.e., more positive view) on the instrumental domains. Finally, the finding showing that whether using variable- or person-approach commanders' evaluations are not related to future orientation suggests that both adjustment and adjustment problems are inner experiences to which commanders have only very limited access and hence inaccurate information.

Midlife Adjustment to Early Retirement: The Case of Non-Commissioned Officers

Wilf's (2008) study focused on the early retirement of mid-life adult men who spent their entire professional career in military service performing semi-professional jobs. Guided by earlier research (Braitwaite & Gibson, 1987; Hogarth, 1988; Westergaard, Noble & Walker, 1989) as well as by her professional experience of working with this group, she constructed a three-step model consisting of antecedents and consequences of coping with early retirement and tested it in a 1-year longitudinal study.

Step 1 consists of four groups of *antecedent* variables: demographic factors (e.g., age, health, and expected income at retirement), situational conditions (retirement readiness), sense of procedural justice, and personal resources (e.g., self esteem, internal control, and future orientation variables subsumed under the three components of work and career and marriage and family domains). Assuming that early retirement is a stressful event, the model draws on Lazarus's theory of stress and coping (Folkman & Lazarus, 1980) and Step 2 includes primary and secondary *cognitive appraisal* and emotion- and problem-focused *coping*. Step 3 comprises *outcomes* defined in terms of subjective quality of life.

The 242 men (average age 45, and 25 years of professional military service) who participated in this study responded to self-report questionnaires (Time 1) and a telephone interview about specific (e.g., psychological, social, and physical health) and overall quality of life (Time 2, 12 months after retirement). Running her model once for work and career future orientation and once for marriage and family future orientation, Wilf's results show the consistent though indirect across-time effect of future orientation on the retirees' sense of quality of life, one year after retirement.

Because results for the various aspects of quality of life are similar here only findings on the retirees' sense of overall quality of life are described. These findings, resulting from multiple regression analyses, show the pivotal role of *expectance*. In both the work and career and the marriage and family models, expectance – that is how optimistic retirees are about fulfilling their hopes, goals, and plans – has a negative effect on the cognitive appraisal of retirement as *threat* and on *emotion-focused* coping, which in turn have negative effects on overall quality of life. Cognitive appraisal of challenge and problem-focused coping are not affected by future orientation variables nor do they affect the respondents' subjective quality of life.

The effect of the two other future orientation variables on emotion-focused coping is domain specific and positive. Exploration of marriage and family options and internal control over the fulfillment of work and career hopes and plans are each related to emotion-focused coping. Although at first sight the positive effect of the two future orientation indices on emotion-focused coping is puzzling, examination of their meaning for midlife men suggests the following interpretation. Exploration of marriage and family at mid-life indicates doubts about the marital bond, and internal control over work and career may reflect the burden of responsibility for finding a new job; consequently both increase emotion-focused coping. The value of these findings comes not only from shedding light on the relevance of future orientation for adults' sense of quality of life but also from highlighting the contextuality of future orientation effects. Specific to this group of retirees, some aspects of future orientation may hinder rather facilitate adjustment to civil life as indicated by their sense of overall quality of life.

In summary, a study of adjustment to early retirement as a major change in the lives of midlife men shows the relevance of future orientation to adjustment as assessed by their sense of overall quality of life. Specifically, three indicators of future orientation – expectance, internal control, and exploration – affect cognitive appraisal of retirement as threat and emotion-focused coping and via them the retirees' sense of overall quality of life. However, the nature of their effect varies. While internal control and exploration weaken it, expectance (indicating optimism about fulfilling hopes, goals, and plans) indirectly promotes the subjective quality of life.

Summary

This chapter examined five outcomes of future orientation: adolescents' academic achievement, emerging adults' identity and the capacity for intimacy, and adjustment to transition for emerging and midlife adults. The effect of future orientation on *academic achievement* is domain specific but not culture specific and interpreted in terms of perceived instrumentality. Specifically, academic achievement is positively affected by instrumental (higher education, work and career) future orientation and with one exception (negative effect on academic achievement of Israeli Arab adolescents) not by the marriage and family future orientation. These findings withstand cultural diversity and apply to Israeli Arab and Jewish girls and boys as well as to ultra-orthodox Jewish girls.

Domain specificity also holds for the effect of future orientation on identity and intimacy, showing that the extent to which specific future orientation variables affect each are domain specific. Moreover, while the behavioral variables of future orientation show a consistent effect on identity, commitment is especially relevant to identity formation and exploration to intimacy. These findings need to be considered in light of the theoretical controversy about the direction of the relation between future orientation and identity and the neglect of cultural consideration. Both are discussed in the chapter.

The effect of future orientation on adjustment to military service and from it to civilian life holds across time (18 months for adjustment to military service, and 1 year for adjustment to civilian life). However, while for emerging adults adjustment to military life is directly affected by future orientation, for midlife adults it reduces cognitive appraisal of retirement as threat and emotion-focused coping and via both improves their sense of quality of life.

Altogether, analyses of the effect of future orientation on the five outcomes show that the underlying processes for each future orientation-outcome link differ by all relevant dimensions, i.e., the nature of the outcome, the future orientation domain, and respondents' characteristics, particularly their gender, age and ethnicity. Overall, the contextuality of future orientation emphasized in each of the previous chapters is reiterated here too.

Chapter 8
Summary, Conclusions and Future Directions for Research and Action

By way of conclusion, this chapter attends to three main topics. The first is a summary. However, instead of recapitulating each of the chapters, it cuts across them and highlights the five main issues that have guided this volume. The second and third topics relate to implications for further research and for the translation of accumulated findings into future orientation guided programs.

Recapitulation: Future Orientation in Light of Five Main Issues

The Five Issues

The first issue concerns future orientation *conceptualization*. Its point of departure is the multiple research approaches studying future thinking and its objective is to examine their commonalities and differences toward understanding the effect of future orientation on development and psychological well-being. The second issue focuses on *developmental* perspectives. It examines the various indicators of future orientation across development from infancy to adolescence, emerging adulthood and adulthood and highlights the different psychological processes facilitating individuals' future thinking. Recent work on future orientation in adulthood and old age, not extensive enough for a separate chapter is reviewed in this section.

The third issue relates to *personality* antecedents. It sums up the effect of each of several self representation aspects and personality characteristics deemed relevant on the construction of future orientation and suggests an integrated view of their effect. The fourth issue concerns the effect of *interpersonal relationships*. It examines relationships with parents, siblings, and peers and focuses on three age-specific questions pertaining to socialization (in early childhood), relationships and beliefs (in adolescence). Finally, the fifth issue relates to culture. It reviews cross-cultural research on future orientation and its effect on developmental outcomes, shows that the answer to the question *does culture matter* is both *yes* and *no*, and specifies the conditions for each.

R. Seginer, *Future Orientation*, The Springer Series on Human Exceptionality,
DOI 10.1007/978-0-387-88641-1_8, © Springer Science+Business Media, LLC 2009

The Conceptual Issue: Future Orientation and Interfacing Approaches

Describing future orientation as an umbrella term indicates that, beyond a shared interest in how individuals see the future (or think about it), the approaches subsumed under it differ in their conceptualization, structure (as athematic or thematic and uni- or multiple-component) and consequently in their research questions and design. Concurrently, several other approaches share interest in future thinking but drawing on different theoretical underpinnings and developing separate research lines have been described in this volume (Chap. 1) as *interfacing approaches*.

In light of their common purpose – to describe how individuals construct the future – and diverse theoretical underpinnings, terminology, and research questions, the aim of this section is to indicate the common core and unique characteristics of each of the various approaches by weighing them against future orientation conceptualizations, in particular vis-á-vis the thematic approach and the three-component model introduced and examined in earlier chapters. Hence, a short recapitulation of the future orientation and the interfacing approaches will be followed by a section indicating the conceptual affinity of all and the unique contribution of each.

Future orientation: the thematic and three component model approaches. The *thematic* approach assesses future orientation by employing a three step procedure. In the first individuals write an essay or list their hopes and fears for the future, in the second these narratives are coded according to their content (themes) into separate hopes and fears future life domains, and in the third domain density scores defined as the number of domain-specific narratives/total number of narratives comprising the hopes and fears (respectively) *future life space* are computed. Research carried out with different age, sex, and socio-cultural groups distinguished between universal and culture-specific domains and between prospective life course and existential domains.

For adolescents and emerging adults, the four *universal* domains are higher education, work and career, marriage and family, and self concerns. *Prospective life course* domains are instrumental, goal-oriented domains which for adolescents and emerging adults pertain to higher education, work and career, and marriage and family, and the existential domains include self concerns ("to be happy", "that all my hopes will be materialized"), others (family members, friends), and collective issues ("world peace").

The three component model describes future orientation as consisting of motivational, cognitive representation, and behavioral aspects whose definitions in terms of manifest variables partly overlap with the variables of Nurmi's (1991) three components model. Also, like Nurmi's model, the three component model is generic (i.e., can be applied to different life domains) and its structure consists of multiple steps. In the three component model the motivational component affects the cognitive representation and the behavioral components and the cognitive representation component affects the behavioral component. Thus, the behavioral component is directly affected by the cognitive component and indirectly (via the cognitive component) by the motivational component.

The motivational component consists of the *value* attributed to a life domain, probability of materializing hopes, goals, and plans related to a life domain (*expectance*), and sense of internal *control* over materialization of domain specific hopes, goals, and plans. The cognitive representation component consists of the salience of domain specific *hopes* and *fears*, and the behavioral component consists of *exploration* of future options by gathering relevant information about each and their suitability for the person. *Commitment* pertains to making a decision about one of the options considered in the process of exploration.

Although the two behavioral variables are described by terms initially used in ego identity research underlying the future orientation and ego identity terms are different processes. Thus whereas in the ego identity theoretical framework exploration and commitment serve as the *observable indicators of intrapsychic processes* of identity formation (Marcia, 1993), in the future orientation conceptualization they indicate active engagement in exploration and commitment that leads toward the materialization of prospective hopes, wishes, and plans. Moreover, while ego identity statuses are defined by the *combined* presence or absence of explorations and commitment (Cote & Levine, 2002; Marcia, 1993) the future orientation conceptualization treats them as separate (though related) variables.

The interfacing approaches. Each of the interfacing approaches shares some commonalities with the future orientation models but also has unique characteristics or characteristics common to the other interfacing approaches but not to the future orientation models. To demonstrate it, after each is briefly summarized, its resemblance to the other approaches and its unique contributions are highlighted.

The future time perspective approach (Lens, Herrera, & Lacante, 2004; Nuttin & Lens, 1985) emphasizes the motivational basis of future thinking. Accordingly, the motivational relevance of the future emanates from the following rationale: human needs are translated into goals and behaviors aimed at achieving these goals, and goals, like plans, hopes, and fears are placed in the future. However, the motivational potential of the future is realized only if individuals perceive the instrumentality of present behavior to future goals and are able to create means-end chains that link the present to the future.

Three approaches – *personal projects* (Little, 1989), *personal strivings* (Emmons, 1989), and *life tasks* (Cantor & Kihlstrom, 1987) – represent the goal or *personal action construct* (Little & Chambers, 2004) approach to personality. Although each draws on a different theoretical framework, they commonly describe the pursuit of projects, strivings, or life tasks as self-generated, intentional, behavior guiding, and meaning giving. Moreover, all three approaches assess the *value* of each project (pertaining to its self benefit, fun, integrity, and support), striving (its valence), or life task (its importance and enjoyment); the personal projects and personal strivings assess internal *control* (indexed as efficacy, effort), and the personal strivings approach also assesses *expectance* (probability of success) and *commitment*.

The personal strivings approach assumes that strivings direct individuals toward some outcomes (approach) and away from others (avoidance), personal projects are analyzed in terms of their *motivational-affective, cognitive*, and *behavioral* aspects, and the personal strivings and life task approaches assess *behavioral* strategies (or ways for materializing strivings).

Of all four interfacing approaches, the *possible selves* conceptualization and research most closely resemble recent work on future orientation. This similarity must be viewed in the context of their different theoretical underpinnings and concurrent development but nonetheless few cross-references. As future orientation research draws on Lewin's (1939, 1942/1948) field theory and Atkinson's (1964) expectancy-value theory, *possible selves* research originated from self theory building on three assumptions: that the self is multifaceted, has motivational capacities, and exists in all time zones. The future self has been described by James (1890/1950) as potential self and by contemporary researchers (Markus & Nurius, 1986) as consisting of three possible selves: the ideal (or desired) self, the real self (what one could probably become), and the feared self (what one is afraid of becoming and hence should avoid).

Possible selves have three functions: motivational, evaluative (by comparing current to hoped for and feared selves), and simulation of the resources and behavioral strategies necessary for materializing desired and avoiding feared selves. However, the probability of achieving a desired goal increases if possible selves are linked to pertinent behavioral strategies (self-regulating), balanced (i.e., consist of both desired and feared possible selves that arouse both approach and avoidance behaviors), and socio-culturally contextualized.

Finally, the fourth approach views future orientation as a stable *personality disposition* (Boyd & Zimbardo, 2005; Zimbardo & Boyd, 1999) reflected in the ability to plan, set future goals, and understand the (present) behavior-(future) outcomes contingency as it applies to the probability that behavior will successfully lead to a particular outcome (similar to the three-components future orientation *expectance*) and confidence in one's ability to reach desired outcome (similar to the three-components future orientation *control*).

Summary: conceptual commonalities and differences. Although they draw on different theoretical framework, common to all approaches to future thinking has been its motivating power, be it because goals, hopes, and fears are located in the future (the *future time perspective* and *future orientation* approaches), because goals instigate and direct behavior into achieving them (*goal* approaches to personality, *personality* approaches), or because the self has a motivational capacity (*possible self* approach).

However, most approaches have also gone one step further and either described the nature of the motivating forces or suggested conditions that enhance the motivating power of future thinking and the likelihood of instigating behavior that will result in achieving a desired end state. The future orientation approaches as well as the goal approaches to personality specify several motivating forces, among them the *value* of a prospective domain specific object (i.e., hopes, goals, plans, strivings, projects, or tasks), the subjective probability of attaining a prospective object (*expectance*), and having *control* over its attainment. Four conditions augment the motivational power of the future and thus increase the probability of achieving a desired end state: perceiving the *instrumentality* of present behavior for achieving a future goal, creating *means-end* chains (future time perspective), developing *both desired and feared* domain specific possible selves, and *evaluating* one's present self vis-á-vis both (possible selves).

Finally, not all domains and not all possible selves are behavior-guiding. In the conceptual framework of future orientation *prospective life course* domains relate to developmental tasks (such as transition to adulthood and adulthood tasks, for adolescents) and hence are behavior guiding whereas the *existential* domains consist of either global future states or specific future states on which they have no control (e.g., world peace). In the *possible selves* framework, possible selves that include strategies for obtaining hoped for possible selves and avoiding feared possible selves *self regulate* behavior and those that do not include strategies provide only a sense of *self enhancement.*

Possibly because some approaches emphasize future thinking and others relate to extension (or projection) into the future, not all approaches include a behavioral aspect. Those that do treat it differently. Thus, the *future time perspective* approach emphasizes the importance of means-end chain, the *three-component model* of future orientation has a behavioral component that subsumes exploration of future options and commitment to one, and the *personal strivings, life tasks,* and *possible selves* approaches include specific goal-achieving behavioral strategies. However, other approaches, particularly the *personal projects* and *personal strivings* approaches, emphasize emotional outcomes. The *personal projects* approach identifies personal projects characteristics leading to psychological well being, and the *personal strivings* approach indicates that self striving pursuit incurs benefits and costs.

Finally, both Nurmi's (1989, 1991) and Seginer's (2005) *three-component* future orientation models describe future orientation as a multiple step process which has both theoretical and empirical levels and predict such adolescent developmental outcomes as academic achievement and emerging adults' tasks as adjustment to new situations, and experienced identity and intimacy. Overall, conceptual diversity notwithstanding, the common interest of the various approaches in the phenomenon and meaning of extension to the future explains their commonalities obscured by the use of different terminologies.

The Developmental Issue: A Case of Non-continuous Indicators

The importance of future thinking for human functioning (Suddendorf & Corballis, 2007; Tulving, 2002) has led researchers to examine future orientation across the life span. Nonetheless, as indicated in earlier chapters, this interest is unevenly distributed across different developmental periods. Ranking it according to number of publications, adolescence and recently also emerging adulthood come first followed by early childhood and infancy. Adulthood and particularly old age come last with relatively little work, although, as maintained in a subsequent section, extant work highlights its meaning for the elderly.

Future orientation in infancy and early childhood. While extension to the future is most clearly assessed by individuals' narratives and other verbal responses to future-related issues, these procedures obviously cannot be used with infants. To overcome it, researchers have turned to eye movement which is fast, controllable from birth, and an indicator closely related to the relevant perceptual systems. Using the visual expectation paradigm, Haith and his colleagues (see Chap. 2) have been able to show that the ability to anticipate object location develops early (2 months of age) and improves with time so that as infants grow older they are able to overcome task demandingness.

Infants' extension into the future is only several seconds long. Nonetheless, researchers assume that this ability speeds up information processing, may provide infants with a sense of control, and finally, serves as an early manifestation of and foundation for more elaborate future orientation. Thus, it may be concluded that by engaging in visual anticipatory behavior, infants introduce themselves to the notion and meaning of "future" long before they can verbally demonstrate it.

As is true of other areas of developmental research (e.g., attachment), children's developmental abilities influence research methods. However, in the area of future orientation they also affect conceptualization and research questions. Thus, as children reach early childhood the focus shifts to the assessment of cognitive abilities underlying future thinking, its verbal representations, and its behavioral consequences particularly indicated by planning behavior.

This research has informed us of three main conclusions: that children's ability to express future thinking depends on their ability to grasp the notion of time, understand the meaning of past and be able to distinguish between events occurring in the past and the future, that future thinking is a necessary condition for planning behaviors, and that clear indications of ability for future thinking appear between the age of 3 and 4. Mothers' time- and future talk is an important socializing factor, and though the relevance of children's literature has not been systematically examined, incidental reading suggests it too serves as an important and adult-mediated socializing factor of future thinking and future talk.

Future orientation in middle childhood, adolescence, and emerging adulthood. As children reach middle childhood they are able to describe their hopes and fears for the future. Although in its early stages their future orientation is infused with fantasy, between 2nd and 4th grades this tendency goes down sharply, children are able to relate to sex-typed adolescent, transition to adulthood, and adulthood developmental tasks. Given the importance of future thinking for adolescents and emerging adults, since Lewin's (1939) analysis these developmental periods have drawn much interest from future orientation researchers employing different approaches.

Among them are the thematic (narrative) approach pertaining to hopes, fears and goals for the future, the possible selves, and the multiple component future orientation approach. Their findings show that across the adolescent and emerging adult years, individuals construct their future in terms of relevant instrumental (e.g., higher education, work and career), relational (e.g., marriage and family), and existential (particularly self concerns) domains, and that the relative weight of these domains in the prospective life *space* is gender-specific so that females put higher emphasis on marriage and family and males on work and career.

However, in recent years the gender divide is narrowing down. Higher education is more salient for females, especially females growing up in transition to modernity cultural settings who view education as a "weapon in women's hands". Conceptualized as a three-component model, future orientation has been found to have an effect on developmental-specific outcomes: academic achievement for adolescents, adjustment to a new situation (i.e., military service for Israeli adolescents), and identity and intimacy development for emerging adults, and adjustment to early retirement for midlife adults.

Future orientation in adulthood and old age. As indicated earlier, research about future orientation in adulthood and old age is sparse. However, this is currently made up for by several studies on the construction and the effect of future orientation on adults' coping, particularly as they deal with transitional experiences. One study uses a longitudinal design to study the effect of adjustment of relevant (child related) goal appraisals during infertility treatment and its effect on depressive symptoms (Salmela-Aro & Suikkari, 2008).

Several studies have focused on the nature of future goals constructed by cancer patients and controls (Pinquart, Frohlich, & Silbereisen, 2007, 2008; Pinquart, Nixdorf-Hanchen, & Silbereisen, 2005), and two other studies examined the effect of future orientation on the psychological wellbeing of early retirees (Wilf, 2008) and on the effect of future orientation on bereavement among parents who lost a son in military action (Shalev, 2009). Work that has been carried out indicates that age-gradedness found among adolescents and emerging adults also applies to adulthood so that across a 10-year longitudinal study educational goals decrease and work, family and health goals increase (Salmela-Aro, Aunola, & Nurmi, 2007).

Research on future orientation in old age is even scarcer, presumably indicating the irrelevance of future thinking to old age. Extant research indicates that older adults' hopes and fears concern their health but their hopes, plans and dreams also relate to retirement, leisure and the world (Nurmi, 1992). Most telling is an interview carried out in a hospital ward with an old person who died shortly after being interviewed. Reflecting on his interest in the future he said:

> Here is what you might call a surprise. Even with the knowledge of what's happening to a person, I still go on dreaming about my future and making all sorts of plans. Nothing foolish, of course, and everything resting on the chance that I'll be getting out of this prison [hospital] one of these days. I have a notion it might be a good idea to straighten up my room and see whether I can't find some friends I know must be in the city, someplace. Lots of them are gone, I'm sure, but I think there would be a lot left, all probably wondering many of the things I'm wondering about. So you see, I'm thinking quite a bit about the future. That doesn't stop. Don't let anybody tell you that it does. (Cottle & Klineberg, 1974, pp. 57–58).

The future thinking of old adults has been studied in recent years by neuropsychologists. Their work shows several differences between future thinking of older and younger adults. Thus, when tested older adults generate closer future events (and more distant past events), and their responses have a larger number of emotional events than those of young adults (Addis, Wong, & Schacter, 2008; Lang & Carstensen, 2002). Moreover, building on work about the relation and neurological similarity between processes of retrieving the past and imagining the future (Addis, Wong, & Schacter, 2007; Schacter & Addis, 2007), research on the elderly has shown that, like in the case of remembering past events, imagining future events is characterized by decreased episodic specificity (Addis et al., 2008; Spreng & Levine, 2006).

This decrease is indicated by less information regarding the main event (internal details) and more information which is of lesser relevance to the main event and the time and place of its occurrence (external details). While the researchers suggest this pattern of imagining future events may be related to their ability to *integrate* information (relational memory), they also suggest it may reflect older adults breadth of knowledge and wisdom and tendency to place events within more meaningful contexts.

In the words that Tennyson poetically strung for Ulysses, past experiences feed future course, and the dialogue between them never ceases:

> . . .
> There lies the port; the vessel puffs
>   her sail:
> there gloom the dark broad seas.
>   My mariners,
> Souls that have toil'd , and wrought,
>   and thought with me –
> That ever with a frolic welcome took
> The thunder and the sunshine, and
>   opposed
> Free hearts, free foreheads – you and
>   I are old;
> Old age hath yet his honor and his
>   toil;
> Death closes all: but something ere
>   the end,
> Some work of noble note, may yet
>   be done,
> Not unbecoming men that strove with
>   Gods.
> The lights begin to twinkle from the
>   rocks:
> The long day wanes: the slow moon
>   climbs: the deep
> Moans round with many voices,
> Come, my friends,
> 'Tis not too late to seek a newer
>   world.
> Push off, and sitting well in order
>   smite
> the sounding furrows; for my pur-
>   pose holds
> To sail beyond the sunset, and the
>   baths
> Of all western stars, until I die.
> It may be that the gulfs will wash us
>   down:
> It may be we touch the Happy
>   Isles,

And see the great Achilles, whom
  we knew.
Tho' much is taken, much abides
  and tho'
we are not now that strength which
  in old days
moved earth and heaven; that which
  we are, we are;
One equal temper of heroic hearts,
Made weak by time and fate, but
  strong in will
To strive, to seek, to find, and not to
  yield. (Tennyson, 1861, pp. 104–105)

Summary. Overall, the relevance of future orientation to the entire life span requires different research designs and results in three kinds of age-related information; visual anticipation in infancy, future talk and planning in early childhood, and several approaches for studying the developmental span from early adolescence to old age. The thematic approach indicates the age-gradedness of future orientation, and the three component approach shows the consistency of the relations among the three components across age from early adolescence to emerging adulthood, and the age-specific relevance of their outcomes. Paucity of research on future orientation in adulthood and old age has recently been made up for indicating changes that future thinking may undergo as individuals reach old age.

The Personality Issue: The Role of the Self and Other Personality Characteristics

Initially, the study of the effect of the self and personality variables on future orientation drew on two considerations. One is that engagement in future orientated thinking and behavior calls for inner strength and optimism and therefore will be more prevalent among individuals who score high on self-evaluation, self empowerment, primary control, and strategic optimism. Conversely, future orientation may have a compensatory function and thus make up for loneliness, be prompted by the need to defend oneself against failure (defensive pessimists), and serve individuals who gain a sense of control by changing themselves (to fit external demands) rather than the environment (secondary control).

Empirical tests support the inner strength rather than the compensation rationale. Future orientation is constructed by individuals able to extend simultaneously to the future and attend to present demands. Underlying it are sense of self worth, psychological empowerment, and optimism about materialization of hopes, goals, and plans.

The moderating effects of culture and gender. As cultural and gender factors are added to our research design, the picture becomes more complex and the moderating effect of gender more pronounced. This is especially notable for the Arab girls who, against a background of traditionalism, challenge approaches of cultural prototypes and demonstrate strategies that intertwine acceptance of tradition with personal aspirations.

This applies particularly to high achieving Arab girls who caught between their aspirations for higher education and family endorsement of traditional women's roles develop high sense of self empowerment. They, like Druze girls, understand higher education as depending on self (psychological empowerment) and the need to control the environment (primary control). Druze boys, on the other hand, more than any of the other groups taking part in our studies treat the environment with deference, humility and obligation as these are reflected in a negative relation between primary control and military service and positive relation between secondary control and work and career.

Effects on future orientation as a three-component construct. As future orientation conceptualization is expanded to the three component model, the greater susceptibility of the motivational than of the cognitive representation and the behavioral variables to personality influences becomes evident. Of particular effect are the intra-personal factors indicating emotional health. However, in light of the effect of the motivational variables on the cognitive and behavioral aspects of future orientation, the emotional health intra-personal factors *indirectly* affect the cognitive and behavioral variables. Altogether, the effect of each of the intrapersonal characteristics examined in our studies has been modest but together they impress the relevance of psychological health and inner strength for engaging in future oriented thinking and behavior.

However, the question about the net effects of each of the inner strength (or psychological health) indicators is only partly answered. Our studies have some indications about the cultural and interpersonal specificity of the mediating effect of *self* constructs on future orientation. Thus, in models including both self esteem and psychological empowerment, for Jewish adolescents both tend to mediate the relation between parenting and peer relationships and future orientation, but only self agency mediates the effect of sibling relations and future orientation. For traditional Arab and ultra-orthodox Jewish girls, psychological empowerment but not self esteem mediates the effect of parenting as well as the effect of sibling and peer relationships.

Summary. Research has shown moderate positive effects of characteristics indicating inner strength and moderate negative effects of loneliness, defensive pessimism, and secondary control. While this tendency is shared by different cultural groups and gender, some analyses also show cultural and gender specificity. Moreover, the unique effect of each of the self and personality characteristics on future orientation needs to be further assessed.

The Interpersonal Relationships Issue: The Effect of Parents, Siblings and Peers

The non-continuity of future orientation conceptualization and research questions across age periods also applies to the effect of interpersonal relationships on the construction of future orientation. Differences pertain to two dimensions: the relationship object (i.e., parents, siblings, peers) and the nature of their effect and will be summarized here in relation to the two developmental periods in which these issues have been studied: early childhood and adolescence.

Early childhood. Early childhood research focuses on parents – particularly mothers – and examines how their socializing behaviors affect future talk and planning behavior. Its findings show that, although mothers devote only a very small part of their talk to time talk in general and future talk in particular, future talk has specific characteristics. It is age dependent, more complex than talk about the present and the past, and engages the child in the conversation. Thus, it is an instance of guided participation, effective when mother and child attend to an aspect brought by the other and take the other's perspective. In other words, underlying it is a process of *intersubjectivity*. However, while intersubjectivity is no doubt facilitated by the motivational-affective nature of mother-child relationships, this aspect has been only infrequently examined. One more sparsely studied issue has been nursery literature, which as shown in Chap. 2 may serve as another rich source of future talk mediated by mothers and other caregivers.

Adolescence. Research on the future orientation of adolescents has examined the effect of parents, siblings and peers by addressing relationships, beliefs, and interaction. However, only the effect of relationships has been examined for all three relationships. The effect of beliefs applies only to parents and of interaction only to peers. Moreover, drawing on the importance psychologists attribute to the *subjective* and their view that it is the environment as *experienced* by individuals that affects how they construct their conception of the self, perform various cognitive and social tasks and maintain relationships with others, the perceived aspect of both relationships and beliefs serves as the basis of all analyses.

These analyses have shown that, although both relationships with parents (parenting) and their perceived beliefs affect adolescents' future orientation, the underlying processes differ. Parenting affects future orientation only indirectly via the self whereas parental beliefs affect future orientation directly. The mediated path also characterizes the effect of relationships with siblings and peers and is maintained when the effect of all three relationships is examined. While this applies to western (Israeli Jewish adolescents), traditional Moslem (Israeli Arab adolescents) and ultra-orthodox Jewish girls, the parenting-future orientation is mediated via self esteem for the western adolescents and via self empowerment for the two traditional groups.

Although plausible that parents, siblings and peers affect the construction of future orientation by discussing, reflecting and bringing relevant information, data on the effect of such interaction exists only for peers. These data, as scarce as they are, indicate the power of the group to encourage but also to deter emerging adults from expressing commitment to high achievement goals.

Summary. Although future orientation has been examined across the life span, interest in the effect of interpersonal relationships has been limited to two periods: early childhood and adolescence. Early childhood research has focused on future talk socialization during mother-child interaction, showing that when mothers speak about the future they use more complex language and engage their child in conversation which prompts intersubjectivity for mother (or other caretakers) and child.

While early childhood research emphasizes cognitive aspects, research carried out with adolescents examines both affective (interpersonal relationships) and social cognitive (beliefs) aspects of interaction with others showing that both result in positive effect but via different paths: beliefs have a direct effect on future orientation whereas interpersonal relationships affect it only indirectly via self appraisal.

The Cultural Context Issue: Does Culture Matter?

The relevance of social context to the construction of future orientation was first examined by Israeli's (1936) work on future autobiographies in different social groups. Cross-cultural differences were first examined by Gillespie and Allport (1955). However, their interest was not prompted by theoretical considerations but rather by a belief in scientists' social responsibilities to world community. Several years after the end of World War II they studied the future images of young people in different countries, believing common hopes about the future would prompt international understanding and world peace.

Only later research conducted from the 1980s on has been guided by theoretical considerations drawing on socio-cultural characteristics. Following Cantril's (1965) distinction between hopes and fears of the future, these studies have shown various cultural differences particularly between adolescents growing up in western and non-western cultural settings. Although research questions and procedures varied, these studies did indicate the effect of cultural settings and orientations.

To illustrate, in an early study (Mehta et al., 1972) American young adolescents listed more self-related future events and Indian adolescents more other-related future events; in a later study (Nurmi et al., 1995) Australian adolescents were higher than Finnish and Israeli adolescents in listing leisure hopes and Israeli adolescents were higher than the two other groups in listing military service. However, differences were more pronounced and yielded a clearer picture when analyses also included sex differences: girls from transition to modernity settings (Indian, Israeli Arab, and Israeli Druze) scored higher on educational hopes and fears than did all other groups (i.e., transition to modernity boys and modern girls and boys).

However, studies conducted over the last 20 years comparing Israeli Arab, Druze, and Jewish adolescents showed three trends worth noting. While in early years, Israeli Arab and Druze adolescents scored lower on the prospective life course domains (pertaining to instrumental and relational behavior-directing narratives related to higher education, work and career, and marriage and family domains) and higher on existential domains (pertaining to non-specific, non-behavior directing narratives related to self concerns, others, and the collective) than Jewish adolescents, these differences have become smaller in recent years mainly due to changes in the future orientation of Arab and Druze adolescents now scoring higher on the prospective life course domains (Seginer, 2001a).

Nonetheless, one difference has been maintained through the years: Israeli Arab and Druze girls score higher on higher education hopes and fears than do all other groups. A third consistent finding qualifies these findings, showing that as future orientation is conceptualized in terms of the three-component model and its empirical fit is assessed across Arab, Jewish, and ultra-orthodox Jewish girls samples, the effect of culture all but disappears. This also applies to models including interpersonal relationships antecedents and academic achievement outcomes. However, with one exception, marriage and family future orientation have a negative effect on the academic achievement of Arab girls while nonsignificant for all other groups.

Thus, the answer to the *Does culture matter* question guiding this section is both *yes* and *no*; the rest of the section is devoted to delineating the conditions under which each applies. These considerations draw on three psychological approaches: Bronfenbrenner's (1979, 1989, 1995, 2005) ecology of human behavior, Gjerde's (2004) person-centered approach to cultural psychology, and McAdams and Pals' (2006) new big five theory. Bronfenbrenner's ecological approach has guided our hypothesis on future orientation cultural differences, Gjerde's person-centered approach has been included to present possible limits of the ecological approach, and McAdams and Pals' approach has been employed after the fact, to explain findings that do and do not support it.

Three approaches to cultural differences. Three aspects of Bronfenbrenner's *ecology of human development* approach are particularly relevant here. All are concerned with the question how culture (or any other instance of the macrosystem such as social class or ethnicity) affects specific aspects of human growth and development? The first contends that it is not culture *in toto*, or the entire cultural setting that affects development, but rather some of its features pertaining to *uniquely relevant* values and beliefs, economic and social resources, and available opportunities for *specific aspects* of personal growth.

The second is that these features are not just *distal* factors. Instead, they *permeate* into every environmental aspect or ecological system – from the exosystem to the microsystem – and conjointly affect children and adolescents' development. The third is that culture – like other aspects of the environment – gains its power over individuals by the manner in which it is being *experienced* by the individual. Most important to the present discussion is that, according to Bronfenbrenner's ecological approach, relevant cultural aspects 'color' all ecological systems and thus all affect the individual's development. However, their effect may take different pace (Silbereisen, 2005), and as a result of social circumstances (Trommsdorff, 2002), personality characteristics and how individuals experience reality result in individual differences (Bronfenbrenner & Morris, 2006).

Currently, at the other end of the continuum is Gjerde's (2004) person-centered approach. Gjerde's critique of existing conventions about culture led him to three conclusions. One is that culture and its ensuing ethnic or national identities have been created in the interest of political systems to maintain their members' loyalty by separating them from the other. In other words, culture is a colonial invention guided by the *separate and rule* dictum.

The second pertains to the power of culture. Given that transmitted cultural values, beliefs and practices are subjectively interpreted by individuals (as also contended by Bronfenbrenner), their influence is lesser than assumed by researchers. Finally, in light of the importance of systems of meaning, the valid unit of analysis should not be culture or ethnicity but rather social class. All in all, Gjerde's person-centered approach contends that culture and collective identity are products of political manipulation and "individuals are always more than their memberships in communities, cultures or any other social aggregates" (p. 153).

While many researchers may contest Gjerde's approach, the viability of the manipulation of social identities has been demonstrated by Sherif's (1976) early social psychological work in which experimentally induced animosity between groups created a within group "we-feeling".

In between the two approaches is McAdams and Pal's (2006) approach presented in their paper *a new big five theory*. As indicated by its title, their approach has been developed in the theoretical context of personality theory and its purpose has been to outline an integrative framework for the study of personality. As indicated by the authors, its aim has been "...to help consolidate the gains personality psychology has made in recent years and to bring its many regions together within an elegant theoretical frame" (p. 205). This is important to emphasize because in the present context the new big five theory is "borrowed" for other purposes than those intended by the authors and used to interpret cultural commonalities and differences found in future orientation studies. Relevant to the present analysis is McAdams and Pal's contention that cultural effects depend on the personality level under consideration.

Specifically, psychological universals designed through evolution to serve basic psychological needs are least dependent on cultural variations. While McAdams and Pals list autonomy, competence, and relatedness as psychological universals, it is here contended that serving as the temporal dimension of motivation in general and goal-setting and planning in particular future orientation is another such psychological universal (Kluckhohn & Strodtbeck, 1961). At the other end of cultural adaptation are surface personality characteristics (Asendorpf & van Aken, 2003) subsuming motivational, social-cognitive and developmental processes indicated by goals, plans, and strivings individuals set for themselves, self-image descriptors, and society set developmental tasks, and even more so life narratives reflecting persons' identity. All these are to a large extent product of cultural settings and the orientations developed in them.

A fourth approach: the developmental niche. The developmental niche (Super & Harkness, 1986, 2002) is adapted to the child's developmental period and like the ecological system aimed at affecting developmental outcomes, consists of several integrated subsystems (the physical and social settings, child rearing customs, and caretakers' psychology) and shaped by cultural characteristics. Especially relevant to findings on the future orientation of transition to modernity girls is the developmental niche function to *preserve the continuity of cultural regularities* via three different mechanisms: redundancy, elaboration, and chaining.

By assuming cultural stability this analysis emphasizes the *challenges* faced by adolescents for whom cultural continuity counteracts adolescents' developmental strivings. Cases in point are American ethnic minority and immigrant adolescents engaged in the task of bridging multiple selves (Cooper, 2003; Cooper, Dominguez,

& Rosas, 2005), lower-class ethnic minority adolescents who do not enjoy automatic cuing of academic self-regulating behaviors provided by the concerted support of parents, school and community (Oyserman, Bybee, & Terry, 2006), and Israeli Arab girls who strive for a new identity combining tradition with modernity and women's independence, extensively discussed in this volume.

Applied to findings on the future orientation of transition to modernity adolescents, and particularly transition to modernity girls, it underscores the conflicting forces underlying their future orientation and their attempt to resolve these conflicts by intertwining *higher education* with *marriage and family, others,* and *collective issues* domains. Thus, while in developing their future orientation western adolescents enjoy a concerted support sustained by individualistic value orientations and made concrete by pertinent information and the availability of role models provided through multiple channels, this is not the case for transition to modernity adolescents and particularly for girls. Under conditions of social change, they may strive for more modern adulthood than accorded by their society, which is stressful for both. From the society's point of view, cultural reproduction (i.e., continuity) is threatened, and from the point of view of the individual, the support ensuing from the developmental niche regularity (Super & Harkness, 2002) is missing. This is attested by Israeli Arab girls' narratives reported in several chapters of this book, particularly Chap. 7.

Summary. Given that findings have indicated an inconsistent picture of the effect of culture on future orientation, the aim of this section has been to show which aspects of future orientation are more and less susceptible to it, and provide an explanation to these differences. Studies conducted in recent years in Israel showed that the three-component future orientation model has been empirically estimated across several socio-cultural groups. These groups differ, however, in the narratives and the density of future life domains.

While hypotheses drawing on the ecological model predict cultural differences across all future orientation aspects and the person-centered approach predicts no cultural differences, the new big five approach, though developed as an integrated personality theory, suits these findings best. It contends that the effect of culture varies from low effect on personality as reflected in basic psychological needs such as autonomy, competence, and relatedness and highest on personality as reflected in life narratives. Applying the differential role of culture principle to future orientation, it is contended that *future orientation is another psychological need that serves both individual and societies and hence its structure (the three-component model) is least susceptible to cultural differences whereas its narratives are culture specific.*

Directions for Future Research

Three directions for future research are suggested here. The first direction pertains to augmentation of extant research. Thus, each of the five issues around which the summary is organized may serve as basis for additional research of three kinds.

One pertains to substantiating existing results by examining additional samples in the same and different socio-cultural and age groups. The second is pursuing longitudinal studies that will show the developmental course of various dimensions of future orientation, examine the continuity of future orientation across age and different indicators and explore the effect of future orientation on various developmental outcomes across time.

The second direction pertains to the study of two developmental periods all but neglected by future orientation research: adulthood and old age. Research pertaining to each period may focus on three issues. The first is to learn how individuals subjectively construct their prospective life space; given that future orientation of adolescents and emerging adults is self-centered, the extent to which adults and old age individuals include in their prospective life space family and non-family members is of special interest. The second is to examine the validity of the three component model for these age groups, and the third is to delineate the developmental course of future orientation across the adulthood and old age periods by employing longitudinal designs.

The third direction pertains to expanding future orientation research by examining questions so far only sparsely investigated. One pertains to the relations between memory and future orientation. The question is not new. Tulving (1985, 2005) has emphasized it in his work, Suddendorf and Corballis (1997, 2007) have coined the *mental time travel* term to capture both memory and future thinking processes, and the relations between personal (episodic) memory and future thinking (personal strivings) of emerging adults has been recently empirically tested (Sutin & Robins, 2008). Working with young children, Friedman's (1990, 2005) findings show that future thinking emerges from their sense of time, and drawing on Tulving's distinction between episodic and semantic memory Atance and O'Neill (2001) assess *episodic future thinking*. Finally, to underscore the parallel nature of memory and future thinking, in this volume (Chap. 1) future orientation has been described as individuals' *prospective* autobiography.

Recently, these issues have taken a new direction by scientists searching for the equivalence of neurological processes underlying memory of past events and imaging of future events (e.g., Addis et al., 2007, 2008; Schacter & Addis, 2007; Spreng & Levine, 2006). While this work is at its initial stages it calls for expanding the perimeter of future orientation research by investigating the neurological processes underlying the construction of future orientation as it applies to the volume, themes, and emotional tone of future orientation across the lifespan.

Theory into Practice: Turning Hopes into Plans and Plans into Outcomes

Intervention programs based on future orientation and possible selves have been scant, though their number has increased in recent years. With one exception, these interventions are intended for adolescents and focus on academic achievement.

The aim of this section is to summarize this work and suggest several more issues that need to be considered to help people of a wide age range to identify goals, develop plans, and commit themselves to implementation. Overall, the aim of these intervention programs has been to encourage future thinking and particularly extension of the self into the future and use it as leverage for enhancing psychological well-being.

The academic achievement pathway. Work aimed at school success has been drawing on the possible selves conceptualizations. While the specific programs (Hock, Deshler, & Schumaker, 2006; Oyserman, Brikman, & Rhodes, 2007; Oyserman et al. 2006; Oyserman, Terry, & Bybee, 2002) varied, they all build on the extended conceptualization of possible selves (Oyserman et al., 1995) that distinguishes between self-regulating and self-enhancing possible selves and contends that to become self-regulating, possible selves must be balanced (i.e., include domain specific possible selves that are both positive and desired and negative and to be avoided) and linked to pertinent behavioral strategies.

All programs have shown better results for "treatment" than for control students ranging in age from middle school (Oyserman et al., 2007, 2006, 2002) to undergraduate university students (Hock et al., 2006). However, the advantages of a program that goes beyond the development of academic possible selves and appropriate behavioral strategies for attaining those academic selves has been indicated in a program implemented by Oyserman and her associates (Oyserman et al., 2007, 2006) with lower class ethnic minority middle school (8th grade) students.

This program includes four additional elements: it guides students to view difficulties as a normative part of attaining desired academic possible selves (inoculation), it integrates possible selves into students' social identity, emphasizes the relevance of academic possible selves to all participants (peers), and translates personal experiences into metamessages (e.g., "we all care about school", "we all want good future"). Thus, altogether, the program is contextualized in personal meanings, interpersonal relationships, and social identity. Its effectiveness has been attested by contrasting the treatment and the control groups at three postinterventional points: end of 8th grade, and the fall and spring of 9th grade.

These analyses show that at the end of 8th grade within each homeroom, adolescents participating in the intervention program scored higher than controls on all three outcomes: academic possible selves (balanced academic possible selves, plausible academic possible selves, and feared possible selves), self-regulatory behaviors (school attendance), and academic outcomes (pertaining to GPA and standardized test scores). By end of 9th grade, the effect of the intervention on self-regulatory behavior and academic outcomes were not only sustained but the differences between students participating in the program and control increased, in fact indicating a decrease of self-regulatory behaviors and academic outcomes among controls. Thus, this program protected participants against academic outcomes decline and facilitated transition to high school.

Building on studies conducted by Oyserman and her associates, Oyserman and James (2008) have recently charted a multiple-step model delineating the path from the construction of possible self in context to persistent self regulation toward achieving expected possible self (and avoiding negative possible self). To successfully reach the final step, several additional steps need to be satisfied: the gap between present and expected possible self is clear, the possible self is attainable (or a feared possible self avoidable), balanced (i.e., consists of expected and its relevant feared possible self), linked to appropriate strategies, corresponds to important social identities, and the goal associated with the possible self is considered important.

Career development. The program designed to improve students' career planning introduced them to future orientation thinking. While using different terminology, in fact the program includes all of the variables subsumed under the three component future orientation model. In the language of its developers the aim of the program has been to "recognize the importance of planning for the future" (*value*), "evaluate the possibilities of achieving their goals" (*expectance*), "anticipate events they can expect to experience" (*control*), "construct a representation of their future life" (*cognitive representation*), and "engage in the process of goal setting" (*exploration* and *commitment*) (Marko & Savickas, 1998, p. 108).

Their participants were high school (10th graders) and community college students randomly divided between treatment and control groups. The treatment groups participated in 5 weekly sessions (40 min) divided into three phases: orientation, differentiation, and integration. The aim of orientation has been to increase awareness of and optimism toward the future, the aim of differentiation has been to concretize the future and encourage goal setting and planning, and the aim of integration to establish links between present behavior and future outcomes, practice planning skills, and prompt career awareness. The control participants received no treatment and all participants were briefed about the program (rationale and aim) and personal score on the Career Maturity Inventory. Tests of the effectiveness of this program showed that, relative to controls, the treatment group participants enhanced their motivation but not the *quality* of their planning skills. It is plausible, however, that given their enhanced motivation, additional training would result also in higher planning skills scores for the treatment than for the controls.

Additional applications. Research (Petry, Bickel, & Arnett, 1998) showing that future orientation serves as a protective factor against consumption, the application of possible selves conceptualization to therapy (Dunkel, Kelts, & Coon, 2006), and studies conducted with adults undergoing personal transitions and reported earlier in this chapter (section on future orientation in adulthood and old age) indicate the breadth of issues to which intervention programs based on future orientation research are relevant.

Theory into Practice: A Generic Scheme of Linking Future Hopes to Present Behavior

Although the programs described above are a modest starting point from which to propose an outline for future orientation intervention programs, the cumulative knowledge on the factors affecting and affected by future orientation at different developmental periods provides a sound basis for such programs. Hence, this section outlines several elements deemed important to the implementation of all such programs. Moreover, although all three components of the future orientation model pertaining to motivational, cognitive representation, and behavioral aspects need to be included in such programs, the sequence may vary.

In other words, programs may first encourage participants to construct their future orientation as it applies to hopes and fears, followed by work on the *value* of and personal meaning of tasks such as student, job-holder and family person, the extent to which one can gain *control* over the materialization of the person's hopes, goals, and plans, and conditions for enhancing the probability of materialization (*expectance*).

In other words, by relating to these motivational aspects the program moves from description into the prerequisites for action-planning that emphasizes the responsibility of the individual together with her or his dependence on the commitment of individuals and institutions to their well-being. Thus, by working on the motivational aspects of future orientation, programs may also emphasize interpersonal reciprocity and the individual's responsibility for obtaining help from individuals and social institutions (psychological empowerment).

The third phase of these programs draws on the behavioral component that includes exploration of each of the hopes translated into a goal and commitment to one domain-specific option. By examining the nature and the requirements of options as well as the extent to which it indeed fits the person, exploration guides the individual to identify and gain the necessary information and skills for developing necessary strategies. This process may also advise individuals whether an option initially deemed feasible indeed fits them and make other options initially considered impractical or unfit attainable. Consequently, exploration may narrow down the number of viable options and thus facilitate the process of commitment.

Obviously, this outline offers guidelines for a *generic* program that needs to be adjusted to the age group, participants' special circumstances and needs, and their cultural setting. Hopes, goals, plans, appropriate strategies for achieving them and the permission to exercise self-empowerment may all be subject to cultural interpretations that need to be considered while developing a specific program.

Finally, although future orientation has been described as a process that involves mainly intrapersonal processes, programs aimed to help individuals develop future orientated thinking and behavior must also attend to two social considerations. One pertains to the role of interpersonal relationships as a source of help and collaboration; the second relates to the community: to gain effectiveness future orientation programs (as well as other intervention programs) must be supported by the social environment. Thus another guideline for designing future orientation based programs draws on *across-system regularity* (Super & Harkness, 2002). For adolescents it implies the inclusion of peers, parents (Oyserman et al., 2007, 2006, 2002) and schools, and for adults, their families and members of their social milieu. Altogether, the contextualization of future orientation emphasized across this book is also relevant to intervention programs based on it.

In Conclusion

While this book has addressed many topics subsumed here under the five themes of conceptual, developmental, personality, interpersonal relationships, and cultural context, underlying them is a common theme: linking hopes, goals and plans situated in the future to present behavior, future oriented thinking and future-guided behavior facilitate development, prompt adjustment and consequently promote individuals' well-being. The findings of studies presented in this volume attest to it, indicating what early future orientation studies have asserted: our future orientation serves our present. Poets say it best:

> Go, go, go, said the bird: human kind
> Cannot bear very much reality.
> Time past and time future
> What might have been and what has been
> Point to one end, which is always present. (T.S. Eliot, 1963)

References

Ablin, E. (2006). *Psychological development and adjustment to military service: A short-term longitudinal study*. Unpublished doctoral dissertation, University of Haifa, Israel.

Abramson, L. Y., Metalsky, G. I., & Alloy, L. B. (1989). Hopelessness depression: A theory-based subtype of depression. *Psychological Review, 96,* 358–372.

Adams, G. R., & Archer, S. L. (1994). Identity: A precursor to intimacy. In S. L. Archer (Ed.), *Interventions for adolescent identity development* (pp. 193–213). Thousand Oaks, CA: Sage.

Addis, D. R., Wong, A. T., & Schacter, D. L. (2007). Remembering the past and imagining the future: Common and distinct neural substrates during event construction and elaboration. *Neuropsychologia, 45,* 1363–1377.

Addis, D. R., Wong, A. T., & Schacter, D. L. (2008). Age-related changes in the episodic simulation of future events. *Psychological Science, 19,* 33–41.

Adler, S. A., & Haith, M. M. (2003). The nature of infants' visual expectations for event content. *Infancy, 4,* 389–421.

Allen, J. P., Hauser, S. T., Bell, K. L,, & O'Connor, T. G. (1994). Longitudinal assessment of autonomy and relatedness in adolescent-family interactions as predictors of adolescent ego development and self-esteem. *Child Development, 65,* 179–194.

Allport, F. H. (1937). Teleonomic description in the study of personality. *Character and Personality, 5,* 202–214.

Allport, G. W. (1937/1949). *Personality: A psychological interpretation.* London: Constable & Company LTD.

Alsaker, F. D., & Olweus, D. (1992). Stability of global self evaluations in early adolescence: A cohort longitudinal study. *Journal of Research on Adolescence, 2,* 123–145.

Anastasi, A. (1958). *Differential psychology: Individual and group differences in behavior.* New York, NY: Mcmillan.

Anderson, J. R. (1983). *The architecture of cognition.* Cambridge, MA: Harvard University Press.

Anderson, K. B., & Wood, M. D. (2005). Considering the future consequences of aggressive acts: Established and potential effects in the context of the general aggression model. In A. Strathman & J. Joireman (Eds.) *Understanding behavior in the context of time: Theory, research, and application* (pp. 243–270). Mahwah, NJ: Erlbaum.

Andriessen, I., Phalet, K., & Lens, W. (2006). Future goal setting, task motivation and learning of minority and non-minority students in Dutch schools. *British Journal of Educational Psychology, 76,* 827–850.

Anthis, K. S., Dunkel, C. S., & Anderson, B. (2004). Gender and Identity status differences in late adolescents' possible selves. *Journal of Adolescence, 27,* 147–152.

Archer, J. (1996). Sex differences in social behavior: Are the social role and evolutionary explanations compatible? *American Psychologist, 51,* 909–917.

Archer, S. L. (1989). Gender differences in identity development: Issues of process, domain, and timing. *Journal of Adolescence, 12,* 117–138.

Archer, S. L., & Waterman, A. S. (1993). Identity status interview: Late adolescent college form. In J. E. Marcia, A. S. Waterman, D. R. Matteson, S. L. Archer, & J. L. Orlofsky (Eds.), *Ego identity: A handbook for Psychological research* (pp. 303–317). New York, NY: Springer-Verlag.

Arnett, J. J. (2000). Emerging adulthood: A theory of development from the late teens through the twenties. *American Psychologist, 55*, 469–480.

Asendorpf, J. B., & van Aken, M. A. G. (2003). Personality-relationship transaction in adolescence: Core vs. surface personality characteristics. *Journal of Personality, 71*, 629–666.

Atance, C. M., & O'Neill, D. K. (2001). Planning in 3-year-olds: A reflection of the future self? In C. Moore & K. Lemmon (Eds.), *The self in time: Developmental perspectives* (pp. 121–140). Mahwah, NJ & London: Erlbaum.

Atance, C. M., & O'Neill, D. K. (2005a). Preschoolers' talk about future situations. *First Language, 25*, 5–18.

Atance, C. M., & O'Neill, D. K. (2005b). The emergence of episodic future thinking in humans. *Learning and Motivation, 36*, 126–144.

Atance, C. M., & Melzoff, A. N. (2005). My future self: Young children's ability to anticipate and explain future states. *Cognitive Development, 20*, 341–361.

Atance, C. M., & Melzoff, A. N. (2006). Preschoolers current desires wrap their choices for the future. *Psychological Science, 17*, 583–587.

Atkinson, J. W. (1964). *An introduction to motivation*. Princeton, NJ: Van Nostrand.

Atkinson, J. W., & Feather, N. T. (1966). Review and appraisal. In J. W. Atkinson & N. T. Feather (Eds.), *A theory of achievement motivation* (pp. 327–370). New York: Wiley.

Austin, J. T., & Vancouver, J. B. (1996). Goal constructs in psychology: Structure, process, and content. *Psychological Bulletin, 120*, 338–375.

Aviezer, O., Sagi, A., Resnick, G., & Gini, M. (2002). School competence in young adolescence: Links to early attachment relationship beyond concurrent self-perceived competence and representations of relationships. *International Journal of Behavioral Development, 26*, 397–409.

Azmitia, M. (1988). Peer interaction and problem solving: When are two heads better than one? *Child Development, 59*, 87–96.

Azmitia, M., & Hesser, J. (1993). Why siblings are important agents of cognitive development: A comparison of siblings and peers. *Child Development, 64*, 430–444.

Azmitia, M., Montgomery, R., & Cruz, S. (1993). Friendship, transactive dialogues, and the development of scientific reasoning. *Social Development, 2*, 202–221.

Bakan, D. (1966). *The duality of human existence: Isolation and communication in western man*. Boston: Beacon Press.

Baker, C. D. (1984). Contemporary of future choosers? A research note. *Journal of Early Adolescence, 4*, 75–81.

Bandura, A. (1977). *Social learning theory*. Englewood Cliffs, NJ: Prentice-Hall.

Bandura, A. (1982). Self-efficacy mechanism in human agency. *American Psychologist, 37*, 122–147.

Bandura, A. (1986). The explanatory and predictive scope of self efficacy theory. *Journal of Social and Clinical Psychology, 4*, 359–373.

Bandura, A. (1993). Perceived self-efficacy in cognitive development and functioning. *Educational Psychologist, 28*, 117–148.

Bandura, A. (1997). *Self-efficacy: The exercise of control*. New York, NY: Freeman.

Bandura, A. (2001). Social cognitive theory: An agentic perspective. *Annual Review of Psychology, 52*, 1–26.

Bank, S. P., & Kahn, M. D. (1982). *The sibling bond*. New York, NY: Basic Books.

Bank, L., Patterson, G. R., & Reid, J. B. (1996). Negative sibling interaction patterns as predictors of later adjustment problems in adolescent and young adult males. In G. H. Brody (Ed.), *Sibling relationships: Their causes and consequences* (pp. 197–230). Norwood, NJ: Ablex.

Barakat, H. (1993). *The Arab world*. Berkeley, CA: University of California Press.

Barndt, R. J., & Johnson, D. M. (1955). Time orientation in delinquents. *The Journal of Abnormal and Social Psychology, 51*, 343–345.

Bauer, P. J., Schwade, J. A., Wewerka, S. S., & Delaney, K. (1999). Planning ahead: Goal-directed problem solving by two-year-olds. *Developmental Psychology, 35,* 1321–1337.

Bem, S. L. (1993). *The lenses of gender: Transforming the debate on sexual inequality.* New Haven & London: Yale university press.

Benson, J. B. (1994). The origins of future orientation in the everyday lives of 9-to 36-month infants. In M. M. Haith, J. B. Benson, R. R. Roberts, & B. Pennington, (Eds.), *The development of future-oriented Processes* (pp. 375–407). Chicago, IL: University of Chicago Press.

Benson, J. B. (1997). The development of planning: Its About Time. In S. Friedman & E. Skolnick (Eds.), *The developmental psychology of planning: Why, how, and when do we plan?* (pp. 43–75). Mahwah, New Jersey: Erlbaum.

Benson, J. B., Talmi, A., & Haith, M. M. (1999). *Adult speech about events in time: A replication.* Poster session presented at the biennial meeting of the Society for Research in Child Development, Albuquerque, NM.

Berkman, S. (1993). *The future orientation of high school students and high school graduates: Age and academic track effects in the context of vocational education.* Unpublished master's thesis, University of Haifa, Israel.

Berzonsky, M. D. (1989). Identity style: Conceptualization and measurement. *Journal of Adolescent Research, 4,* 267–281.

Berzonsky, M. D. (2003). Identity style and well-being: Does commitment matter? *Identity, 3,* 131–142.

Berzonsky, M. D. (2005). Ego identity: A personal standpoint in a postmodern world. *Identity, 5,* 125–136.

Berzonsky, M. D., & Adams, G. R. (1999). Reevaluating the identity status paradigm: Still useful after 35 years. *Developmental Review, 19,* 557–590.

Beyers, W., & Goossens, L. (1999). Emotional autonomy, psychosocial adjustment and parenting: Interactions, moderating, and mediating effects. *Journal of Adolescence, 22,* 753–769.

Blasi, A., & Glodis, K. (1995). The development of identity. A critical analysis from the perspective of the self as subject. *Developmental Review, 15,* 404–433.

Blatt, S. J., D'-Afflitti, J. P., & Quinlan, D. M. (1976). Experiences of depression in normal young adults. *Journal of Abnormal Psychology, 85,* 383–389.

Blatt, S. J., Hart, B., Quinlan, D. M., Leadbeater, B., & Auerbach, J. (1993). Interpersonal and self-critical dysphoria and behavioral problems in adolescents. *Journal of Youth and Adolescence, 22,* 253–269.

Boivin, M., Hymel, S., & Bukowski, W. M. (1995). The role of social withdrawal, peer rejection, and victimization by peers in predicting loneliness and depressed mood in childhood. *Development and Psychopathology, 7,* 765–785.

Booth, M. (2002). Arab adolescents facing the future: Enduring ideals and pressures to change. In B. B. Brown, R. W. Larson, & T. S. Saraswathi (Eds.), *The world's youth: Adolescence in eight regions of the globe* (pp. 207–242). New York, NY: Cambridge University Press.

Bosma, H. A., & Kunnen, E. S. (2001). Determinants and mechanisms in ego identity development: A review and synthesis. *Developmental Review, 21,* 39–66.

Bowlby, J. (1973). *Attachment and loss: Vol. 2. Separation: Anxiety and anger.* New York, NY: Basic Books.

Boyd, J. N., & Zimbardo, P. G. (2005). Time perspective, health, and risk taking. In A. Strathman & J. Joireman (Eds.), *Understanding behavior in the context of time: Theory, research, and application* (pp. 85–107). Mahwah, NJ: Erlbaum.

Braitwaite, V. A., & Gibson, D. M. (1987). Adjustment to retirement: What we know and what we need to know. *Aging and Society, 7,* 1–18.

Briggs, S. R. (1989). The optimal level of measurement for personality constructs. In D. M. Buss & N. Cantor (Eds.), *Personality psychology: Recent trends and emerging directions* (pp. 246–260). New York: Springer Verlag.

Brittain, C. V. (1963). Adolescent choices and parent-peer cross pressures. *American Sociological Review, 28,* 385–391.

Brock, T. C., & Giudice, C. D. (1963). Stealing and temporal orientation. *Journal of Abnormal and Social Psychology, 66,* 91–94.

Brody, G. H. (1998). Sibling relationship quality: Its cause and consequences. *Annual Review of Psychology, 49,* 1–24.

Brody, G. H., & Stoneman, Z. (1995). Sibling relationships in middle childhood. In R. Vasta (Ed.), *Annals of child development* (Vol. 11, pp. 73–93). London and Bristol, PA: Kingsley Publishers.

Brody, G. H., Stoneman, Z., & Burke, M. (1987). Child temperament, maternal differential behavior, and sibling relationships. *Developmental Psychology, 23,* 354–362.

Bromberg, P. M. (2006). "Ev'ry time we say goodbye I die a little": Commentary on Holly Levenkorn's "Love (and hate) with proper stranger". *Psychoanalytic Inquiry, 26,* 182–201.

Bronfenbrenner, U. (1979). *The ecology of human development: Experiments by nature and design.* Cambridge, MA: Harvard University Press.

Bronfenbrenner, U. (1989). Ecological systems theory. In R. Vasta (Ed.), *Annals of Child Development: Vol. 6. Six theories of child development: Revised formulations and current issues* (pp. 187–249). Greenwich, CT: JAI Press.

Bronfenbrenner, U. (1995). Developmental ecology through space and time: A future perspective. In P. Moen, G. H. elder, & K. Lüscher (Eds.), *Examining lives in context: Perspectives on the ecology of human development* (pp. 619–647). Washington, DC: American Psychological Association.

Bronfenbrenner, U. (Ed.). (2005). *Making human beings human: Bioecological perspectives on human development.* Thousand Oaks, CA: Sage.

Bronfenbrenner, U., & Morris, P. (2006). The bioecological model of human development. In W. Damon & R. M. Lerner (Eds.), *Handbook of child psychology* (6th ed., Vol. 1, pp. 793–828). Hoboken, NJ: John Wiley & Sons.

Brown, B. B. (2004). Adolescents' relationships with peers. In R. M. Learner & L. Steinberg (Eds.), *Handbook of adolescent psychology* (2nd Ed., pp. 363–393). Location: John Wiley & Sons, Inc.

Brown, K. W., & Ryan, R. M. (2003). The benefits of being present: Mindfulness and its role in psychological well-being. *Journal of Personality and Social Psychology, 84,* 822–848.

Brunia, C. H. M., & van Boxtel, G. J. M. (2001). Wait and see. *International Journal of Psychophysiology, 43,* 59–75.

Bryant, B. K. (1992). Sibling caretaking: Providing emotional support during middle adolescence. In F. Boer & J. Dunn (Eds.), *Children's sibling relationships: Developmental and clinical issues* (pp. 55–69). Hillsdale, NJ: Erlbaum.

Buhrke, R. A. (1988). Factor dimensions across different measures of sex role ideology. *Sex Roles, 18,* 309–321.

Busby, J., & Suddendorf, T. (2005). Recalling yesterday and predicting tomorrow. *Cognitive Development, 20,* 362–372.

Buss, D. M. (1994). *The evolution of desire: Strategies of human mating.* New York, NY: Basic Books.

Buss, D. M. (1995a). Psychological sex differences: Origins through sexual selection. *American Psychologist, 50,* 164–168.

Buss, D. M. (1995b). Evolutionary psychology: A new paradigm for psychological science. *Psychological Inquiry, 6,* 1–30.

Buss, D. M. (2004). *Evolutionary psychology: The new science of the mind.* Boston: Pearson.

Buss, D. M., Abbott, M., Angleitner, A., Asherian, A., Biaggio, A., Blanco-Villasenor, A., et al. (1990). International perspectives in selecting mates: A study of 37 cultures. *Journal of Cross-Cultural Psychology, 21,* 5–47.

Buss, D. M., & Schmitt, D. P. (1993). Sexual strategies theory: An evolutionary perspective on human mating. *Psychological Review, 100,* 204–232.

Cacciopo, J. T., Ernst, J. M., Burleson, M. H., McClintock, M. K., Malarkey, W. B., Hawkley, et al. (2000). Lonely traits and concomitant physiological processes: The MacArthur social neuroscience studies. *International Journal of Psychophysiology, 35,* 143–154.

Cantor, N. (1990). From thought to behavior: "Having" and "doing" in the study of personality and cognition. *American Psychologist, 45,* 735–750.

Cantor, N., Acker, M., & Cook-Flannagan, C. (1992). Conflict and preoccupation in the intimacy life task. *Journal of Personality and Social Psychology, 63,* 644–655.

Cantor, N., & Harlow, R. E. (1994). Personality, strategic behavior, and daily-life problem solving. *Current Directions in Psychological Science, 3,* 169–172.

Cantor, N., Kemmelmeier, M., Basten, J., & Prentice, D. A. (2002). Life task pursuit in social groups: Balancing self exploration and social integration. *Self and Identity, 1,* 177–184.

Cantor, N., & Kihlstrom, J. F. (1987). *Personality and social intelligence.* Englewood, NJ: Prentice-Hall.

Cantor, N., & Langston, C. A. (1989). Ups and downs of life tasks in a life transition. In L. A. Pervin (Ed.), *Goal concept in personality and social psychology* (pp. 127–168). Hillsdale, NJ: Erlbaum.

Cantor,N., & Norem, J. K. (1989). Defensive pessimism and stress and coping. *Social Cognition, 7,* 92–112.

Cantor, N., Norem, J. K., & Brower, A. M. (1987). Life tasks, self concept ideals, and cognitive strategies in a life transition. *Journal of Personality and Social Psychology, 53,* 1178–1191.

Cantor, N., Norem, J. K., Langston, C. A., Zirkel, S., Fleeson, W., & Cook-Flannagan, C. (1991). Life tasks and daily life experience. *Journal of Personality, 59,* 425–451.

Cantor, N., Norem, J. K., Niedenthal, P. M., Langston, C. A., & Brower, A. M. (1987). Life tasks, self-concept ideals, and cognitive strategies in a life transition. *Journal of Personality and Social Psychology, 53,* 1178–1191.

Cantor, N., & Sanderson, C. A. (1998). The functional regulation of adolescent dating relationships and sexual behavior: An interaction of goals, strategies, and situations. In J. Heckhausen & C. S. Dweck (Eds.), *Motivation and self-regulation across the life span* (pp. 185–215). New York, NY: Cambridge University Press.

Cantril, H. (1965). *The pattern of human concerns.* New Brunswick, NJ: Rutgers University Press.

Carver, C. S., & Scheier, M. F. (2001). Optimism, pessimism and self regulation In E. C. Chang (Ed.), *Optimism and pessimism: Implications for theory, research, and practice* (pp. 31–51). Washington, DC: American Psychological association.

Carver, C. S., & Scheier, M. F. (2002). Optimism. In C. R. Snyder & S. J. Lopez (Eds.), *Handbook of positive psychology* (pp. 231–243). New York, NY: Oxford University Press.

Cashmore, J. A., & Goodnow, J. J. (1985). Agreement between generations: A two-process approach. *Child Development, 56,* 493–501.

Cervone, D. (2005). Personality architecture: Within-person structures and processes. *Annual Review of Psychology, 56,* 423–452.

Chao, R. K. (2001). Extending research on the consequences of parenting style for Chinese Americans and European Americans. *Child Development, 72,* 1832–1843.

Chen, X., Chang, L., He, Y., & Liu, H. (2005). The peer group as a context: Moderating effects on relations between maternal parenting and social and school adjustment in Chinese children. *Child Development, 76,* 417–434.

Chodorow, N. (1978). *The reproduction of mothering: Psychoanalysis and the sociology of gender.* Berkley, Los Angeles, CA: University of California Press.

Clark, K. E., & Ladd, G. W. (2000). Connectedness and autonomy support in parent-child relationships: Links to children's socioemotional orientation and peer relationships. *Developmental Psychology, 36,* 485–498.

Cleveland, E. S., & Reese, E. (2005). Maternal structure and autonomy support in conversations about the past: Contributions to children's autobiographical memory. *Developmental Psychology, 41,* 276–388.

Coleman, J., Herzberg, J., & Morris, M. (1977). Identity in adolescence: Present and future self concepts. *Journal of Youth and Adolescence, 6,* 63–75.

Collins, W. A., & Laursen, B. (2004). Parent-adolescent relationships and influences. In R. M. Lerner & L. Steinberg (Eds.), *Handbook of adolescent psychology* (2nd ed., pp. 331–361). New York, NY: John Wiley & Sons, Inc.

Constantinople, A. (1969). An Eriksonian measure of personality development in college students. *Developmental Psychology, 1,* 357–372.

Cooley, C. H. (1902). *Human nature and the social order.* Glencoe, IL: Free press.

Cooper, C. R. (2003). Bridging multiple worlds: Immigrant youth identity and pathways to college. *International Society for the Study of Behavioral Development Newsletter,* No. 2, Serial No. 38, 1–4.

Cooper, C. R. (in press). *The weaving of maturity: Cultural perspectives on adolescent development.* New York, NY: Oxford University Press.

Cooper, C. R., & Cooper, R. G. (1992). Links between adolescents' relationships with their parents and peers: Models, evidence and mechanisms. In R. D. Parke & G. W. Ladd (Eds.), *Family-peer relationships: Modes of linkage* (pp. 135–158). Hillsdale, NJ: Erlbaum.

Cooper, C. R., Dominguez, E., & Rosas, S. (2005). Soledad's dream: How immigrant children bridge multiple worlds and build pathways to college. In C. R. Cooper, C. T. Garcia Coll, W. T. Bartko, H. Davis, & C. Chatman (Eds.), *Developmental pathways through middle childhood* (pp. 235–260). Mahwah, NJ: Erlbaum.

Coopersmith, S. (1967). *The antecedents of self esteem.* San Francisco: Freeman.

Cote, J. E., & Levine, C. G. (2002). *Identity formation, agency and culture.* Mahwah, NJ: Erlbaum.

Cottle, T. J., & Klineberg, S. L. (1974). *The present of things future: Explorations in the time of human experience.* New York, NY: The Free Press.

Craig-Bray, L., & Adams, G. R. (1986). Measuring social intimacy in same-sex and opposite-sex contexts. *Journal of Adolescent Research, 1,* 95–101.

Creten, H., Lens, W., & Simons, J. (2001). The role of perceived instrumentality in student motivation. In A. Efklides, J. Kuhl, & R. M. Sorrentino (Eds.), *Trends and prospects in motivation research* (pp. 37–45). Dordrecht: Kluwer Academic Publishers.

Cronin, H. (1991). *The ant and the peacock.* Cambridge, UK: Cambridge University Press.

Cross, S., & Markus, H. (1990). The willful self. *Personality and Social Psychological Bulletin, 16*(4), 726–742.

Csikszentmihalyi, M., & Larson, R. (1984). *Being adolescent.* New York, NY: Basic Books, Inc.

Cummings, E. M., & Smith, D. (1993). The impact of anger between adults on sibling emotions and social behavior. *Journal of Child Psychology and Psychiatry, 34,* 1425–1433.

Daly, M., & Wilson, M. (1994). Evolutionary psychology of male violence. In J. Archer (Ed.), *Male violence* (pp. 253–288). London: Routledge.

Dar, Y., & Kimhi, S. (2001). Military service and self-perceived maturation among Israeli youths. *Journal of Youth and Adolescence, 30,* 427–448.

Day, J. D., Borkowski, J. G., Punzo, D., & Howespian, B. (1994). Enhancing possible selves in. Mexican American students. *Motivation and Emotion, 18,* 79–103.

Deaux, K., & Major, B. (1987). Putting gender into context: An interactive model of gender-related behavior. *Psychological Review, 94,* 369–389.

Deaux, K., & Major, B. (2004). A social-psychological model of gender. In M. S. Kimmel (Ed.), *The gendered society reader* (pp. 72–81). New York, NY: Oxford University Press.

Dekel, S. (2009). *The world of ultra-orthodox girls: An ecological analysis of women's roles and future orientation.* Unpublished doctoral dissertation. University of Haifa, Israel.

Dekovic, M., & Meeus, W. (1997). Peer relations in adolescence: Effects of parenting and adolescents' self concept. *Journal of Adolescence, 20,* 163–176.

De Volder, M., & Lens, W. (1982). Academic achievement and future time perspective as a cognitive-motivational concept. *Journal of Personality and Social Psychology, 42,* 566–571.

DiLalla, L. F., Thompson, L. A., Plomin, R., Phillips, K., Fagan, J. F. III, Haith, M. M., et al. (1990). Infant predictors of preschool and adult IQ: A study of infant twins and their parents. *Developmental Psychology, 26,* 759–769.

Douvan, E., & Adelson, J. (1966). *The Adolescent experience.* New York, NY: Wiley.

Dr. Seuss. (1990). *Oh, the places you'll go!*. New York, NY: Random House.

Dudai, Y., & Carruthers, M. (2005). Memory: Some systems in the brain may be better equipped to handle the future than the past. *Nature, 434*, 567.

Dunkel, C. S. (2000). Possible selves as a mechanism for identity exploration. *Journal of Adolescence, 23*, 519–529.

Dunkel, C. S., & Anthis, K. S. (2001). The role of possible selves in identity formation: A short-term longitudinal study. *Journal of Adolescence, 24*, 765–776.

Dunkel, C. S., Kelts, D., & Coon, B. (2006). Possible selves as mechanisms of change in therapy. In C. Dunkel & J. Kerpelman (Eds.), *Possible selves: Theory, research, and applications* (pp. 187–204). New York, NY: Nova.

Dunn, J. (1983). Sibling relationships in early childhood. *Child Development, 54*, 787–811.

Dunn, J. (1992). Sisters and brothers: Current issues in developmental research. In F. Boer & J. Dunn (Eds.) *Children's sibling relationships: Developmental and clinical issues* (pp. 1–17). Hillsdale, NJ: Erlbaum.

Dunn, J. (2005). Commentary: Siblings in their families. *Journal of Family Psychology, 19*, 654–657.

Dunn, J., Slomkowski, C., & Beardsall, L. (1994). Sibling relationships from the preschool period through middle childhood and early adolescence. *Developmental Psychology, 30*, 315–324.

Dyk, P. A., & Adams, G. R. (1987). The association between identity development and intimacy during adolescence: A theoretical treatise. *Journal of Adolescent Research, 2*, 223–235.

Dyk, P. A., & Adams, G. R. (1990). Identity and intimacy: An initial investigation of three theoretical models using cross-lag panel correlations. *Journal of Youth and Adolescence, 19*, 91–110.

Eagly, A. H. (1987). *Sex differences in social behavior: A social-role interpretation*. Hillsdale, NJ: Erlbaum.

Eagly, A. H. (1995). The science and politics of comparing women and men. *American Psychologist, 50*, 145–158.

Eagly, A. J., & Crowley, M. (1986). Gender and helping behavior: A meta-analytic review of the social psychological literature. *Psychological Bulletin, 100*, 283–308.

Eagly, A. H., & Johnson, B. T. (1990). Gender and leadership style: A meta-analysis. *Psychological Bulletin, 110*, 109–128.

Eagly, A. H., Karau, S. J., & Makhijani, M. G. (1995). Gender and the effectiveness of leaders: A meta-analysis. *Psychological Bulletin, 117*, 125–145.

Eagly, A. H., & Mitchell, A. A. (2004). Social role theory of sex differences and similarities: Implications for the sociopolitical attitudes of women and men. In M. A. Paludi (Ed.), *Praeger guide to the psychology of gender* (pp. 183–206). Westport, CT: Praeger.

Eagly, A. H., & Steffen, V. J. (1984). Gender stereotypes stem from the distribution of women and men into social roles. *Journal of Personality and Social Psychology, 46*, 735–754.

Eagly, A. H., & Wood, W. (1999). The origins of sex differences in human behavior: Evolved dispositions versus social roles. *American Psychologist, 54*, 408–423.

East, P. L., & Rook, K. S. (1992). Compensatory patterns of support among children's peer relationships: A test using school friends, nonschool friends, and siblings. *Developmental Psychology, 28*, 163–172.

Eccles, J. S., Adler, T. F., & Meece, J. L (1984). Sex differences in achievement: A test of alternate theories. *Journal of Personality and Social Psychology, 46*, 26–43.

Eccles, J. S., & Wigfield, A. (1995). In the mind of the actor: The structure of adolescents' achievement, task value and expectancy related beliefs. *Personality and Social Psychology Bulletin, 21*, 215–225.

Eccles, J. S., & Wigfield, A. (2002). Motivation, beliefs, and goals. *Annual Review of Psychology, 53*, 109–132.

Ekman, G., & Lundberg, U. (1971). Emotional reaction to past and future events as a function of. temporal distance. *Acta Psychologica, 35*, 430–441.

Elder, G. H. Jr. (1974). *Children of the Great Depression: Social Change in Life Experience*. Chicago, London: University of Chicago Press.

Elder, G. H. Jr. (1986). Military times and turning points in men's lives. *Developmental Psychology, 22,* 233–245.

Elder, G. H., Jr., Caspi, A., & Burton, L. M. (1988). Adolescent Transitions in Developmental Perspective: Sociological and Historical Insights. In M. R. Gunnar & W. A. Collins (Eds.), *Development During the Transition to Adolescence* (pp. 151–179). Hillsdale, NJ: Erlbaum.

Elder, G. H., Jr., Modell, J., & Parke, R. S. (Eds.). (1993). *Children in Time and Place: Developmental and Historical Insights.* New York: Cambridge University Press.

Eliot, T. S. (1963). *Four quartets.* London: Faber.

Emmons, R. A. (1989). The personal striving approach to personality. In L. A. Pervin (Ed.), *Goal concepts in personality and social psychology* (pp. 87–126). Hillsdale, NJ: Erlbaum.

Emmons, R. A. (1992). Abstract versus concrete goals: Personal striving level, physical illness, and psychological well-being. *Journal of Personality and Social Psychology, 62*(2), 292–300.

Emmons, R. A. (1996). Striving and feeling: Personal goals and subjective well-being. In J. Bargh & P. Gollwitzer (Eds.), *The psychology of action: Linking motivation and cognition to behavior* (pp. 314–337). New York: Guilford.

Emmons, R. A. (1999). *The psychology of ultimate concerns: Motivation and spirituality in personality.* New York: Guilford.

Emmons, R. A., & King, L. A. (1988). Conflict among personal strivings: Immediate and long-term implications for psychological and physical well-being. *Journal of Personality and Social Psychology, 54,* 1040–1048.

Engels, R. C. M. E., Deković, M., & Meeus, W. (2002). Parenting practices, social skills and peer relationships in adolescence. *Social Behavior and Personality, 30,* 3–18.

Epley, D., & Ricks, D. R. (1963). Foresight and hindsight in the TAT. *Journal of Projective Techniques, 27,* 51–59.

Erikson, E. H. (1950). *Childhood and society.* New York, NY: Norton.

Erikson, E. H. (1958). *Young man Luther.* New York, NY: Norton.

Erikson, E. H. (1963). *Childhood and society* (2nd ed.). New York, NY: Norton.

Erikson, E. H. (1964). *Insight and responsibility.* New York, NY: Norton.

Erikson, E. H. (1968). *Identity, youth and crisis.* New York, NY: Norton.

Eronen, S., Nurmi, J. E., & Salmela-Aro, K. (1998). Optimistic, defensive-pessimistic, impulsive and self-handicapping strategies in university environments. *Learning and Instruction, 8,* 159–177.

Evans, G. W., Shapiro, D. H., & Lewis, M. A. (1993). Specifying dysfunctional mismatches between different control dimensions. *British Journal of Psychology, 84,* 255–273.

Eysenck, M., & Payne, S. (2006). Anxiety and depression: Past, present, and future events. *Cognition & Emotion, 20,* 274–294.

Ezrahi, Y., & Gal, R. (1995). *World views and attitudes of high school students toward social, security and peace issues.* Zichron Ya'akov, Israel: The Carmel Institute for Social Studies. (Hebrew)

Farruggia, S. P, Chen, C., Greenberger, E., Dmitrieva, J., & Macek, P. (2004). Adolescent self-esteem in cross-cultural perspective: Testing measurement equivalence and a mediation model. *Journal of Cross-Cultural Psychology, 35,* 719–733.

Feingold, A. (1992). Gender differences in mate selection preferences: A test of the parental investment model. *Psychological Bulletin, 112,* 125–139.

Fischer, J. L., Munsch, J., & Greene, S. M. (1996). Adolescence and intimacy. In G. R. Adams, R. Montemayor, & T. P. Gullotta (Eds.), *Psychosocial development during adolescence* (pp. 95–129). Thousand Oaks, CA: Sage.

Flum, H., & Blustein, D. L. (2000). Reinvigorating the study of vocational exploration: A framework for research. *Journal of Vocational Behavior, 56,* 380–404.

Folkman, S., & Lazarus, R. S. (1980). Analysis of coping in a middle-aged community sample. *Journal of Health and Social Behavior, 21,* 219–239.

Frank, L. K. (1939). Time perspectives. *Journal of Social Philosophy, 4,* 293–312.

Friedlmeier, W., & Trommsdorff, G. (1998). Japanese and German mother-child interactions in early childhood. In G. Trommsdorff, W. Friedlmeier, & H. J. Kornadt (Eds.), *Japan in transition: Sociological and psychological aspects* (pp. 217–230). Berlin: Pabst Science Publishers.

Friedman, W. J. (1990). Children's representation of the. pattern. of. daily. activities,. *Child Development, 61*, 1399–1412.

Friedman, W. J. (2000). The development of children's knowledge of the times of future events. *Child Development, 71*, 913–932.

Friedman, W. J. (2005). Developmental and cognitive perspectives on humans' sense of the times of past and future events. *Learning and Motivation, 36*, 145–158.

Friedman, W. J., & Kemp, S. (1998). The effects of elapsed time and retrieval of young children's judgments of the temporal distances of past events. *Cognitive Development, 13*, 335–367.

Friedman, S. L., & Scholnick, E. K. (Eds.). (1997). *The developmental psychology of planning: Why, how, and when do we plan?* Mahwah, NJ & London: Lawrence Erlbaum Associates.

Fromm, E. (1941). *Escape from freedom.* New York, NY: Greenwood Press.

Frost, R. (1960). *A pocket book of Robert Frost's poems.* New York: Washington Square Press.

Gal, R. (1986). *A portrait of the Israeli soldier.* New York, NY: Greenwood Press.

Gardner, W., & Rogoff, B. (1990). Children's deliberateness of planning according to task circumstances. *Developmental Psychology, 26*, 480–487.

Gass, K., Jenkins, J., & Dunn, J. (2007). Are sibling relationships protective? A longitudinal study. *Journal of Child Psychology and Psychiatry, 48*, 167–175.

Gauvain, M. (1999). Everyday opportunities for the development of planning skills: Sociocultural and family influences. In A. Goncu (Ed.), *Children's engagement in the world: Sociocultural perspectives*, (pp. 173–201). New York, NY: Cambridge University Press.

Gauvain, M., & Perez, S. M. (2008). Mother-child planning and child compliance. *Child Development, 79*, 761–775.

Gauvain, M., & Rogoff, B. (1989). Collaborative problem solving and children's planning skills. *Developmental Psychology, 25*, 139–151.

Gelberg, Y. (1996). *Development of future orientation in pre-adolescence: Age and sex differences during middle childhood.* Unpublished master's thesis, University of Haifa, Israel.

Gillespie, J. M., & Allport, G. W. (1955). *Youth's outlook on the future; a cross-national study.* Garden City, New York: Doubleday.

Gini, M., Oppenheim, D., & Sagi-Schwartz, A. (2007). Negotiation styles in mother-child narrative co-construction in middle childhood: Associations with early attachment. *International Journal of Behavioral Development, 31*, 149–160.

Gjerde, P. F. (2004). Culture, power, and experience: Toward a person-centered cultural psychology. *Human Development, 47*, 138–157.

Gjesme, T. (1983). On the concept of future time orientation: Considerations of some functions' and measurements' implications. *International Journal of Psychology, 18*, 443–461.

Goldstein, S. E., Davis-Kean, P. E., & Eccles, J. S. (2005). Parents, peers, and problem behavior: A longitudinal investigation of the impact of relationship perceptions and characteristics on the development of adolescent problem behavior. *Developmental Psychology, 41*, 401–413.

Goodnow, J. J. (1997). The interpersonal and social aspects of planning. In S. L. Friedman & E. K. Scholnick (Eds.), *The developmental psychology of planning: Why, how, and when do we plan?* (pp. 339–357). Mahwah, NJ & London: Lawrence Erlbaum Associates.

Goodnow, J. J., & Collins, W. A. (1990). *Development according to parents: The nature, sources, and consequences of parents' ideas.* Hillsdale, NJ: Erlbaum.

Gordon, R. M., Aron, L., Mitchell, S. A., & Davies, J. M. (1998). Relational psychoanalysis. In R. Langs (Ed.), *Current theories of psychoanalysis* (pp. 31–58). Madison, CT: International Universities Press.

Goossens, L. (2006). Emotion, affect, and loneliness in adolescence. In S. Jackson & L. Goossens (Eds.), *Handbook of adolescent development* (pp. 51–70). New York: Psychology Press.

Goossens, L., Luyckx, K., Lens, W., & Smits, I. (2008, July). Time perspective and identity formation: Short-term longitudinal dynamics in emerging adulthood. Paper presented in T. Shirai & W. Lens (Chairs), *Future time perspective in adolescence and emerging adulthood.* Symposium conducted at the meeting of the 29th International Congress of Psychology, Berlin, Germany.

Goossens, L., & Marcoen, A. (1999). Adolescent loneliness, self-reflection, and identity: From individual differences to developmental processes. In K. J. Rotenberg & S. Hymel (Eds.), *Loneliness in Childhood and Adolescence* (pp. 225–243). Cambridge, UK: Cambridge University Press.

Gray, M. R., & Steinberg, L. (1999). Unpacking authoritative parenting: Reassessing a multidimensional construct. *Journal of Marriage and the Family, 61*, 574–587.

Greene, A. L. (1986). Future-time perspective in adolescence: The present of things future revisited. *Journal of Youth and Adolescence, 15*, 99–113.

Greene, A. L. (1990). Great expectations: Constructions of the life course during adolescences. *Journal of Youth and Adolescences, 19*, 289–306.

Greene, A. L., & Wheatley, S. M. (1992). "I've got a lot to do and I don't think I'll have the time": Gender differences in late adolescents' narratives of the future. *Journal of Youth and Adolescences, 21*, 667–687.

Greene, B. A., & DeBacker, T. K. (2004). Gender and orientations toward the future: links to motivation. *Educational Psychology Review, 16*, 91–120.

Grotevant, H. D. (1987). Toward a process model of identity formation. *Journal of Adolescent Research, 2*, 203–222.

Grotevant, H. D. (1998). Adolescent development in family contexts. In W. Damon (Series Ed.) & N. Eisenberg (Vol. Ed.), *Handbook of child psychology Vol. 3. Social, emotional, and personality development* (5th ed., pp. 1097–1149). New York: Wiley.

Grotevant, H. D., & Adams, G. R. (1984). Development of an objective measure to assess ego identity in adolescence: Validation and replication. *Journal of Youth and Adolescence, 13*, 419–438.

Grotevant, H. D., & Cooper, C. R. (1985). Patterns of interaction in family relationships and the development of identity exploration in adolescence. *Child Development, 56*, 415–428.

Grotevant, H. D., & Cooper, C. R. (1986). Individuation in family relationships: A perspective on individual differences in the development of identity and role-taking skill in adolescence. *Human Development, 29*, 82–100.

Grotevant, H. D., & Cooper, C. R. (1998). Individuality and connectedness in adolescent development: Review and prospects for research on identity, relationships, and context. In E. E. Aspaas Skoe & A. L. Vonder Lippe (Eds.), *Personality development in adolescence: A cross national and life span perspective* (pp. 3–37). London: Routledge.

Guter, S. (1995). *Transition to adulthood during military service: Future orientation, self image, and control orientations among Israeli adolescents.* Unpublished master's thesis, University of Haifa, Israel.

Haith, M. M. (1994). Visual expectations as the first step toward the development of. future-oriented processes. In M. Haith, J. Benson, B. Pennington, & R. Roberts (Eds.), *The Development of Future-oriented Processes* (pp. 11–38). Chicago: University of Chicago Press.

Haith, M. M. (1997). The development of future thinking as essential for the emergence of skill in planning. In S. L. Friedman & E. K. Scholnick (Eds.), *The developmental psychology of planning: Why, how, and when do we plan?* (pp. 25–42). Mahwah, NJ: Erlbaum.

Haith, M., Benson, J., Roberts, R., & Pennington, B. (1994). *The development of future-oriented processes* (pp. 293–321). Chicago and London: The University of Chicago Press.

Haith, M. M., Hazan, C., & Goodman, G. S. (1988). Expectation and anticipation of dynamic visual events by 3.5-month-old babies. *Child Development, 59*, 467–479.

Haith, M. M., Wentworth, N., & Canfield, R. (1993). The formation of expectations in early infancy. In C. Rovee-Collier & L. P. Lipsitt (Eds.), *Advances in infancy research.* Norwood, NJ: Ablex.

Haj-Yahia, M. M (2002). Beliefs of Jordanian women about wife-beating. *Psychology of Women Quarterly, 26*, 282–291.

Halabi-Kheir, H. (1992). *Cultural and personality contexts of adolescent future orientation.* Unpublished master's thesis, University of Haifa, Israel.

Hampton, E., & Moffat, S. D. (2004). The psychobiology of gender: Cognitive effects of the reproductive hormones in the adult nervous system. In A. H. Eagly, A. E. Beal, & R. J. Sternberg (Eds.), *The psychology of Gender* (2nd ed., pp. 38–64). New York, NY: Guilford.

Harter, S. (1982). The perceived competence scale for children. *Child Development*, *53*, 87–97.

Harter, S. (1996). Developmental changes in self-understanding. across the 5 to 7 shift. In A. J. Sameroff & M. M. Haith (Eds.), *The five to seven year shift: The age of reason and responsibility* (pp. 207–236). Chicago and London: University of Chicago Press.

Harter, S. (1999). *The construction of the self: A developmental perspective*. New York: Guilford.

Harter, S. (2003). The development of self-representations during childhood and adolescence. In M. R. Leary & J. P. Tangney (Eds.), *Handbook of Self and Identity* (pp. 610–642). New-York, London: The Guilford Press.

Hartup, W. W. (1992). Conflict and friendship relations. In C. U. Shanz & W. W. Hartup (Eds.), *Conflict in child and adolescent development* (pp. 186–215). New York: Cambridge University Press.

Hartup, W. W. (1996). The company they keep: Friendships and their developmental significance. *Child Development*, *67*, 1–13.

Heckhausen, H. (1977). Achievement motivation and its constructs: A cognitive model. *Motivation and Emotion*, *1*, 283–329.

Heckhausen, J. (1999). *Developmental regulation in adulthood: Age-normative and sociostructural constraints as adaptive challenges*. New York, NY: Cambridge University Press.

Heckhausen, J., & Schulz, R. (1995). A life-span theory of control. *Psychological Review*, *102*, 284–304.

Heckhausen, J., & Schulz, R. (1999). The primacy of primary control is a human universal: A reply to Gould's (1999) critique of the life span theory of control. *Psychological Review*, *106*, 605–609.

Higgins, E. T. (1991). Development of self-regulatory and self-evaluative processes: Cost, benefits, and tradeoffs. In M. R. Gunnar & L. A. Sroufe (Eds.), *Self processes and development: The Minnesota Symposia on Child Development* (Vol. 23, pp.125–166). Hillsdale, NJ: Erlbaum.

Hines, M. (2004). Androgen, estrogen, and gender: Cognitive Contributions of the early hormone environment to gender-related behavior. In A. H. Eagly, A. E. Beal, & R. J. Sternberg (Eds.), *The psychology of gender* (2nd ed., pp. 9–37). New York: Guilford.

Hock, M. F., Deshler, D. D., & Schumaker, J. B. (2006). Enhancing student motivation through the pursuit of possible selves. I. N. C. Dunkel & J. Kerlpelman (Eds.), *Possible selves: Theory, research, and applications* (pp. 205–221). New York, NY: Nova.

Hoffman, H. (1845/1935). *Struwwelpeter*. New York, NY: Harper & Brothers (Translated by Mark Twain).

Hogarth, J. M. (1988). Accepting an early retirement bonus: An empirical study. *Journal of Human Resources*, *23*, 22–33.

Horen, H. (1985). *Hello, Hello daddy*. Tel-Aviv, Israel: Yesod (Hebrew).

Hudson, J. A. (2001). The anticipated self: Mother-child talk about future events. In C. Moore & K. Lemmon (Eds.), *The self in time: Developmental perspectives* (pp. 53–74). Mahwah, NJ & London: Lawrence Erlbaum Associates.

Hudson, J. A. (2002). "Do you know what we're going to do this summer?": Mothers' talk to preschool children about future events. *Journal of Cognition and Development*, *3*, 49–71.

Hudson, J. A. (2006). The development of future time concepts through mother-child conversation. *Merrill-Palmer Quarterly*, *52*, 70–95.

Hudson, J. A, & Fivush, R. (1991). Planning in the preschool years: The emergence of plans from general event knowledge. *Cognitive Development*, *6*, 393–415.

Hudson, J. A., Shapiro, L. R., & Sosa, B. B. (1995). Planning in the real world: Preschool children's scripts and plans for familiar events. *Child Development*, *66*, 984–998.

Hudson, J. A., Sosa, B. B., & Shapiro, L. R. (1997). Scripts and Plans: The development of preschool children's event knowledge and event planning. In S. L. Friedman & E. K. Scholnick (Eds.), *The developmental psychology of planning: Why, how, and when do we plan?* (pp. 77–102). Mahwah, NJ & London: Lawrence Erlbaum Associates.

Husman, J., & Lens, W. (1999). The role of the future in student motivation. *Educational Psychologist*, *34*, 113–125.

Husman, J., & Shell, D. F. (2008). Beliefs and perceptions about the future: A measurement of future time perspective. *Learning and Individual Differences, 18,* 166–175.

Hyde, J. S. (1996). Where are the gender differences? Where are the gender similarities? In D. M. Buss & N. M. Malamuth (Eds.), *Sex, power, conflict: Evolutionary and feminist perspectives* (pp. 107–118). New York, NY: Oxford University Press.

Hyde, J. S. (2005). The gender similarities hypothesis. *American Psychologist, 60,* 581–592.

Hyde, J. S., & Plant, E. A. (1995). Magnitude of psychological gender differences: Another side of the story. *American Psychologist, 50,* 159–161.

Inhelder, B., & Piaget, J. (1958). *The growth of logical thinking from childhood to adolescence.* New York: Basic Books.

Israeli Defense Forces (IDF). (1983). *Adjustment problems questionnaire.* Department of Behavioral Sciences (Hebrew).

Israeli, N. (1930). Some aspects of the social psychology of futurism. *Journal of Abnormal and Social Psychology, 25,* 121–132.

Israeli, N. (1933a). The social psychology of time, comparative rating of and emotional reactions of the past, present, and future. *Abnormal and Social Psychology, 27,* 209–213.

Israeli, N. (1933b). The measurement of attitudes and reactions to the future. *Journal of Abnormal and Social Psychology, 28,* 181–193.

Israeli, N. (1936a). The psychology of prediction: Judgments relating of the past and future. *Psychological Exchange, 4,* 129–132.

Israeli, N. (1936b). Political and scientific outlook of superiors (Scotland): Method of future autobiography. *Psychological Exchange, 4,* 166–169.

Jacklin, C. N., & Reynolds, C. (1993). Gender and childhood socialization. In A. E. Beall & R. J. Sternberg (Eds.), *The psychology of gender* (pp. 197–214). New York, London: Guilford Press.

Jacobson, S. W., Jacobson, J. L., O'Neill, J. M., Padgett, R. J., Frankowski, J. J., & Bihun, J. T. (1992). Visual expectation and dimensions of infant information processing. *Child Development, 63,* 711–724.

James, W. (1910). *Psychology: A briefer course.* New York: Holt.

James, W. (1890/1950). *The principles of psychology.* New York, NY: Dover Publications.

Jenkins, J. (1992). Sibling relationships in disharmonious homes: Potential difficulties and protective effect. In F. Boer & J. Dunn (Eds.). *Children's sibling relationships: Developmental and clinical issues* (pp. 126–138). Hillsdale, NJ: Erlbaum.

Joireman, J., Anderson, J., & Strathman, A. (2003). The aggression paradox: Understanding links among aggression, sensation seeking, and the consideration of future consequences. *Journal of Personality and Social Psychology, 84,* 1287–1302.

Jones, E. E., & Nisbett, R. E. (1971). The actor and the observer: Divergent perceptions of the causes of behavior. In E. E. Jones, D. E. Kanouse, H. H. Kelley, R. E. Nisbett, S. Valins, & B. Weiner (Eds.), *Attribution: Perceiving the causes of behavior* (pp. 79–94). Morristown, NJ: General Learning Press.

Josselson, R. (1987). *Finding herself: Pathways to identity development in women.* San Francisco: Jossey Bass.

Kagitcibasi, C. (1996). *Family and human development across cultures: A view from the other side.* Hillsdale, NJ, England: Lawrence Erlbaum Associates, Inc.

Kandel, D. B. (1978). Similarity in real-life adolescent friendship pairs. *Journal of Personality and Social Psychology, 36,* 306–312.

Kandel, D. B. (1986). Processes of peer influences in adolescence. In R. K. Silbereisen, K. Eyferth, & G. Rudinger (Eds.), *Development as action in context: Problem behaviors and normal youth development* (pp. 203–227). Heidelberg: Germany: Springer Verlag.

Karoly, P. (1993). Goal systems: An organizing framework for clinical assessment and treatment planning. *Psychological assessment, 5,* 273–280.

Kelley, H. H. (1967). Attribution theory in social psychology. In D. Levine (Ed.), *Nebraska Symposium on Motivation* (Vol. 15, pp. 192–238). Lincoln, NE: University of Nebraska Press.

Kelly, G. A. (1955). *The psychology of personal constructs*. New York: Norton.

Kendall, M. B., & Sibley, R. F. (1970). Social class differences in time orientation: Artifact? *The Journal of Social Psychology, 82*, 187–191.

Keniston, K. (1970). Youth as a stage of life. *American Scholar, 39*, 631–654.

Kerpelman, J. L., & Mosher, L. S. (2004). Rural African American adolescents' future orientation: The importance of self efficacy, control and responsibility, and identity development. *Identity: An International Journal of Theory and Research, 4*, 187–208.

Kerpelman, J. L., & Schvaneveldt, P. L. (1999). Young adults' anticipated identity importance of career, marital, and parental roles: Comparisons of men and women with different role balance orientation. *Sex Roles, 41*, 189–217.

Kim, J., & Cicchetti, D. (2006). Longitudinal trajectories of self-system processes and depressive symptoms among maltreated and non-maltreated children. *Child Development, 77*, 624–639.

Kim, J. E., Hetherington, E. M., & Reiss, D. (1999). Associations among family relationships, antisocial peers, and adolescents' externalizing behaviors: Gender and family type differences. *Child Development, 70*, 1209–1230.

Klineberg, S. L. (1967). Changes in outlook on the future between childhood and adolescence. *Journal of Personality and Social Psychology, 7*, 185–193.

Kluckhohn, F. R., & Strodtbeck, F. L. (1961). *Variations in value orientations*. Evanston, Il: Row, Peterson, & Co.

Knox, M. H., Funk, J., Elliott, R., & Bush, E. G. (1998). Adolescents' possible selves and their relationship to global self-esteem. *Sex Roles, 39*, 61–80.

Knox, M., Funk, J., Elliott, R., & Bush, E. G. (2000). Gender differences in adolescents' possible selves. *Youth & Society, 31*, 287–309.

Koenig, L. J., & Abrams, R. F. (1999). Adolescent loneliness and adjustment: A focus on gender differences. In K. J. Rotenberg & S. Hymel (Eds.), *Loneliness in Childhood and Adolescence* (pp. 296–322). Cambridge, UK: Cambridge University Press.

Koenig, L. J., Isaacs, A. M., & Schwartz, J. A. J. (1994). Sex differences in adolescent depression and loneliness: Why are boys lonlier if girls are more depressed? *Journal of Research in Personality, 28*, 27–43.

Kowal, A., & Kramer, L. (1997). Children's understanding of parental differential treatment. *Child Development, 68*, 113–126.

Kracke, B. (2002). The role of personality, parents and peers in adolescents career. exploration. *Journal of Adolescence, 25*, 19–30.

Kracke, B., & Schmitt-Rodermund, E. (2001). Adolescent career exploration in the context of educational and occupational transitions. In J. -E. Nurmi (Ed.), *Navigating through adolescence: European perspectives* (pp. 137–161). New York, NY: Garland.

Kramer, L., & Kowal, A. K. (2005). Sibling relationship quality from birth to adolescence: The enduring contributions of friends. *Journal of Family Psychology, 19*, 503–511.

Kreppner, K. (1994). William L. Stern: A neglected founder of developmental psychology. In R. D. Parke, P. A. Ornstein, J. J. Reiser, & C. Zahn-Waxler (Eds.), *A century of developmental psychology* (pp. 311–331). Washington, DC: American Psychological Association.

Kupersmidt, J. B., Sigda, K. B., Sedikides, C., & Voegler, M. E. (1999). In K. J. Rotenberg & S. Hymel (Eds.), *Loneliness in childhood and adolescence*, (pp. 263–279). Cambridge, UK: Cambridge University Press.

Laible, D. J., Carlo, G., & Roesch, S. C. (2004). Pathways to self-esteem in late adolescence: The role of parent and peer attachment, empathy, and social behaviors. *Journal of Adolescence, 27*, 703–716.

Lam, A. G., & Zane, N. W. S. (2004). Ethnic differences in coping with interpersonal stressors: A test of self-construals as cultural mediators. *Journal of cross-cultural, 35*, 446–459.

Lamb, M. E. (1978). Interactions between 18-months-olds and their pre-school siblings. *Child Development, 49*, 51–59.

Lamb, M. E., & Sutton-Smith, B. (1982). *Sibling relationships: Their nature and significance across the life-span*. Hillsdale, NJ: Erlbaum.

Lamm, H., Schmidt, R. W., & Trommsdorff, G. (1976). Sex and social class as determinants of future orientation (time perspective) in adolescence. *Journal of Personality and Social Psychology, 34*, 317–326.

Lansford, J. E., Criss, M. M., Pettit, G. S., Dodge, K. A., & Bates, J. E. (2003). Friendship quality, peer group affiliation, and peer antisocial behavior as moderators of the link between negative parenting and adolescent externalizing behavior. *Journal of Research on Adolescence, 13*, 161–184.

Lang, F. R., & Carstensen, L. L. (2002). Time counts: Future time perspective, goals, and social relationships. *Psychology and aging, 17*, 125–139.

Lanz, M., Rosnati, R., Marta, E., & Scabini, E. (2001). Adolescents' future: A comparison of adolescents' and their parents' views. In J. -E. Nurmi (Ed.), *Navigating through adolescence: European perspectives* (pp. 169–198). New York, NY: Routledge.

Lanz, M., Scabini, E., Vermulst, A. A., & Gerris, J. R. M. (2001). Congruence on child rearing families with early adolescent and middle adolescent children. *International Journal of Behavioral Development, 25*, 133–139.

Larson, R. W., Moneta, G., Richards, M. H., Holmbeck, G. H., & Duckett, E. (1996). Changes in adolescents' daily interactions with their families from ages 10 to 18: Disengagement and transformation. *Developmental psychology, 32*, 744–754.

Larson, R. W., & Richards, M. H. (1991). Daily companionship in late childhood and early adolescence: Changing developmental contexts. *Child Development, 62*, 284–300.

Laursen, B., Furman, W., & Mooney, K. S. (2006). Predicting interpersonal competence and self-worth from adolescent relationships and relational networks: Variable-centered and person-centered perspectives. *Merrill-Palmer Quarterly, 52*, 572–600.

Lawrence, J. A., & Dodds, A. (2003). Goal directed activities and life-span development. In J. Valsiner & K. J. Connoly (Eds.), *Handbook of developmental psychology* (pp. 517–533). London: Sage.

Lazarus, R. S., & Folkman, S. (1984). *Stress, appraisal, and coping.* New York, NY: Springer.

Lefcourt, H. M. (1966). Internal versus external control of reinforcement. *Psychological Bulletin, 65*, 206–220.

Lens, W. (1986). Future time perspective: A cognitive-motivational concept. In D. R. Brown & J. Veroff, (Ed.), *Frontiers of Motivational Psychology* (pp. 173–190). New York, NY: Springer-Verlag.

Lens, W. (2006). Future time perspective: A psychological approach. In Z. Uchhnast (Ed.), *Psychology of time: Theoretical and empirical approaches* (pp. 51–64). Lublin, Poland: Wydawnictwo KUL.

Lens, W., Herrera, D., & Lacante, M. (2004). The role of motivation and future time perspective in educational counseling. *Psychologia, 169–180.*

Lens, W., Simons, J., & Dewitte, S. (2002). From duty to desire: The role of students' future time perspective and instrumentality perceptions for study motivation and self-regulation. In F. Pajares & T. Urdan (Eds.). *Academic motivation of adolescents* (Vol. 2 in the Adolescence and education Series, pp. 221–245). Greenwich, CT: Information Age Publishing.

Leseman, P. P. M., Rollenberg, L., & Rispens, J. (2001). Playing and working in kindergarten: Cognitive co-construction in two educational situations. *Early Childhood Research Quarterly, 16*, 363–384.

Lessing, E. E. (1968). Demographic, developmental, and personality correlates of length of future time perspective (FTP). *Journal of Psychology, 36*, 183–201.

Lessing, E. E. (1972). Extension of personal future time perspective, age and life satisfaction of children and adolescents. *Developmental Psychology, 6*, 457–468.

Levinson, D. J. (1978). *The seasons of a man's life.* New York, NY: Ballentine Books.

Lewin, K. (1936). *Principles of topological psychology.* New York, NY: McGraw-Hill.

Lewin, K. (1939). Field theory and experiment in social psychology. *American Journal of Sociology, 44*, 868–896.

Lewin, K. (1942/1948). Time perspective and morale. In K. Lewin (Ed.), *Resolving social conflict* (pp. 103–124). New York, NY: Harper & Brothers Publishers.

Lieblich, A., & Perlow, M. (1988). Transition to adulthood during military service. *The Jerusalem Quarterly, 47*(Summer), 40–78.

Lilach, E. (1996). *Future orientation of adolescents who experience loneliness.* Unpublished master's thesis, University of Haifa, Israel.

Linn, R. (1996). When the individual soldier says 'no' to war: A look at selective refusal during the Intifada. *Journal of Peace Research, 33*, 421–431.

Little, B. R. (1983) Personal projects: A rationale and method for investigation. *Environment and behavior, 15*, 273–277.

Little, B. R. (1987). Personal projects and fuzzy selves: Aspects of self-identity in adolescence. In T. Honess & K. Yardley (Eds.), *Self and identity: Perspectives across the life span.* London: Routledge & Kegan Paul.

Little, B. R. (1989). Personal projects analysis: Trivial pursuits, magnificent obsessions, and the search for coherence. In D. Buss & N. Cantor (Eds.), *Personality psychology: Recent trends and emerging directions* (pp. 15–31). New York, NY: Springer-Verlag.

Little, B. R. (1996). Free traits, personal projects and idio-tapes: Three tiers for personality research. *Psychological Inquiry, 8*, 340–344.

Little B. R. (2000). Free traits and personal contexts: Expanding a social ecological model of well-being. In W. B. Walsh, K. H. Craik, & R. H. Price (Eds.), *Person-environment psychology: New directions and perspectives* (2nd ed., pp. 87–116). Mahwah: Erlbaum.

Little, B. R. (2006). Personal projects as integrative units: Comment. *Applied Psychology: An international Review, 55*, 419–427.

Little, B. R. (2007). Prompt and circumstance: The generative contexts of personal projects analysis. In B. R. Little, K. Salmela-Aro, & S. D. Phillips (Eds.), *Personal project pursuit: Goals, action, and human flourishing* (pp. 3–49). Mahwah, NJ: Erlbaum.

Little, B. R., & Chambers, N. C. (2004). Personal projects pursuit: On human doings and well-beings. In W. M. Cox & E. Klinger (Eds.), *Handbook of motivational counseling: Concepts, approaches, and assessment* (pp. 65–82). New York, NY: John Wiley & Sons.

Loftus, E. F. (2003). Make-believe memories. *American Psychologist, 58*, 867–873.

Luyckx, K., Goossens, L., Soenens, B., & Beyers, W. (2006). Unpacking commitment and exploration: Preliminary validation of an integrative model of late adolescent identity formation. *Journal of Adolescence, 29*, 361–378.

Maatta, S., Nurmi, J.-E., & Stattin, H. (2007). Achievement orientations, school adjustment, and well-being: A longitudinal study. *Journal of Research on Adolescence, 17*, 789–812.

Maccoby, E. E. (1990). Gender and relationships: A developmental account. *American Psychologist, 45*, 513–520.

Maccoby, E. E. (1992a). The role of parents in the socialization of children: An historical review. *Developmental Psychology, 28*, 1006–1017.

Maccoby, E. E. (1992b). Trends in the study of socialization: Is there a Lewinian heritage? *Journal of Social issues, 48*, 171–185.

Maccoby, E. E. (1994). The role of parents in the socialization of children: An historical view. In R. S. Parke, P. A. Ornstein, J. J. Rieser, & C. Zahn-Waxler (Eds.), *A century of developmental psychology* (pp. 589–615). Washington, DC: American Psychological Association.

Maccoby, E. E., & Jacklin, C. N. (1974). *The psychology of sex differences.* Stanford: Stanford University Press.

Mahajna, S. (2000). *Socio-cultural correlates of future orientation: The case of Arab adolescent girls.* Unpublished master's thesis, University of Haifa, Israel.

Mahajna, S. (2007). *Future orientation: Its nature and meaning among girls from different Israeli Arab settings.* Unpublished doctoral dissertation, University of Haifa, Israel.

Malka, A., & Covington, M. V. (2005). Perceiving school performance as instrumental to future goal attainment: Effects on graded performance. *Contemporary Educational Psychology, 30*, 60–80.

Malmberg, L. -E., Ehrman, J., & Lithen, T. (2005). Adolescents' and parents' future beliefs. *Journal of Adolescence, 28*, 709–723.

Malmberg, L. E., & Trempata, J. (1997). Anticipated transition to adulthood: The effect of educational track, gender, and self-evaluation on Finnish and Polish adolescents' future orientation. *Journal of Youth and Adolescences, 26,* 517–537.

Marcia, J. E. (1983). Some directions for the investigation of ego development in early adolescence. *Journal of Early Adolescence, 3,* 215–223.

Marcia, J. E. (1993). The ego identity status approach to ego identity. In J. E. Marcia, A. S. Waterman, D. R. Matteson, S. L. Archer, & J. L. Orlofsky (Eds.), *Ego identity: A handbook for Psychological research* (pp. 3–21). New York, NY: Springer-Verlag.

Marcia, J. E., & Archer, S. L. (1993). Identity status in late adolescents: Scoring criteria. In J. E. Marcia, A. S. Waterman, D. R. Matteson, S. L. Archer, & J. L. Orlofsky. *Ego identity: A handbook for Psychological research* (pp. 205–240). New York, NY: Springer-Verlag.

Marcia, J. E., Waterman, A. S., Matteson, D. R., Archer, S. L., & Orlofsky, J. L. (1993). *Ego identity: A handbook for Psychological research* (pp. 3–21). New York, NY: Springer.

Margieh, I. (2007). *Future orientation in social context: The case of Israeli Palestinian college students.* Masters thesis in preparation. University of Haifa, Israel.

Mar'i, M. M. (1983). *Sex Role perceptions of Palestinian males and females in Israel.* Unpublished doctoral dissertation. Michigan State University, East Lansing, MI.

Marko, K. W., & Savickas, M. L. (1998). Effectiveness of a career time perspective intervention. *Journal of Vocational Behavior, 52,* 106–119.

Markus, H. (1977). Self-schemata and processing information about the self. *Journal of Personality and Social Psychology, 35,* 63–78.

Markus, H. (1983). Self knowledge: An expended view. *Journal of Personality, 51,* 543–565.

Markus, H., Cross, S., & Wurf, E. (1990). The role of the self-system in competence. In R. J. Sternberg & J. Kolligian, Jr. (Eds.), *Competence considered* (pp. 205–225). New Haven, CT: Yale University Press.

Markus, H., & Nurius, P. (1986). Possible selves. *American Psychologist, 41,* 954–969.

Markus, H., & Ruvolo, A. (1989). Possible selves: Personalized representations of goals. In L. Pervin (Ed.), *Goal concepts in personality and social psychology* (pp. 211–241). Hillsdale, NJ: Erlbaum.

Markus, H., & Wurf, E. (1987). The dynamic self-concept: A social psychological perspective. *Annual Review of Psychology, 38,* 299–337.

Marsh, H. W. (1986). Global self esteem: Its relation to specific facets of self concept and their importance. *Journal of Personality and Social Psychology, 51,* 1224–1236.

Marsh, H. W., & Hattie, J. (1996). Theoretical perspectives on the structure of self concept. In B. A. Bracken (Ed.), *Handbook of self concept: Developmental, social, and clinical considerations* (pp. 38–90). New York: Wiley.

Martin, A. J., Marsh, H. W., & Debus, R. L. (2001a). A quadripolar need achievement representation of self-handicapping and defensive pessimism. *American Educational Research Journal, 38,* 583–610.

Martin, A. J., Marsh, H. W., & Debus, R. L. (2001b). Self-handicapping and defensive pessimism: Exploring a model of predictors and outcomes from a self protection perspective. *Journal of Educational Psychology, 93,* 87–102.

Martin, A. J., Marsh, H. W., & Debus, R. L. (2003). Self handicapping, defensive pessimism, and goal orientation: A qualitative study of university students. *Journal of Educational Psychology, 95,* 617–628.

Mayseless, O., & Hai, I. (1998). Leaving home transition in Israel: Changes in parent-adolescent relationships and adolescents' adaptation to military service. *International Journal of Behavioral Development, 22,* 589–609.

Mayseless, O., Scharf, M., & Sholt, M. (2003). From authoritative parenting to an authoritarian context: Exploring the person-environment fit. *Journal of Research on Adolescence, 13,* 427–456.

McAdams, D. P. (1996). Personality, modernity, and the storied self: A contemporary framework for studying persons. *Psychological Inquiry, 7,* 295–321.

McAdams, D. P., & Pals, J. L. (2006). A new big five: Fundamental principles for an integrative science of personality. *American Psychologist, 61*, 204–217.

McCallion, A., & Trew, K. (2000). A longitudinal study of Northern Irish children's hopes, aspirations, and fears for the future. *The Irish Journal of Psychology, 21*, 227–236.

McClure, E. B. (2000). A meta-analytic review of sex differences in facial expression processing and their development in infants, children and adolescents. *Psychological Bulletin, 126*, 424–453.

McGillicuddy-DeLisi, A. V., & Sigel, I. E. (1995). Parental beliefs. In M. H. Bornstein (Ed.), *Handbook of parenting: Vol. 3. Status and social conditions of parenting* (pp. 333–358). Mahwah, NJ: Lawrence Erlbaum Associates.

McGregor, I., & Little, B. R. (1998). Personal projects, happiness and meaning: On doing well and being yourself. *Journal of Personality and Social Psychology, 74*, 494–512.

McHale, S. M., & Crouter, A. C. (1996). The family contexts of children's sibling relationships. In G. H. Brody (Ed.), *Sibling relationships: Their causes and consequences* (pp. 173–195). Norwood, NJ: Ablex Publishing Corporation.

McHugh, M. C., & Frieze, I. H. (1997). The measurement of gender-role attitudes: A review and commentary. *Psychology of Women Quarterly, 21*, 1–16.

Mead, G. H. (1934). *Mind, self and society.* Chicago: University of Chicago Press.

Meeus, W., Iedema, J. Helsen, M., & Vollebergh, W. (1999). Patterns of adolescent identity development: Review of literature and longitudinal analysis. *Developmental Review, 19*, 419–461.

Mehta, P. H., Sundberg, N. D., Rohila, P. K., & Tyler, L. E. (1972). Future time perspectives of adolescents in India and in the United States. *Journal of Cross-Cultural Psychology, 3*, 293–302.

Melges, F. T. (1982). Time and the inner future: A temporal approach to psychiatric disorders. New York, NY: Wiley.

Mello, Z. R. (2008). Gender variation in developmental trajectories of educational and occupational expectations and attainment from adolescence to adulthood. *Developmental Psychology, 44*, 1069–1080.

Melzer, Y. (2000). *Parenting style, autonomy granting, parental acceptance, and future orientation of adolescents.* Unpublished master's thesis, University of Haifa, Israel.

Miceli, M., & Castelfranchi, C. (2002). The mind and the future: The (negative) power of expectation. *Theory & Psychology, 12*, 335–366.

Miller, R. B., & Brickman, S. J. (2004). A model of future-oriented motivation and self-regulation. *Educational Psychology Review, 16*, 9–33.

Miller, R. B., DeBaker, T. K., & Greene, B. A. (1999). Perceived instrumentality and academics: The link to task valuing. *Journal of Instructional Psychology, 26*, 250–260.

Mischel, W. (1968). *Personality and assessment.* New York, NY: Wiley.

Mischel, W. (2004). Toward an integrative science of the person. *Annual Review of Psychology, 55*, 1–22.

Mischel, W., Grusec, J., & Masters, J. C. (1969). Effects of expected delay time on the subjective value of rewards and punishments. *Journal of Personality and Social Psychology, 11*, 363–373.

Mischel, W., & Shoda, Y. (1995). A cognitive-affective system theory of personality: Reconceptualizing the in variance in personality and the role of situations. *Psychological Review, 102*, 246–286.

Mönks, F. (1968). Future time perspective in adolescents. *Human Development, 11*, 107–123.

Montemayor, R. (1983). Parents and adolescents in conflict: All families some of the time and some families most of the time. *Journal of Early Adolescence, 3*, 83–103.

Moore, C., & Lemmon, K. (2001). The nature and utility of the temporally extended self. In C. Moore & K. Lemmon (Eds.), *The self in time: Developmental perspectives,* (pp. 1–13). Mahwah, NJ & London: Lawrence Erlbaum Associates.

Morling, B., & Evered, S. (2006). Secondary control reviewed and defined. *Psychological Bulletin, 132*, 269–296.

Morling, B., & Evered, S. (2007). The construct formerly known as secondary control: Reply to Skinner (2007). *Psychological Bulletin, 133*, 917–919.

Murray, H. A. (1938). *Explorations in personality.* New York, NY: Oxford University Press.

Murray, H. A. (1959). Preparation for a scaffold of a comprehensive system. In S. Koch (Ed.) *Psychology: A study of science* (Vol. 3, pp. 7–54). New York, NY: McGraw-Hill.

Nakamura, Y., & Flammer, A. (1998). Control orientations of Japanese adolescents. In G. Trommsdorff, W. Friedlmeier, & H. J. Kornadt (Eds.), *Japan in transition: Sociological and psychological aspects* (pp. 173–182). Berlin: Pabst Science Publishers.

Nakash, R. (2000). *Future orientation of adolescents who immigrated to Israel without parents.* Unpublished master's thesis, University of Haifa, Israel.

Nelson, K. (1986). *Event knowledge: Structure and function in development.* Hillsdale, NJ: Lawrence Erlbaum Associates.

Nelson, K. (1993). The psychological and social origins of autobiographical memory. *Psychological research, 4*, 7–14.

Nelson, K. (1996). Memory development from 4 to 7 years. In A. J. Sameroff & M. M. Haith (Eds.), *The five to seven year shift: The age of reason and responsibility* (pp. 141–160). Chicago and London: The University of Chicago Press.

Nelson, K. (2000). Narrative, time, and the emergence of the encultured self. *Culture and Psychology, 6*, 183–196.

Nelson, K. (2001). Language and the self: From the "Experiencing I" to the "Continuing Me". In C. Moore & K. Lemmon (Eds.), *The self in time: Developmental perspectives* (pp. 15–33). Mahwah, NJ: Erlbaum.

Nelson, K., & Fivush, R. (2004). The emergence of autobiographical memory: A social-cultural developmental theory. *Psychological review, 111*, 486–511.

Newson, J., & Newson, E. (1975). Intersubjectivity and the transmission of culture: On the social origins of symbolic functioning. *Bulletin of the British Psychological Society, 28*, 437–446.

Norem, J. K. (2008). Defensive pessimism as a positive self-critical tool. In E. C. Chang (Ed.), *Self criticism and self-enhancement: Theory, research, and clinical implications* (pp. 89–104). Washington, DC: American Psychological association.

Norem, J. K., & Cantor, N. (1986a). Anticipatory and post hoc cushioning strategies: Optimism and defensive pessimism in "risky" situations. *Cognitive Therapy and Research, 10*, 347–362.

Norem, J. K., & Cantor, N. (1986b). Defensive pessimism: Harnessing anxiety as motivation. *Journal of Personality and Social Psychology, 51*, 1208–1217.

Norem, J. K., & Cantor, N. (1990). Capturing the "flavor" of behavior: Cognition, affect, and interpretation. In B. S. Moore & A. M. Isen (Eds.), *Affect and social behavior* (pp. 39–63). Cambridge: Cambridge University Press.

Norem, J. K., & Chang, E. C. (2002). The positive psychology of negative thinking. *Journal of Clinical Psychology, 58*, 993–1001.

Norem, J. K., & Illingworth, K. S. S. (1993). Strategy-dependent effects of reflecting on self and tasks: Some implications of optimism and defensive pessimism. *Journal of Personality and Social Psychology, 65*, 822–835.

Norton, D. G. (1993). Diversity, early socialization, and temporal development: The dual perspective revisited. *Social Work, 38*, 82–90.

Noyman, M. (1998). *Future orientation and identity.* Unpublished master's thesis, University of Haifa, Israel.

Nurmi, J. E. (1987). Age, sex, social class, and quality of family interaction as determinants of adolescents' future orientation: A developmental task interpretation. *Adolescence, 22*, 977–991.

Nurmi, J. E. (1989). Development of orientation to the future during early adolescence: A four-year longitudinal study and two cross-sectional comparisons. *International Journal of Psychology, 24*, 195–214.

Nurmi, J. E. (1991). How do adolescents see their future? A review of the development of future orientation and planning. *Developmental Review, 11*, 1–59.

Nurmi, J. E. (1992). Age differences in adult life goals, concerns, and their temporal extension: A life course approach to future-oriented motivation. *The International Society for the Study of Behavioral Development, 15*, 487–508.

Nurmi, J. E. (1993). Adolescent development in age-graded context: The role of personal beliefs, goals, and strategies in the tackling of developmental tasks and standards. *International Journal of the Study of Behavioral Development, 16*, 169–189.

Nurmi, J.-E. (2008). Self and socialization: How do young people navigate through adolescence? In H. W. Marsh, R. G. Craven, & D. M. McInerney (Eds.), *Self-processes, learning, and enabling human potential: Dynamic new approaches* (pp. 305–328). Charlotte, NC: Information Age Publishing.

Nurmi, J. E., Poole, M. E., & Kalakoski, V. (1993). Age differences in adolescent future-oriented goals, concerns, and related temporal extension in different sociocultural contexts. *Journal of Youth and Adolescence, 23*, 471–487.

Nurmi, J. E., Poole, M. E., & Seginer, R. (1995). Tracks and transitions – A comparison of adolescent future-oriented goals, explorations, and commitments in Australia, Israel, and Finland. *International Journal of Psychology, 30*, 355–375.

Nurmi, J. E., & Pulliainen, H. (1991). The changing parent-child relationship, self-esteem, and intelligence as determinants of orientation to the future during early adolescence. *Journal of Adolescence, 14*, 35–51.

Nurmi, J. -E., Seginer, R., & Poole, M. (1995). Searching for the future in different environments: A comparison of Australian, Finnish and Israeli adolescents' future orientation, explorations and commitments. In P. Noack, M. Hofer, & J. Youniss (Eds.), *Psychological responses to social change: Human development in changing environments* (pp. 219–238). Berlin: De Gruyter.

Nurmi, J. E., Toivonen, S., Salmela-Aro, K., & Eronen, S. (1996). Optimistic approach-oriented and avoidance strategies in social situations: Three studies on loneliness and peer relationships. *European Journal of Personality, 10*, 201–219.

Nuttin, J. (1984). *Motivation, planning, and action: A relational theory of behavior dynamics.* Louvain: Lawrence Erlbaum Associates.

Nuttin, J., & Lens, W. (1985). *Future time perspective and motivation: Theory and research method.* Location: Erlbaum.

Ochse, R., & Plug, C. (1986). Cross-cultural investigation of the validity of Erikson's theory of personality development. *Journal of Personality and Social Psychology, 50*, 1240–1252.

Offer, D., Ostrov, E., Howard, K. I., & Atkinson, R. (1988). *The teenage world: Adolescents' self-image in ten countries.* New York, NY: Plenum.

Orlev, U. (1985/2005). *Journey to the age of four.* Or Yehuda, Israel: Kinneret, Zmora-Bitan, Dvir Publishing House (Hebrew).

Orlofsky, J. L. (1993). Intimacy status: Theory and research. In J. E. Marcia, A. S. Waterman, D. R. Matteson, S. L. Archer, & J. L. Orlofsky (1993). *Ego identity: A handbook for Psychological research* (pp. 111–133). New York, NY: Springer-Verlag.

Orlofsky, J. L., Marcia, J. E., & Lesser, I. M. (1973). Ego identity status and intimacy versus isolation crisis in young adulthood. *Journal of Personality and social Psychology, 27*, 211–219.

Osgood, C. E., Suci, G. J., & Tannenbaum, P. H. (1971). *The measurement of meaning.* Urbana, IL: The University of Chicago Press.

Oyserman, D., Brikman, D., & Rhodes, M. (2007). School success, possible selves, and parent involvement. *Family relations, 56*, 479–489.

Oyserman, D., Bybee, D., & Terry, K. (2006). Possible selves and academic outcomes: How and when possible selves impel action. *Journal of Personality and Social Psychology, 91*, 188–204.

Oyserman, D., Bybee, D., Terry, K., & Hart-Johnson, T. (2004). Possible selves as roadmaps. *Journal of Research in Personality, 38*, 130–149.

Oyserman, D., Gant, L., & Ager, J. (1995). A socially contextualized model of African American identity: School persistence and possible selves. *Journal of Personality and Social Psychology, 69*, 1216–1232.

Oyserman, D., & James, L. (2008). Possible selves: From content to process. In K. D. Markman, W. M. P. Klein, & J. A. Suhr (Eds.), *The handbook of imagination and mental simulation* (pp. 393–394). Psychology Press.

Oyserman, D., & Markus, H. (1990). Possible Selves and Delinquency. *Journal of Personality and Social Psychology, 59*, 112–125.

Oyserman, D., & Saltz, E. (1993). Competence, delinquency, and attempts to attain possible selves. *Journal of Personality and Social Psychology, 65*, 360–374.

Oyserman, D., Terry, K., & Bybee, D. (2002). A possible selves intervention to enhance school involvement. *Journal of Adolescence, 25*, 313–326.

Page, R. M. (1990). High school size as a factor in adolescent loneliness. *High School Journal, 73*, 150–153.

Parsons, T., & Bales, R. F. (1955). *Family, socialization, and interaction processes.* Glencoe, IL: Free Press.

Perkins, D. D., & Zimmerman, M. A. (1995). Empowerment theory, research, and application. *American Journal of Community Psychology, 23*, 569–579.

Pervin, L. A. (1989). Goals concepts: Themes, issues, and questions. In L. A. Pervin (Ed.), *Goal concepts in personality and social psychology* (pp. 473–478). Hillsdale, NJ: Erlbaum.

Petry, N. M., Bickel, W. K., & Arnett, M. (1998). Shortened time horizons and insensitivity to future consequences in heroin addicts. *Addiction, 93*, 729–738.

Piaget, J. (1926). *The language and thought of the child.* New York, NY: Harcourt, Brace.

Piaget, J. (1932). *The moral judgment of the child.* New York, NY: Harcourt, Brace.

Piaget, J. (1955). The development of time concepts in the child. In P. H. Hoch & J. Zubin (Eds.), Psychopathology of childhood (pp. 34–44). New York, NY: Grune & Stratton.

Pinquart, M., Frohlich, C., & Silbereisen, R. K.(2007). Optimism, pessimism, and change of psychological well-being in cancer patients. *Psychology, Health and Medicine, 12*, 421–432.

Pinquart, M., Frohlich, C., & Silbereisen, R. K. (2008). Testing models of change in life goals after cancer diagnosis. *Journal of Loss and Trauma, 13*, 330–351.

Pinquart, M., Nixdorf-Hanchen, J. C., & Silbereisen, R. K. (2005). Association of age and cancer with individual goal commitment. *Applied Developmental Science, 9*, 54–66.

Pomerantz, E. M., Fei-Yin Ng, F., & Wang, Q. (2004). Gender socialization: A parent x child model. In A. H. Eagly, A. E. Beall, & R. J. Sternberg (Eds.), *The psychology of gender* (2nd ed., pp. 120–144). New York, NY: Guilford.

Poole, M. E., & Cooney, G. H. (1987). Orientation to the future: A comparison of adolescents in Australia and Singapore. *Journal of Youth and Adolescence, 16*, 129–151.

Pulkkinen, L. (1990). Home atmosphere and adolescent future orientation. *European Journal of Psychology of Education, 5*, 33–43.

Pulkkinen, L., & Rönkä, A. (1994). Personal control over development, identity formation, and future orientation as components of life orientation: A developmental approach. *Developmental Psychology, 30*, 260–271.

Putnam, F. W. (1994). Dissociation and disturbance of self. In S. Toth & D. Cicchetti (Eds.), *Disorders and dysfunctions of the self* (pp. 251–265). Rochester, NY: University of Rochester Press.

Rappaport, H., Enrich, K., & Wilson, A. (1985). Relation between ego identity and temporal perspective. *Journal of Personality and Social Psychology, 48*, 1609–1620.

Raynor, J. O., & Entin, E. E. (1982). *Motivation, career striving, and aging.* New York, NY: Hemisphere

Raynor, J. O., & Entin, E. E. (1983). The function of future orientation as a determinant of human behavior in a step-path theory of action. *International Journal of Psychology, 18*, 463–487.

Reis, O., & Youniss, J. (2004). Patterns of identity change and development in relationships with mothers and friends. *Journal of Adolescent Research, 19*, 31–44.

Reznick, J. S. (1994). In search of infant expectation. In M. Haith, J. Benson, B. Pennington, & R. Roberts (Eds.), *The Development of Future - oriented Processes* (pp. 39–59). Chicago: University of Chicago Press.

Ridgeway, C. (1997). Interaction and the conversation of gender inequality: Considering employment. *American Sociological Review, 62*, 218–235.

Riegel, K. (1977). Toward a dialectical interpretation of time and change. In B. S. Gorman & A. E. Wessmanz (Eds.), *The personal experience of time* (pp. 59–108). New York, NY: Plenum.

Rogoff, B. (1990). *Apprenticeship in thinking: Cognitive developments in social context*, New York, NY: Oxford University Press.

Rokeach, M., & Bonier, R. (1960). Time perspective, dogmatism, and anxiety. In M. Rokeach (Ed.), *The open and closed mind* (pp. 366–375). New York, NY: Basic Books.

Rommetveit, R. (1985). Language acquisition as increasing linguistic structuring of experience and symbolic behavior control. In J. V. Wertsch (Ed.), *Culture, communication, and cognition: Vygotskian perspectives* (pp. 183–204). London: Cambridge University Press.

Roney, C. J., Higgins, E. T., & Shah, J. (1995). Goals and framing: How outcome focus influences motivation and emotion. *Personality and Social Psychology Bulletin, 21*, 1151–1160.

Rosenberg, M. (1965). *Society and the adolescent self-image*. Princeton, NJ: Princeton University Press.

Rosenberg, M. (1979). *Conceiving the self*. New York, NY: Basic Books.

Rosenberg, M. (1986). Self concept from middle childhood through adolescence, In J. Suls & A. G. Greenwald (Eds.), *Psychological perspectives on the self* (Vol. 3, pp. 107–135). Mahwah, NJ: Erlbaum.

Rosenthal, D. A., Gurney, R. M., & Moore, S. M. (1981). From trust to intimacy: A new inventory for examining Erikson's stages of psychosocial development. *Journal of Youth and Adolescence, 10*, 525–537.

Rotenberg, K. J. (1999). Parental antecedents of children's loneliness. In K. J. Rotenberg & S. Hymel (Eds.), *Loneliness in childhood and adolescence* (pp. 325–347). Cambridge, UK: Cambridge University Press.

Rothbaum, F., Weisz, J. R., & Snyder, S. S. (1982). Changing the world and changing the self: A two-process model of perceived control. *Journal of Personality and Social Psychology, 42*, 5–37.

Rothspan, S., & Read, S. (1996). Present versus future time perspective and HIV risk among heterosexual college students. *Health Psychology, 15*, 131–134.

Rotter, J. B. (1954). *Social learning and clinical psychology*. Englewood Cliffs, NJ: Prentice-Hall.

Rotter, J. B. (1966). Generalized expectancies for internal versus external control of reinforcement. *Psychological Monographs: General and Applied, 80*, 1–28.

Rotter, J. B. (1981). The psychological situation in social learning theory. In D. Magnusson (Ed.), *Toward the psychology of situations: An interactional perspective* (pp. 169–178). Hillsdale, NJ: Erlbaum.

Rotter, J. B. (1990). Internal versus external control of reinforcement: A case history of variable. *American Psychologist, 45*, 489–493.

Rubenstein, C. M., & Shaver, P. (1982). The experience of loneliness. In L. A. Peplau & D. Perlman (Eds.), *Loneliness – A sourcebook of current theory, research and therapy* (pp. 206–223). New York, NY: John Wiley & Sons.

Russell, D. W. (1996). UCLA Loneliness Scale (Version 3): Reliability, validity, and factor structure. *Journal of Personality Assessment, 66*, 20–40.

Russell, D. W., Peplau, L. A., & Cutrona, C. E. (1980). The revised UCLA loneliness scale: Concurrent and discriminant validity evidence. *Journal of Personality and Social Psychology, 39*, 472–480.

Salmela-Aro, K., Aunola, K., & Nurmi, J.-E. (2007). Personal goals during emerging adulthood: A 10-year follow up. *Journal of Adolescent Research, 22*, 690–715.

Salmela-Aro, K., Nurmi, J. -E., Saisto, T., & Halmesmäki, E. (2001). Goal construction and depressive symptoms during transition to motherhood: Evidence from two longitudinal studies. *Journal of Personality and Social Psychology, 81*, 1144–1159.

Salmela-Aro, K., & Suikkari, A. -M. (2008). Letting go your dreams – Adjustment of child-related goal appraisals and depressive symptoms during infertility treatment. *Journal of Research in Personality, 42*, 988–1003.

Salmela-Aro, K., Vuori, J., & Koivisto, P. (2007). Adolescents' motivational orientations, school-subject values, and well-being: A person-centered approach. *Hellenic Journal of Psychology, 4*, 310–330.

Sanna, L. J. (1996). Defensive pessimism, optimism, and simulating alternatives: Some ups and downs of prefactual and counterfactual thinking. *Journal of personality and Social Psychology, 71*, 1020–1036.

Scabini, E., Marta, E., & Lanz, M. (2006). *The transition to adulthood and family relations: An intergenerational perspective.* New York, NY: Psychology press.

Scarr, S. (1988). Race and gender as psychological variables: Social and ethical issues. *American psychologist, 43*, 56–59.

Schacter, D. L., & Addis, D. R. (2007). The ghosts of past and future. *Nature, 445*, 27–28.

Schaefer, E. S. (1965). A configurational analysis of children's reports on parents. *Journal of Consulting Psychology, 29*, 552–557.

Scharf, M., Mayseless, O., & Kivenson-Baron, I. (2004). Adolescents' attachment representations and developmental tasks in emerging adulthood. *Developmental Psychology, 40*, 430–444.

Schlesinger, R. (2001). *Family environment and adolescent future orientation: A model of direct and self-mediated links.* Unpublished doctoral dissertation, University of Haifa, Israel.

Schmitt-Rodermund, E., & Silbereisen, R. K. (1998). Career maturity determinants: Individual development, social context, and historical time. *The Career Development Quarterly, 47*, 16–31.

Schroeder, J. E. (1980). Imaginary representations of time cycles. *Perceptual and Motor Skills, 50*, 723–734.

Sebald, H. (1986). Adolescents' shifting orientation toward parents and peers: A curvilinear trend over recent decades. *Journal of Marriage and Family, 48*, 5–13.

Seginer, R. (1986a). Jewish-Arab relations in Israel: A psychology of adolescence perspective. *Journal of Psychology, 120*, 557–566.

Seginer, R. (1986b). Mothers' behavior and boys' performance: An initial test of an academic achievement path model. *Merrill Palmer Quarterly, 32*, 153–166.

Seginer, R. (1988a). Adolescents facing the future: Cultural and socio-political perspectives. *Youth and Society, 19*, 314–333.

Seginer, R. (1988b). Adolescents' orientation toward the future: Sex role differentiation in a socio-cultural context. *Sex Roles, 18*, 739–757.

Seginer, R. (1988c). Social milieu and future orientation: The case of kibbutz vs. urban adolescents. *International Journal of Behavioral Development, 11*, 247–273.

Seginer, R. (1992a). Future orientation: Age related differences among adolescent females. *Journal of Youth and Adolescence, 21*, 421–437.

Seginer, R. (1992b). Sibling relationships in early adolescence: A study of Israeli Arab sisters. *Journal of Early Adolescence, 12*, 96–110.

Seginer, R. (1995). The hopes and fears of anticipated adulthood: Adolescent future orientation in cross-cultural context. In G. Trommsdorff (Hsg.), *Kinderheit und Jugend im Kulturvergleich* (pp. 225–247). Weinheim, Germany: Juventa.

Seginer, R. (1998a). Adolescents' perception of relationships with older sibling in the context of other close relationships. *Journal of Research on Adolescence, 8*, 287–308.

Seginer, R. (1998b). Primary and secondary control in interpersonal and cultural settings. In G. Trommsdorff, W. Friedlmeier, & H. J. Kornadt (Eds.), *Japan in transition: Sociological and psychological aspects* (pp. 183–196). Berlin: Pabst Science Publishers.

Seginer, R. (1999). Beyond the call of duty: The service of Israeli youth in military and civic contexts. In M. Yates & J. Youniss (Eds.), *Community service and civic engagement in youth: International perspectives* (pp. 205–224). New York, NY: Cambridge.

Seginer, R. (2000). Defensive pessimism and optimism correlates of adolescent future orientation: A domain specific analysis. *Journal of Adolescent Research, 15*, 307–326.

Seginer, R. (2001a). Young people chart their path into adulthood: The future orientation of Israeli Druze, Arab and Jewish adolescents. Special Issue: The child in Israel (Eds., C. Greenbaum & I. Levin), *Megamot, 41*, 97–112 (Hebrew).

Seginer, R. (2001b). Emotional distress, personal resources and developmental tasks: Personality correlates of adolescent future orientation. Special Issue: School of Education 25th anniversary (Ed., M. Ben Perez) *Iyunim Bechinuch, 5*, 7–44 (Hebrew).

Seginer, R. (2003). Adolescent future orientation: An integrated cultural-ecological perspective. In W. J. Lonner, D. L. Dinnel, & S. A. Hayes (Eds.), *Online readings in psychology and culture.* Bellingham, WA: Center for Cross Cultural Research.www.ac.wwu.edu/~culture/readings.htm

Seginer, R. (2005). Adolescent future orientation: Intergenerational transmission and intertwining tactics in culture and family settings. In W. Friedelmeier, P. Chakkarath, & B. Schwarz (Eds.), *Culture and human development: The importance of cross-cultural research to the social sciences* (pp. 231–251). Hove, UK: Psychology Press.

Seginer, R. (2006). Parents' educational involvement: A developmental ecology perspective. *Parenting: Science and Practice, 6,* 1–48.

Seginer, R. (2008). Future orientation in times of threat and challenge: How resilient adolescents construct their future. *International Journal of Behavioral Development, 32,* 272–282.

Seginer, R., Dan, O., & Zeliger, R. (1998). *Toward graduation: Mabar special educational project in 12th grade, and from start (10th grade) to completion (12th grade).* Follow up report to the Israeli Ministry of Education and Culture (Hebrew).

Seginer, R., & Golan, M. S. (2007, August). *Family and Schooling model: How parent- and sibling-relationships affect academic achievement.* Paper presented at the 13th European Conference on Developmental Psychology. Jena, Germany.

Seginer, R., & Halabi, H. (1991). Cross cultural variations of adolescents' future orientation: The case of Israeli Druze vs. Israeli Arab and Jewish males. *Journal of Cross-Cultural Psychology, 22,* 224–237.

Seginer, R., & Halabi-Kheir, H. (1998). Adolescent passage to adulthood: Future orientation in the context of culture, age, and gender. *International Journal of Intercultural relations, 22,* 309–328.

Seginer, R., Karayanni, M., & Mar'i, M. M. (1990). Adolescents' attitudes toward women's roles: A comparison between Israeli Jews and Arabs. *Psychology of Women Quarterly, 14,* 119–133.

Seginer, R., & Lilach, E. (2004). How adolescents construct their future: The effect of loneliness on future orientation. *Journal of Adolescence, 27,* 625–643.

Seginer, R., & Mahajna, S. (2003). 'Education is a weapon in women's hands': How Arab girls construct their future. *Journal of Sociology of Education and Socialization. Zeitschrift fur Soziologie der Erziehung und Socialisation, 23,* 200–214.

Seginer, R., & Mahajna, S. (2004). How the future orientation of traditional Israeli Palestinian girls link beliefs about women's roles and academic achievement. *Psychology of Women Quarterly, 28,* 122–135.

Seginer, R., Mahajna, S., & Shoyer, S. (2007, August). *Adolescent future orientation: Does culture matter?* Paper presented at the 13th European Conference on Developmental Psychology. Jena, Germany.

Seginer, R., & Noyman, M. S. (2005). Future orientation, identity and intimacy: Their relations in emerging adulthood. *European Journal of Developmental Psychology, 2,* 17–37.

Seginer, R., Nurmi, J. -E., & Poole, M. (1991). *Adolescent future orientation in cross-cultural perspectives.* Paper presented in the 11th meeting of International Society for the Study of Behavioral Development. Minneapolis, MN.

Seginer, R., & Schlesinger, R. (1998). Adolescents' future orientation in time and place: The case of the Israeli kibbutz. *International Journal of Behavioral Development, 22,* 151–167.

Seginer, R., & Shoyer, S. (2005). *Future orientation and interpersonal relationships of Israeli Jewish girls and boys.* Unpublished raw data.

Seginer, R., Shoyer, S., Hossessi, R., & Tannous, H. (2007). Adolescent family and peer relationships: Does culture matter? In R. W. Larson & L. A. Jensen (Series Eds.), *New Directions for Child and Adolescent Development* (No. 116). B. B. Brown & N. S. Mounts (Vol. Eds.), *Linking parents and family to adolescent peer relations: Ethnic and cultural considerations* (pp. 83–99). San Francisco: Jossey Bass.

Seginer, R., Shoyer, S., & Mahajna, S. (2008, March). Diversity and commonality: Relationships with parents and peers among Israeli Arab and Jewish adolescents. In B. Schwarz (Chair), *The role of parents and peers for adolescent development: A cross-cultural perspective.* Symposium conducted at the 12th Biennial meeting of the Society for Research on Adolescence. Chicago, IL.

Seginer, R., Trommsdorff, G., & Essau, C. (1993). Adolescent control beliefs: Cross-cultural variations of primary and secondary orientations. Special Issue: Planning and control processes across the life span, *International Journal of Behavioral Development, 16,* 243–260.

Seginer, R., & Vermulst, A. A. (2001). The intergenerational transmission of child rearing stress: Congruence, psychological mediators, and ecological moderators. In J. R. M. Gerris (Ed.), *Dynamics of parenting* (pp. 157–178). Leuven, Belgium: Garant.

Seginer, R., & Vermulst, A. (2002). Family environment, educational aspirations, and academic achievement in two cultural settings. *Journal of Cross-Cultural Psychology, 33,* 540–558.

Seginer, R., Vermulst, A., & Shoyer, S. (2004). The indirect link between perceived parenting and adolescent future orientation: A multiple-step analysis. *International Journal of Behavioral Development, 28,* 365–378.

Seymour, P. H. K. (1980). Internal representation of the months, An experimental analysis of spatial forms. *Psychological Research, 42,* 255–273.

Shalev, R. (2009). *Bereaved parents: Change of self, future orientation, functioning and adaptation to loss.* Unpublished PhD dissertation, University of Haifa, Israel.

Shapiro, L. R., & Hudson, J. A., (1991). Tell me a make-believe story: Coherence and cohesion in young children's picture-elicited narratives. *Developmental Psychology , 27,* 960–974.

Shapiro, L. R., & Hudson, J. A. (2004). Effects of internal and external supports on preschool children's event planning. *Journal of Applied Developmental Psychology, 25,* 49–73.

Sharabany, R. (1994). Intimate Friendship scale: Conceptual underpinnings, psychometric properties and construct validity. *Journal of Social and Personal Relationships, 11,* 449–469.

Sharabany, R., Gershoni, R., & Hofman, J. (1981). Girl-friend, boy-friend: Age and sex differences in intimate friendship. *Developmental Psychology, 17,* 800–808.

Shek, D. T. L. (2007). A longitudinal study of perceived parental psychological control and psychological well-being in Chinese adolescents in Hong Kong. *Journal of Clinical Psychology, 63,* 1–22.

Sheldon, K. N., & Vansteenkiste, M. (2005). Personal goals and time travel: How are future places visited and is it worth it? In A. Strathman & J. Joireman (Eds.), *Understanding behavior in the context of time: Theory, research, and application* (pp. 143–163). Mahwah, NJ: Erlbaum.

Shell, D. F., & Husman, J. (2008). Motivation, affect, and strategic self – regulation in the college classroom: A multidimensional phenomena. *Journal of Educational Psychology, 100,* 443–459.

Sherif, C. W. (1976). *Orientation in social psychology.* New York, NY: Harper & Row.

Shirai, T. (2002). Women's transition from school to work in Japan in the 1990s. In U. Teichler & G. Trommsdorff (Eds.), *Challenges of the 21st century in Japan and Germany* (pp. 79–89). Berlin, Germany: Pabst science Publishers.

Shirai, T., & Beresneviciene, D. (2005). Future orientation in culture and socio-economic changes: Lithuanian adolescents in comparison with Belgian and Japanese. *Baltic Journal of Psychology, 6,* 21–30.

Showers, C. (1988). The effects of how and why thinking on perceptions of future negative events. *Cognitive Therapy and Research, 12,* 225–240.

Showers, C. (1992). The motivational and emotional consequences of considering positive or negative possibilities for an upcoming event. *Journal of Personality and Social Psychology, 63,* 474–484.

Showers, C., & Ruben, C. (1990). Distinguishing defensive pessimism from depression: Negative expectations and positive coping mechanisms. *Cognitive Therapy Research, 14,* 385–399.

Shoyer, S. (2001). *Constructed autonomy and provided autonomy: Two correlates of adolescent future orientation.* Unpublished master's thesis, University of Haifa, Israel.

Shoyer, S. (2006). *The construction of future orientation in the context of adolescent-parent relationships as viewed by adolescents and parents*. Unpublished PhD dissertation, University of Haifa, Israel.

Silbereisen, R. K. (2005). Social change and human development: Experiences from German unification. *International Journal of Behavioral Development, 29*, 2–13.

Silk, J. S., Morris, A. S., Kanaya, T., & Steinberg, L. (2003). Psychological control and autonomy granting: Opposite ends of a continuum or distinct constructs? *Journal of Research on Adolescence, 13*, 113–128.

Silverman, I., & Eals, M. (1992). Sex differences in spatial abilities: Evolutionary theory and data. In J. H. Barkow, L. Cosmides, & J. Tooby (Eds.), *The adapted mind* (pp. 533–549). New York, NY: Oxford University Press.

Simons, J., Dewitte, S., & Lens, W. (2000). Wanting to have versus wanting to be: The effect of perceived instrumentality on goal orientation. *British Journal of Psychology, 91*, 335–351.

Simons, J., Vansteenkiste, M., Lens, W., & Lacante, M. (2004). Placing motivation and future time perspective theory in a temporal perspective. *Educational Psychology Review, 16*, 121–139.

Sippola, L. K., & Bukowski, W. M. (1999) Self, other and loneliness from a developmental perspective. In K. J. Rotenberg & S. Hymel (Eds.), *Loneliness in childhood and adolescence* (pp. 280–295). Cambridge, UK: Cambridge University Press.

Sircova, A., Mitina, O. V., Boyd, J., Davidiva, I. S., Zimbardo, P. G., Nepryaho, T. L. et al. (2008). The phenomenon of time perspective across different cultures: Review of research using ZTPI scale. *Cultural Historical Psychology, 2007/4* [Russian Journal; English Abstract obtained from PsycINFO no. 2008-05850-003].

Skinner, E. (2007). Secondary control critiqued: Is it secondary? Is it control? Comment on Morling and Evered. *Psychological Bulletin, 133*, 911–916.

Snyder, C. R., Harris, C., Anderson, J. R., Holleran, S. A., Irving, L. M., Sigmon, S. T., et al. (1991). The will and the ways: Development and validation of an individual differences measure of hope. *Journal of Personality and Social Psychology, 60*, 570–585.

Spence, T. J., & Hahn, E. D. (1997). The Attitudes toward Women Scale and attitude change in college students. *Psychology of Women Quarterly, 21*, 17–34.

Spreng, R. N., & Levine, B. (2006). The temporal distribution of past and future autobiographical events across the lifespan. *Memory & Cognition, 34*, 1644–1651.

Sroufe, L. A., & Fleener, J. (1986). Attachment and the construction of relationships. In W. W. Hartup & Z. Rubin (Eds.), *Relationships and development* (pp. 51–72). Hillsdale, NJ: Erlbaum.

Stanton-Salazar, R. D., & Dornbusch, S. M. (1995). Social capital and the reproduction of inequality: Information networks among Mexican-origin high school students. *Sociology of Education, 68*, 116–135.

Stanton-Salazar, R. D., & Spina, S. U. (2000). The network orientations of highly resilient urban minority youth: A network analytic account of minority socialization and its educational implications. *The Urban Review, 32*, 227–261.

Stein, K. B., Sarbin, T. R., & Kulik, J. A. (1968). Future time perspective: Its relation to the socialization process and the delinquent role. *Journal of Consulting & Clinical Psychology, 32*, 257–264.

Steinberg, L., Lamborn, S. D., Dornbusch, S. M., & Darling, N. (1992). Impact of parenting practices on adolescent achievement: Authoritative parenting, school involvement, and encouragement to succeed. *Child Development, 63*, 1266–1281.

Steinberg, L., & Monahan, K. C. (2007). Age differences in resistance to peer pressure. *Developmental Psychology, 43*, 1531–1543.

Steinberg, L., & Silk, J. S. (2002). Parenting adolescents. In M. H. Bornstein (Ed.), *Handbook of parenting, 2nd Edition, Vol. 1: Children and parenting*. (pp. 103–133). Mahwah, NJ: Erlbaum.

Stern, D. (1985). *The interpersonal world of the infant*. New York, NY: Basic Books.

Sternberg, R. J. (1993). What is the relation of gender to biology and environment? An evolutionary model of how what you answer depends on just what you ask. In A. E. Beall & R. J. Sternberg (Eds.), *The psychology of gender* (pp. 1–6). New York, London: Guilford Press.

Stewart, A. J., & Healy, J. M. (1989). Linking individual development and social changes, *American Psychologist, 44,* 30–42.

Strathman, A., Gleicher, F., Boninger, D. S., & Edwards, C. S. (1994). The consideration of future consequences: Weighing immediate and distant outcomes of behavior. *Journal of Personality and Social Psychology, 66,* 742–752.

Strickland, B. R. (1989). Internal-external control expectancies: From contingency to creativity. *American Psychologist, 44,* 1–12.

Suddendorf, T., & Busby, J. (2005). Making decisions with the future in mind: Developmental and comparative identification of mental time travel. *Learning and Motivation, 36,* 110–125.

Suddendorf, T., & Corballis, M. C. (1997). Mental time travel and the evolution of the human mind. *Genetic Social and General Psychology Monographs, 123,* 133–167.

Suddendorf, T., & Corballis, M. C. (2007). The evolution of foresight: What is mental time travel and is it unique to humans? *Behavioral and Brain Sciences, 30,* 299–313.

Suh, E. J., Moskowitz, D. S., Fournier, M. A., & Zuroff, D. C. (2004). Gender and relationships: Influences on agentic and communal behaviors. *Personal Relationships, 11,* 41–59.

Suleiman, M. A. (2000). *Parental style and future orientation among Arab adolescents.* Unpublished master's thesis, University of Haifa, Israel.

Sundberg, N. D., Poole, M. E., & Tyler, L. E. (1983). Adolescents' expectations of future events – A cross-cultural study of Australians, Americans, and Indians. *International Journal of Psychology, 18,* 415–427.

Super, C. M., & Harkness, S. (1986). The developmental niche: A conceptualization at the interface of child and culture. *International Journal of Behavioral Development, 9,* 545–569.

Super, C. M., & Harkness, S. (2002). Culture structures the environment for development. *Human Development, 45,* 270–274.

Sutin, A. R., & Robins, R. W. (2008). Going forward by drawing from the past: Personal strivings, personally meaningful memories, and personality traits. *Journal of Personality, 76,* 631–663.

Tashakkori, A., & Thompson, V. (1991). Social change and change in intentions of Iranian youth regarding education, marriage, and careers. *International Journal of Psychology, 26,* 203–217.

Teahan, J. E. (1958). Future time perspective, optimism, and academic achievement. *Journal of Abnormal and Social Psychology, 57,* 379–380.

Tennyson, A. (1861). *The poems of Alfred Tennyson: From the latest London edition.* New York, NY: A. L. Burt Company.

Tesser, A. (1988). Toward a self-evaluation maintenance model of social behavior. In L. Berkowitz (Ed.), *Advances in experimental social psychology* (Vol. 21, pp. 181–227). New York, NY: Academic Press.

Thomas, W. J. (1928). *The child in America.* New York, NY: Knopf.

Toren-Kaplan, N. (1995). *Adolescent future orientation in the context of immigration and absorption: The case of former USSR immigration to Israel.* Unpublished master's thesis, University of Haifa, Israel.

Trivers, R. L. (1972). Parental investment and sexual selection. In B. Campbell (Ed.), *Sexual selection and the descent of man: 1871–1971* (pp. 136–179). Chicago: Aldine.

Trommsdorff, G. (1982). Group influences on judgments concerning the future. In M. Irle (with L. B. Katz) (Eds.), *Studies in Decision Making* (pp. 145–165). Berlin, New York, NY: Walter de Gruyter.

Trommsdorff, G. (1983). Future orientation and socialization. *International Journal of Psychology, 18,* 381–406.

Trommsdorff, G. (1986). Future time orientation and its relevance for development as action. In R. K. Silbereisen, K. Eyferth, & G. Rudinger (Eds.), *Development as action in context: Problem behavior and normal youth development* (pp. 121–136). Berlin, Heidelberg, New-York, Tokyo: Springer-Verlag.

Trommsdorff, G. (1994). Future time perspective and control orientation: Social conditions and consequences. In Z. Zaleski (Ed.), *Psychology of future orientation* (pp. 39–62). Lublin, Poland: Towarzystwo Naukowe KUL.

Trommsdorff, G. (2002). Effects of social change on individual development: The role of social and personal factors and the timing of events. In R. K. Silbereisen & L. J. Crockett (Eds.), *Negotiating adolescence in times of social change* (pp. 58–68). New York, NY: Cambridge University Press.

Trommsdorff, G., Burger, C., & Füchsle, T. (1982). Social and psychological aspects of future orientation. In M. Irle (with L. B. Katz) (Eds.), *Studies in decision making* (pp. 167–194). Berlin, New York, NY: Walter de Gruyter.

Trommsdorff, G., & Friedlmeier, W. (1993). Control behavior and responsiveness in Japanese and German mothers. *Early Development and Parenting, 2,* 65–78.

Trommsdorff, G., & Lamm, H. (1980), Future orientation of institutionalized and noninstitutionalized delinquents and nondelinquents. *European Journal of Social Psychology, 10,* 247–278.

Trommsdorff, G., Lamm, H., & Schmidt, R. W. (1979). A longitudinal study of adolescents' future orientation (time perspective). *Journal of Youth and Adolescence, 8,* 131–147.

Tucker, C. J., Barber, B. L., & Eccles, J. S. (1997). Advice about life plans and personal problems in late adolescent sibling relationships. *Journal of Youth and Adolescence, 26,* 63–77.

Tulving, E. (1972). Episodic and semantic memory. In E. Tulving & W. Donaldson (Eds.), *Organization of memory* (pp. 382–403). Oxford, UK: Academic Press.

Tulving, E. (1985). Memory and consciousness. *Canadian Psychology, 26*(1), 1–12.

Tulving, E. (2002). Episodic memory: From mind to brain. *Annual Review of Psychology, 53,* 1–25.

Tulving, E. (2005). Episodic memory and autonoesis: Uniquely human? In H. S. Terrance & J. Metclafe (Eds.), *The missing link in cognition: Origins of self-reflective consciousness* (pp. 3–56). New York, NY: Oxford University Press.

United Nations Development Program (1995). *Human development report, 1995.* New York: Oxford University Press.

Van Buskirk, A. M., & Duke, M. P. (1991). The relationship between coping style and loneliness in adolescents: Can "Sad passivity" be adaptive? *The Journal of Genetic Psychology, 152,* 144–157.

Van Calster, K., Lens, W., & Nuttin, J. R. (1987). Affective attitude toward the personal future: Impact on motivation in high school boys. *American Journal of Psychology, 100,* 1–13.

Van IJzendoorn, M. H. (1992). Intergenerational transmission of parenting: A review of studies in nonclinical populations. *Developmental Review, 12,* 76–99

Vansteenkiste, J., Simons, J., Lens, W., Soenens, B., & Matos, L. (2005). Examining the impact of intrinsic versus extrinsic goal framing and internally controlling versus autonomy-supportive communication style upon early adolescents' academic achievement. *Child Development, 76,* 483–501.

Vansteenkiste, J., Simons, J., Soenens, B., & Lens, W. Soenens, B. (2004). How to become a persevering exerciser? Providing a clear, future intrinsic goal in an autonomy supportive way. *Journal of Sport and Exercise Psychology, 26,* 232–249.

Vermulst, A. A., Van Leeuwe, J. F. J., & Lanz, M. (2003). *Measuring and testing congruence in dyads.* Unpublished manuscript, University of Nijmegen, The Netherlands.

Vigotsky, L. S. (1978). *Mind in society: The development of higher psychological processes.* Cambridge, MA: Harvard University Press.

Wallace, M., & Rabin, A. I. (1960). Temporal experience. *Psychological Bulletin, 57,* 213–236.

Waterman, A. S. (1982). Identity development from adolescence to adulthood: An extension of theory and a review of research. *Developmental Psychology, 18,* 342–358.

Waterman, A. S. (1999). Identity, the identity statuses, and identity status development: A contemporary statement. *Developmental Review, 19,* 591–621.

Weiner, B. (1972). *Theories of motivation: From mechanism to cognition.* Chicago: Markham Publishing Company.

Weiner, B. (1974). An attributional interpretation of expectancy-value theory. In B. Weiner (Ed.), *Cognitive views of human motivation* (pp. 51–69). New York, NY: Academic Press.

Weiner, B. (1985). An attributional theory of achievement motivation and emotions. *Psychological Bulletin, 92*, 548–573.

Weiner, B. (1996). *Human motivation: Metaphors, theories and research*. Newbury Park, CA: Sage.

Weist, R. M. (1989). Time concepts in language and thought: Filling the Piagetian void from two to five years. In I. Levin & D. Zakay (Eds.), *Time and Human Cognition: A Life-Span Perspective*, (pp. 63–118). Amsterdam, New York, Oxford & Tokyo: North-Holland.

Weisz, J. R., Rothbaum, F. M., & Blackburn, T. C. (1984). Standing out and standing in: The psychology of control in America and Japan. *American Psychologist, 39*, 955–969.

Wentworth, N., & Haith, M. M. (1992). Event-specific expectations of 2- and 3-month-old infants. *Developmental Psychology, 28*, 842–850.

Wentworth, N., Haith, M. M., & Hood, R. (2002). Spatiotemporal regularity and interevent contingencies as information for infants' visual expectations. *Infancy, 3*, 303–321.

Wentworth, N., Haith, M. M., & Karrer, R. (2001). Behavioral and cortical measures of infant visual expectations. *Infancy, 2*, 175–195.

Westen, D. (1993). The impact of sexual abuse on self structure. In D. Cicchetti & S. L. Toth (Eds.), *Rochester symposium on developmental psychopathology: Disorders and dysfunctions of the self* (Vol. 5, pp. 223–250). Rochester, NY: University of Rochester Press.

Westergaard, J., Nable, I., & Walker, A. (1989). *After redundancy: The experience of economic insecurity*. Cambridge, UK: Polity Press.

Whitman, W. (1892/1983). *Leaves of grass*. New York: Bantam.

Wigfield, A. (1994). Expectancy-value theory of achievement motivation: A developmental perspective. *Educational Psychology Review, 6*, 49–78.

Wilf, M. (2008). *A window to the future: A longitudinal study examining the effect of personal and environmental resources on quality of life of IDF retirees*. Unpublished PhD dissertation, University of Haifa, Israel.

Wiseman, H. (1997). Interpersonal relatedness and self-definition in the experience of loneliness during the transition to university. *Personal Relationships, 4*, 285–299.

Wiseman, H., Guttfreund, D. G, & Lurie, I. (1995). Gender differences in loneliness and depression of university students seeking counseling. *British Journal of Guidance and Counseling, 23*, 231–243.

Wohlford, P. (1968). Extension of personal time in TAT and story completion stories. *Journal of Projective Techniques and Personality Assessment, 32*, 267–280.

Worrell, F. C., & Mello, Z. R. (2007). The reliability and validity of Zimbardo time perspective inventory scores in academically talented adolescents. *Educational and Psychological Measurement, 67*, 487–504.

Wrosch, C., Heckhausen, J., & Lachman, M. E. (2000). Primary and secondary control strategies for managing health and financial stress across adulthood. *Psychology and Aging, 15*, 387–399.

Yeh, H. C., & Lempers, J. D. (2004). Perceived sibling relationships and adolescent development. *Journal of Youth and Adolescence, 33*, 133–147.

Young, R. A., Antal, S., Bassett, M. E., Post, A., DeVries, N., & Valach, L. (1999). The joint action of adolescents in peer conversations about career. *Journal of Adolescence, 22*, 527–538.

Youniss, J., & Smollar, J. (1985). *Adolescent relations with mothers, fathers, and friends*. Chicago: The University of Chicago Press.

Yowell, C. M. (2000). Possible selves and future orientation: Exploring hopes and fears of Latino boys and girls. *Journal of Early Adolescence, 20*, 245–280.

Zaleski, Z. (2005). Future orientation and anxiety. In A. Strathman & J. Joireman (Eds.), *Understanding behavior in the context of time: Theory, research, and application* (pp. 125–141). Mahwah, NJ: Erlbaum.

Zeira, A., & Dekel, R. (2005). The self-image of adolescents and its relationship to their perceptions of the future. *International Social Work, 48*, 177–191.

Zimbardo, P. G., & Boyd, J. N. (1999). Putting time in perspective: A valid, reliable individual differences metric. *Journal of Personality and Social Psychology, 77*, 1271–1288.

Zimmerman, M. A. (1995). Psychological empowerment: Issues and Illustrations. *American Journal of Community Psychology, 23,* 581–599.

Zimmerman, M. A. (2000). Empowerment theory: Psychological, organizational and community levels of analysis. In J. Rappaport & E. Seidman (Eds.), *Handbook of community psychology* (pp. 43–63). New-York, NY: Kluwer Academic/Plenum Publishers.

Zirkel, S., & Cantor, N. (1990). Personal construal of life tasks: Those who struggle for independence. *Journal of Personality and Social Psychology, 58,* 172–18.

Appendix

Future Orientation Questionnaires

These questionnaires consist of questions relating to your thoughts about the future.

The questions have no right or wrong answers. Therefore, we would like you to respond in a way that exactly corresponds to your personal beliefs.

It is very important to the success of this research that you be as open and honest as possible in answering these questions. *The information you give us is confidential and used only by the researchers.*

Thank you for your cooperation.

Future Orientation Questionnaire

1. People often think about the future. In the lines below please write down the *hopes* you have for the future. In the right hand end please write *the age* you believe you will be, or the year when theses hopes will come true.

AGE/YEAR

----

2. Now we would like you to think about *fears* concerning the future and write them down in the lines below. In the right hand end please write *the age* you believe you will be, or the year when theses may happen.

AGE/YEAR

THANK YOU

Prospective Life Course Questionnaire

This questionnaire consists of questions regarding your opinions and thoughts about the future. These questions have no right or wrong answers. Therefore, we would like you to respond in a way that exactly corresponds to your personal beliefs.

The following questions address work and career and marriage and family. Previous research has shown these are two life domains adolescents consider when thinking about the future. Since we are interested in comparing among life domains, the questions repeat themselves (with minor differences) in the two domains. Despite repetition, we ask you to answer patiently.

It is very important for the success of this research that you be as open and honest as possible in answering these questions. The information you give us is confidential and used only by the researchers.

Answer the questions in the blank space provided or circle the most suitable answer. Answer the questions in the order in which they are presented.

Please, fill out this form carefully and accurately. THANK YOU.

Future Work and Career

1. How often do you think about or plan your future career?

1	2	3	4	5
Never	Rarely	Sometimes	Often	Daily

2. How well does each of the following sentences describe you?

	Definitely does not				Definitely describes
a. Looking into several career options I am now focusing on one	1	2	3	4	5
b. I have made up my mind concerning my career	1	2	3	4	5
c. Considering the materialization of my career plans, I am optimistic	1	2	3	4	5

3. Have you actually been seeking information about different careers? How often do you try to get this information?

1	2	3	4	5
Never	Rarely	Sometimes	Often	Daily

What career are you considering? If you are considering several serious possibilities list them all.

----

4. How often do you find yourself thinking about your career?

1	2	3	4	5
Never	Rarely	Sometimes	Often	Daily

5. How well does each of the following sentences describe you?

	Definitely does not				Definitely describes
a. I am making serious preparations to enter a specific career	1	2	3	4	5
b. I have clear plans concerning my career	1	2	3	4	5
c. I think I know which career I will choose	1	2	3	4	5

6. How determined are you to fulfill your plans about your future career?

1	2	3	4	5
Definitely Not	Probably Not	Maybe yes Maybe not	Probably Yes	Definitely Yes

7. How likely do you think it is that your career plans will materialize?

1	2	3	4	5
Definitely will not happen	Quite sure will not happen	Maybe yes Maybe not	Quite sure will happen	Completely sure will happen

8. Which of the following things have you been doing now to get you closer to realizing of your career plans?

	None At all	Very Little	Somewhat	Quite A bit	A lot
a. Talking to people	1	2	3	4	5
b. Collecting information from different sources	1	2	3	4	5
c. Checking whether this career fits me	1	2	3	4	5
d. Consulting with other people	1	2	3	4	5
e. Imagining myself in one career or another	1	2	3	4	5

9. What effect will each of the factors below have on the realization of your plans
    concerning your future career?

	None At all	Very Little	Somewhat	Quite A bit	A lot
a. Personal ability	1	2	3	4	5
b. Personal effort	1	2	3	4	5
c. Self esteem	1	2	3	4	5
d. Other people	1	2	3	4	5
e. Social pressure	1	2	3	4	5
f. Economic conditions	1	2	3	4	5
g. Luck	1	2	3	4	5
h. Drive to succeed	1	2	3	4	5

10. What feelings are aroused when you think about your future career?
    Refer to *each* of the 5 word pairs and put an X in the space which most accu-
    rately describes your feelings.

a. Worries	í	í	í	í	í	Confidence
b. Negative feelings	í	í	í	í	í	Positive feelings
c. Good mood	í	í	í	í	í	Bad Mood
d. Despair	í	í	í	í	í	Hope
e. Courage	í	í	í	í	í	Fear
f. Failure	í	í	í	í	í	Success
	(1)	(2)	(3)	(4)	(5)	

11. How do you *evaluate* your future career? Refer to *each* of the 5 word pairs and
    put an X in the space which most closely describes your evaluation.

a. Important	í	í	í	í	í	Unimportant
b. Useless	í	í	í	í	í	Useful
c. Worth my effort	í	í	í	í	í	Not worth my effort
d. Marginal to life	í	í	í	í	í	Central to my life
e. Enriching	í	í	í	í	í	Of no value
	(1)	(2)	(3)	(4)	(5)	

Marriage and Family

12. How often do you think about or plan your future marriage and family?

1	2	3	4	5
Never	Rarely	Sometimes	Often	Daily

13. To what extent does each of the following sentences describe you?

	Definitely Does not				Definitely Describes
a. I think I know who will be my partner	1	2	3	4	5
b. I have definite plans regarding getting married and having a family	1	2	3	4	5
c. I have a clear picture about my marriage and family life					
d. Considering the materialization of my marriage and family plans, I am optimistic	1	2	3	4	5

14. How determined are you to fulfill your plans about your future marriage and family life?

1	2	3	4	5
Definitely Not	Probably Not	Maybe yes Maybe not	Probably Yes	Definitely Yes

15. How often do you find yourself thinking about your marriage and family life?

1	2	3	4	5
Never	Rarely	Sometimes	Often	Daily

16. How likely do you think it is that your marriage and family plans will materialize?

1	2	3	4	5
Definitely will not happen	Quite sure will not happen	Maybe yes Maybe not	Quite sure will happen	Completely sure will happen

17. Which of the following things have you been doing now to get you closer to realizing of your marriage and family plans?

	None At all	Very Little	Somewhat	Quite A bit	A lot
a. Talking to people	1	2	3	4	5
b. Collecting information from different sources	1	2	3	4	5
c. Checking getting married fits me	1	2	3	4	5
d. Consulting with other people	1	2	3	4	5
e. Imagining myself getting married and having a family	1	2	3	4	5

18. What effect will each of the factors below have on the realization of your plans concerning your future marriage and family?

	None At all	Very Little	Somewhat	Quite A bit	A lot
a. Personal ability	1	2	3	4	5
b. Personal effort	1	2	3	4	5
c. Self esteem	1	2	3	4	5
d. Other people	1	2	3	4	5
e. Social pressure	1	2	3	4	5
f. Economic conditions	1	2	3	4	5
g. Luck	1	2	3	4	5
h. Drive to succeed	1	2	3	4	5

19. What feelings are aroused when you think about your future marriage and family?
Refer to *each* of the 5 word pairs and put an X in the space which most accurately describes your feelings.

a. Worries	í	í	í	í	í	Confidence
b. Negative feelings	í	í	í	í	í	Positive feelings
c. Good mood	í	í	í	í	í	Bad mood
d. Despair	í	í	í	í	í	Hope
e. Courage	í	í	í	í	í	Fear
f. Failure	í	í	í	í	í	Success
	(1)	(2)	(3)	(4)	(5)	

20. How do you *evaluate* your future marriage and family? Refer to *each* of the 5 word pairs and put an X in the space which most closely describes your evaluation.

a. Important	í	í	í	í	í	Unimportant
b. Useless	í	í	í	í	í	Useful
c. Worth my effort	í	í	í	í	í	Not worth my effort
d. Marginal to life	í	í	í	í	í	Central to my life
e. Enriching	í	í	í	í	í	Of no value
	(1)	(2)	(3)	(4)	(5)	

My Future Hopes

Thinking about your future, how often does each of the following issues make you think **hopefully** about it? If you consider it **hopefully** every day, circle 5. If you do not think about this issue at all, circle 1. Circle one of the intermediate scores if one of them describes you more accurately.

	Never	Rarely	Some times	Often	Every day
01 My education	1	2	3	4	5
02 My major subject in college	1	2	3	4	5
03 My job/occupation	1	2	3	4	5
04 My professional career	1	2	3	4	5
05 My romantic partner	1	2	3	4	5
06 My future spouse	1	2	3	4	5
07 My children	1	2	3	4	5
08 My financial situation (income, property, etc.)	1	2	3	4	5
09 What will be with me, in general	1	2	3	4	5
10 My country and the world	1	2	3	4	5
11 My parents and other family members	1	2	3	4	5
12 My close friend	1	2	3	4	5
13. Any other issue.	1	2	3	4	5

My Future Fears

Thinking about your future, how often does each of the following issues make
you **worry** about it? If you **worry** about it every day, circle 5. If you do not think
about this issue at all, circle 1. Circle one of the intermediate scores if one of them
describes you more accurately.

	Never	Rarely	Some times	Often	Every day
01 My education	1	2	3	4	5
02 My major subject in college					
03 My job/occupation	1	2	3	4	5
04 My professional career	1	2	3	4	5
05 My romantic partner	1	2	3	4	5
06 My future spouse	1	2	3	4	5
07 My children	1	2	3	4	5
08 My financial situation (income, property, etc.)	1	2	3	4	5
09 What will be with me, in general	1	2	3	4	5
10 My country and the world	1	2	3	4	5
11 My parents and other family members	1	2	3	4	5
12 My close friend	1	2	3	4	5
13. Any other issue.	1	2	3	4	5

THANK YOU for PARTICIPATING in this STUDY

Coding Instructions for the Hopes and Fears Questionnaire

The Hopes and Fears Open-ended Orientation is analyzed according to content categories (life domains). Across different cultural groups we found the following categories apply:

Education. Depending on the age of respondents you may want distinguish between school and higher education; working with junior and senior high school students we found this distinction useful, although high school senior don't regard school as part of their future.

Examples: *Hopes* – Complete high school, move to a better school, A grade in Physics. *Fears* – That I flunk my final exams, that I will not be admitted to the Science program.

Work & Career. Any statement regarding job, occupation, profession.

Examples: *Hopes* – Become an architect, I would like to be a lawyer, a job that will earn me money and high social position, find a job. *Fears* – That I will not become a lawyer (because I am not a good student), that I will be unemployed, that I will not be allowed to work.

Marriage & Family. Future spouse (romantic partner is included here for transition-to-adulthood and adults, but also depends on the content of the statement), and children.

Examples: *Hopes* – To marry my boyfriend Danny, get married, have an understanding husband and beautiful children, have three children, have a big family. *Fears* – That I will be childless, that I will not marry the right person for me, that after we get married my husband will treat me harshly, that something bad will happen to my children.

Self Concerns. General statements about self like "to be happy", "to have good life", and personality characteristics like "to be honest", "to have courage".

Examples: *Hopes* – That people will love me, to be a respectable person, that all my hopes be fulfilled, to be a good girl, to be beautiful. *Fears* – That I will have unhappy life, that I will not be the happy and respectful woman I wish to become, many disappointments, that other people won't give the respect I really deserve.

Others. Peers, friends, romantic partner if not included in Marriage, parents and other family members.

Examples: *Hopes* – That my mother gets her college degree, that my parents be proud of me, that my father will not die (my mother died of cancer), that my sister recovers from her illness. *Fears* – That terrible things happen to my mother and father and other family members, that my sister's engagement will be annulled, that my parents will not have enough money to send my brother to college.

Collective Issues. Statements pertaining to community, country, and world affairs.

Examples: *Hopes* – World peace, that we will not have nuclear war, that my village will get a new road, that my favorite football team will win the cup, that the Jews will stop discriminating against Arabs. Fears – Nuclear war, that the Palestinians will not get their rights, that the world will be a bad place for people to live in.

Density scores are ratio scores = number of statements for each life domain/total number of items, for Hopes and Fears, respectively.

Coding Instructions for Prospective Life Course Questionnaire

Value	Motivational component			Cognitive component		Behavioral component	
	Expectance	Internal control	External control	Cognitive representation	My future	Exploration	Commitment
Career Domain Scales 11a*, b, c*,d, e*	2c, 7, 10a, b, c*, d, e*	9a, b, c, h	9d, e, f, g	1, 4	03, 04, 08	3, 8a, b, c, d, e	2a, b, 5a, b, c, 6
Family Domain Scales 20a*, b, c*,d, e*	13d, 16, 19a, b, c*, d, e*, f	18a, b, c, h	13d, e, f, g	12, 15	05, 06, 07	17a, b c, e,	13a, b, c, 14

*Recode (1 = 5, 2 = 4, 3 = 3, 4 = 2, 1 = 5)

Index